HANDBOOK OF PLATELETS

Systematic Approach to Thrombocytopenia, Thrombocytosis, and Antithrombotic Pharmacotherapy for Hematology Fellows

Ramon C. Henson, MD

the use, misuse, or application of any information, recommendation, protocol, or clinical guidance contained in this publication.

TABLE OF CONTENT

PREFACE 16
CHAPTER 1: MEGAKARYOPOIESIS, THROMBOPOIESIS, AND PLATELET PRODUCTION 18
Megakaryocyte Development and Differentiation 19
Thrombopoietin Physiology and Regulation 22
THE PLATELET CRISIS DECISION COMPASS — Isolated Thrombocytosis on a Routine Panel 23
Platelet Formation and Release 24
Platelet Kinetics, Lifespan, and Clearance 26
THE PLATELET CRISIS DECISION COMPASS — A Disappointing Platelet Count Rise After Transfusion 28
Megakaryopoiesis Across the Lifespan: Fetal, Neonatal, Pregnancy, and Aging Physiology 28
Disorders of Platelet Production: an Overview and Roadmap 31
THE PLATELET CRISIS DECISION COMPASS — Foundations of Platelet Production 35
Summary and Key Concepts 35
CHAPTER 2: PLATELET ULTRASTRUCTURE, GRANULES, AND RECEPTOR BIOLOGY 36
Platelet Membrane Architecture and Surface Receptors 37
THE PLATELET CRISIS DECISION COMPASS — Prolonged Bleeding Time with a Normal Platelet Count 39
The Cytoskeleton and Platelet Shape Change 40
Granule Biology: Alpha Granules, Dense Granules, and Lysosomes 41
THE PLATELET CRISIS DECISION COMPASS — A Platelet Function Panel Suggesting a Storage Pool Disorder 43
Platelet Receptors in Immune Surveillance and Inflammation 44
Platelet Metabolism, Mitochondria, and Energy Supply for Activation 45
Platelet Membrane Remodeling With Circulating Age 47
Structural Basis of Inherited Platelet Disorders: an Integrative Roadmap 48
THE PLATELET CRISIS DECISION COMPASS — Structural Foundations of Platelet Function 53
Summary and Key Concepts 53

CHAPTER 3: PLATELET ACTIVATION, SIGNALING, AND AGGREGATION MECHANISMS.. 54
Initial Adhesion and Tethering at the Site of Injury 55
Intracellular Signaling Cascades and Amplification..... 56
Platelet Activation Across Arterial, Venous, and Microvascular Contexts..... 58
Aggregation, Integrin Activation, and Thrombus Growth..... 59
THE PLATELET CRISIS DECISION COMPASS — Bleeding on Dual Antiplatelet Therapy..... 61
Platelet Aggregate Architecture: the Core-Shell Model of Thrombus Structure..... 61
Negative Regulation: Keeping Platelet Activation Contained..... 62
Platelet-Leukocyte Interactions and Immunothrombosis 64
Shear-Dependent Regulation of Platelet Aggregation..... 65
Platelets and Coagulation: The Procoagulant Platelet 67
THE PLATELET CRISIS DECISION COMPASS — Early Recognition of Platelet-Driven Microvascular Thrombosis 68
THE PLATELET CRISIS DECISION COMPASS — Activation, Signaling, and the Antiplatelet Drug Map 70
Summary and Key Concepts..... 70
CHAPTER 4: PRIMARY HEMOSTASIS AND PLATELET-VESSEL WALL INTERACTIONS...... 72
The Sequence of Primary Hemostasis 73
The Endothelium as an Active Hemostatic Regulator..... 74
Large-Vessel Versus Microvascular Hemostasis..... 76
Vascular Contributions to Bleeding: Beyond the Platelet 78
THE PLATELET CRISIS DECISION COMPASS — Unexplained Easy Bruising with Normal Platelet Studies..... 79
The Bleeding Time and Its Modern Replacements..... 80
Platelet-Vessel Wall Interaction in Special Clinical Contexts..... 81
Platelets Beyond Hemostasis: Wound Healing and Tissue Repair..... 83
Hemostatic Reserve and Periprocedural Risk Assessment..... 84
THE PLATELET CRISIS DECISION COMPASS — Periprocedural Assessment of a Mild, Borderline Platelet Count..... 85
THE PLATELET CRISIS DECISION COMPASS — Vascular Integration and Hemostatic Reserve 87
Summary and Key Concepts..... 87

CHAPTER 5: CLINICAL APPROACH TO THE PATIENT WITH SUSPECTED PLATELET DISORDER 89
The Structured Bleeding History 90
Standardized Bleeding Assessment Tools 91
Differential Diagnostic Framework: Localizing the Bleeding Tendency 92
THE PLATELET CRISIS DECISION COMPASS — Recognizing a Bleeding History That Requires Same-Day Evaluation 94
Physical Examination in Suspected Platelet Disorders 95
Incidental Versus Symptomatic Thrombocytopenia 97
THE PLATELET CRISIS DECISION COMPASS — A Markedly Low Platelet Count in an Asymptomatic Patient 99
Constructing an Efficient Initial Evaluation 99
Special Populations in the Initial Clinical Encounter 101
Point-of-Care Tools and Communicating Uncertainty to the Patient 102
THE PLATELET CRISIS DECISION COMPASS — Clinical Recognition and Triage 105
Summary and Key Concepts 105
CHAPTER 6: LABORATORY EVALUATION: PLATELET COUNT, MORPHOLOGY, AND PSEUDOTHROMBOCYTOPENIA 107
Automated Platelet Counting: Technology and Limitations 108
Peripheral Blood Smear Examination and Platelet Morphology 109
THE PLATELET CRISIS DECISION COMPASS — An Analyzer Flag Accompanying a Low Platelet Count 111
Pseudothrombocytopenia: Mechanism, Recognition, and Resolution 111
THE PLATELET CRISIS DECISION COMPASS — Resolving a Suspected Pseudothrombocytopenia Result 113
Platelet Indices and Their Clinical Utility 114
Reference Ranges and Interpretation Across Populations 115
Confirming and Trending an Abnormal Platelet Count 117
Special Analytic Circumstances: Severe Thrombocytopenia, Macrothrombocytopenia, and Interfering Samples 118
Quality Assurance and Laboratory-Clinician Communication 120
Historical Methods and the Evolution of Platelet Counting Technology 121

THE PLATELET CRISIS DECISION COMPASS — Laboratory Confirmation and Interpretation 123

Summary and Key Concepts 123

CHAPTER 7: PLATELET FUNCTION TESTING: AGGREGOMETRY, FLOW CYTOMETRY, AND POINT-OF-CARE ASSAYS 125

Light Transmission Aggregometry: Principles and Technique 126

Agonist Panels and Pattern Interpretation 127

THE PLATELET CRISIS DECISION COMPASS — An Aggregometry Pattern Suggesting Glanzmann Thrombasthenia 128

Preanalytic Variables Affecting Aggregometry 129

Flow Cytometric Assessment of Platelet Function 130

Point-of-Care Platelet Function Assays 132

THE PLATELET CRISIS DECISION COMPASS — A Discordant Point-of-Care Closure Time in a Patient on Antiplatelet Therapy 133

Genetic and Molecular Testing for Platelet Function Disorders 134

Interpreting Discordant or Borderline Results 135

Constructing an Efficient Platelet Function Testing Strategy 136

Quality Assurance, Standardization, and Emerging Technologies 137

Special Considerations in Pediatric and Perioperative Testing 139

THE PLATELET CRISIS DECISION COMPASS — Functional Testing Interpretation 141

Summary and Key Concepts 141

CHAPTER 8: DIAGNOSTIC APPROACH TO THROMBOCYTOPENIA IN ADULTS 143

A Mechanistic Framework for Thrombocytopenia 144

Localizing the Mechanism: Decreased Production Versus Increased Destruction 145

Distributional Thrombocytopenia: Splenic Sequestration 146

THE PLATELET CRISIS DECISION COMPASS — New Thrombocytopenia with Accompanying Cytopenias 147

Bone Marrow Examination: Indications and Interpretation 148

Algorithmic Approach to New-Onset Thrombocytopenia 150

Thrombocytopenia in the Hospitalized Patient 151

THE PLATELET CRISIS DECISION COMPASS — Sequencing the Evaluation of New Thrombocytopenia in a Hospitalized Patient 152

Chronic and Recurrent Thrombocytopenia: A Longitudinal Approach 153
Congenital and Inherited Thrombocytopenia in the Adult Differential..... 154
Special Populations in the Thrombocytopenia Evaluation 155
When to Refer and How to Sequence Subspecialty Involvement 157
THE PLATELET CRISIS DECISION COMPASS — Mechanistic Diagnosis and Triage 158
Summary and Key Concepts..... 159
CHAPTER 9: IMMUNE THROMBOCYTOPENIA..... 160
Definition, Classification, and Epidemiology..... 161
Pathophysiology: Antibody-Mediated Destruction and Impaired Production..... 162
Clinical Presentation in Children and Adults..... 163
Diagnostic Criteria and the Exclusion of Secondary Causes 165
THE PLATELET CRISIS DECISION COMPASS — Determining Urgency of First-Line Treatment in Newly Diagnosed Immune Thrombocytopenia 166
Secondary Immune Thrombocytopenia: Associated Conditions..... 167
First-Line Management: Corticosteroids and Immunoglobulin 168
Second-Line and Refractory Management 169
THE PLATELET CRISIS DECISION COMPASS — Sequencing Second-Line Therapy After First-Line Treatment Failure..... 171
Splenectomy and Its Alternatives 171
Immune Thrombocytopenia in Special Populations..... 173
Long-Term Monitoring and Quality of Life 174
THE PLATELET CRISIS DECISION COMPASS — Immune Thrombocytopenia Management Sequencing..... 176
Summary and Key Concepts..... 177
CHAPTER 10: DRUG-INDUCED THROMBOCYTOPENIA..... 178
Epidemiology and Clinical Significance 179
Mechanisms of Drug-Induced Platelet Destruction..... 180
Common Culprit Medications and Their Recognition Patterns..... 181
THE PLATELET CRISIS DECISION COMPASS — Recognizing the Characteristic Timing Pattern of Drug-Induced Thrombocytopenia..... 183
Quinine and Quinine-Like Drug-Induced Thrombocytopenia 183
Vancomycin-Induced Thrombocytopenia 185

Glycoprotein IIb/IIIa Inhibitor-Induced Thrombocytopenia 186
THE PLATELET CRISIS DECISION COMPASS — Managing an Inadvertent Rechallenge with a Previously Implicated Medication 187
Diagnostic Approach and Causality Assessment 188
Management: Discontinuation, Supportive Care, and Rechallenge Considerations 189
Prevention and Documentation for Future Care 191
Special Considerations in Oncology and Chemotherapy-Adjacent Contexts 192
THE PLATELET CRISIS DECISION COMPASS — Drug-Induced Thrombocytopenia Recognition and Prevention 194
Summary and Key Concepts 195
CHAPTER 11: HEPARIN-INDUCED THROMBOCYTOPENIA 196
Epidemiology and Risk Factors 197
Pathophysiology: Platelet Factor 4-Heparin Complex Immunogenicity 198
Clinical Presentation and Timing Patterns 199
Pretest Probability: The 4Ts Score 201
THE PLATELET CRISIS DECISION COMPASS — Applying the 4Ts Score to Guide Immediate Management 202
Laboratory Diagnosis: Immunoassay and Functional Testing 203
Thrombotic Complications and Their Recognition 204
Management: Alternative Anticoagulation Strategies 206
THE PLATELET CRISIS DECISION COMPASS — Managing Confirmed Heparin-Induced Thrombocytopenia with Thrombosis 207
Special Clinical Scenarios 208
Transitioning to Long-Term Anticoagulation 209
THE PLATELET CRISIS DECISION COMPASS — Heparin-Induced Thrombocytopenia Recognition and Management 211
Summary and Key Concepts 212
CHAPTER 12: THROMBOTIC MICROANGIOPATHIES: TTP, SHIGA TOXIN-ASSOCIATED HUS, AND ATYPICAL HUS 213
Overview and Classification of Thrombotic Microangiopathy 214
Thrombotic Thrombocytopenic Purpura: ADAMTS13 Deficiency 215
Clinical Presentation and the Classic Pentad 217

Diagnostic Evaluation and ADAMTS13 Testing 218
THE PLATELET CRISIS DECISION COMPASS — Recognizing Thrombotic Microangiopathy as Requiring Same-Day Treatment 220
Shiga Toxin-Associated Hemolytic Uremic Syndrome 220
Atypical Hemolytic Uremic Syndrome and Complement Dysregulation 222
Distinguishing TTP, STEC-HUS, and Complement-Mediated TMA 223
Management of Thrombotic Thrombocytopenic Purpura 225
THE PLATELET CRISIS DECISION COMPASS — Distinguishing TTP from Atypical HUS While ADAMTS13 Results Are Pending 226
Management of Atypical HUS: Complement Inhibition 227
Long-Term Monitoring and Relapse Prevention 228
THE PLATELET CRISIS DECISION COMPASS — Thrombotic Microangiopathy Recognition and Treatment Sequencing 231
Summary and Key Concepts 231
CHAPTER 13: THROMBOCYTOPENIA IN PREGNANCY AND THE NEONATE 232
Physiologic Platelet Changes in Normal Pregnancy 232
Gestational Thrombocytopenia 234
Hypertensive Disorders of Pregnancy: Preeclampsia and HELLP Syndrome 235
Immune Thrombocytopenia in Pregnancy 237
THE PLATELET CRISIS DECISION COMPASS — Distinguishing Benign Gestational Thrombocytopenia from a Pregnancy Emergency 238
Thrombotic Microangiopathy in Pregnancy 239
Delivery Planning and Anesthesia Considerations 240
Neonatal Alloimmune Thrombocytopenia 242
THE PLATELET CRISIS DECISION COMPASS — Recognizing Neonatal Alloimmune Thrombocytopenia Risk in a Subsequent Pregnancy 243
Neonatal Thrombocytopenia: Broader Differential and Approach 244
Postpartum Considerations and Long-Term Follow-Up 245
THE PLATELET CRISIS DECISION COMPASS — Maternal-Fetal Thrombocytopenia Recognition and Planning 247
Summary and Key Concepts 248
CHAPTER 14: THROMBOCYTOPENIA IN CRITICAL ILLNESS, SEPSIS, DIC, AND LIVER DISEASE 249

Multifactorial Pathophysiology of Critical Illness Thrombocytopenia 250
Disseminated Intravascular Coagulation: Diagnosis 251
THE PLATELET CRISIS DECISION COMPASS — Recognizing Evolving Disseminated Intravascular Coagulation Before Overt Criteria Are Met 253
Disseminated Intravascular Coagulation: Management 253
Thrombocytopenia in Advanced Liver Disease 255
A Systematic Approach to New Thrombocytopenia in the ICU 256
THE PLATELET CRISIS DECISION COMPASS — Distinguishing Chronic Liver Disease Thrombocytopenia from a Superimposed Acute Process 258
Prognostic Significance and Long-Term Considerations 258
Extracorporeal Circuits and Mechanical Circulatory Support 260
Massive Transfusion and Dilutional Thrombocytopenia 261
Nutritional and Metabolic Contributors in Critical Illness 263
THE PLATELET CRISIS DECISION COMPASS — Critical Illness Thrombocytopenia Recognition and Management 265
Summary and Key Concepts 265
CHAPTER 15: INHERITED THROMBOCYTOPENIA SYNDROMES 267
Classification by Platelet Size 268
MYH9-Related Disorders 269
Wiskott-Aldrich Syndrome and X-Linked Thrombocytopenia 271
THE PLATELET CRISIS DECISION COMPASS — Recognizing a Macrothrombocytopenia Pattern Warranting Genetic Evaluation 272
Thrombocytopenia-Absent Radius Syndrome and Congenital Amegakaryocytic Thrombocytopenia 273
Malignancy Predisposition Syndromes: ANKRD26 and RUNX1 274
Diagnostic Approach: Genetic Testing Strategy 276
Malignancy Surveillance in Predisposition Syndromes 277
THE PLATELET CRISIS DECISION COMPASS — Establishing Malignancy Surveillance After Confirming a Predisposition Syndrome 279
Management and Genetic Counseling 279
Additional and Emerging Inherited Thrombocytopenia Syndromes 281
Transitioning Care From Pediatric to Adult Hematology 283

THE PLATELET CRISIS DECISION COMPASS — Inherited Thrombocytopenia Recognition and Surveillance 285
Summary and Key Concepts 285
CHAPTER 16: INHERITED AND ACQUIRED PLATELET FUNCTION DISORDERS 286
Classification of Platelet Function Disorders by Mechanism 286
Glanzmann Thrombasthenia and Disorders of the GPIIb/IIIa Complex 287
THE PLATELET CRISIS DECISION COMPASS — Aggregometry Pattern Recognition Arc .. 289
Bernard-Soulier Syndrome and Disorders of Platelet Adhesion 289
Platelet Storage Pool Disorders and Secretion Defects 291
Additional Rare Inherited Platelet Function Disorders 292
Acquired Platelet Dysfunction 293
THE PLATELET CRISIS DECISION COMPASS — Acquired Dysfunction Recognition Arc .. 295
Diagnostic Approach to Suspected Platelet Function Disorders 295
Laboratory Considerations: Preanalytic Variables and Emerging Assays 296
Perioperative and Acute Bleeding Management 297
Pediatric Presentation and the Diagnostic Odyssey 299
Special Populations and Long-Term Considerations 300
THE PLATELET CRISIS DECISION COMPASS — Platelet Function Disorder Pattern Recognition 301
Summary and Key Concepts 301
CHAPTER 17: THE THROMBOCYTOSES: REACTIVE AND CLONAL DISEASE 303
Definition and Classification of Thrombocytosis 303
Reactive Thrombocytosis 304
Essential Thrombocythemia: Diagnosis 305
THE PLATELET CRISIS DECISION COMPASS — Reactive Versus Clonal Recognition Arc 306
Essential Thrombocythemia: Risk Stratification and Management 307
Essential Thrombocythemia in Pregnancy and Young Patients 308
THE PLATELET CRISIS DECISION COMPASS — Extreme Count Dual-Risk Arc 309
Extreme Thrombocytosis and Its Complications 310
Laboratory and Diagnostic Pitfalls in Thrombocytosis Evaluation 311
Essential Thrombocythemia: Natural History and Disease Transformation 313

Perioperative and Procedural Management of Essential Thrombocythemia 314
Splanchnic Vein Thrombosis in Myeloproliferative Neoplasms 315
Quality of Life and Psychosocial Considerations 317
Long-Term Monitoring and Patient Communication 318
THE PLATELET CRISIS DECISION COMPASS — Thrombocytosis Recognition and Risk Stratification 320
Summary and Key Concepts 320
CHAPTER 18: ANTITHROMBOTIC PHARMACOLOGY, REVERSAL, AND PERIPROCEDURAL MANAGEMENT 321
Pharmacology of Aspirin and Cyclooxygenase Inhibition 321
P2Y12 Inhibitors: Clopidogrel, Prasugrel, and Ticagrelor 322
THE PLATELET CRISIS DECISION COMPASS — Antiplatelet Recovery Timeline Arc 324
Periprocedural Risk Stratification 324
Anticoagulant Pharmacology and Periprocedural Management 326
Reversal Strategies for Antiplatelet-Associated Bleeding 327
THE PLATELET CRISIS DECISION COMPASS — Reversal Agent Selection Arc 328
Reversal Strategies for Anticoagulant-Associated Bleeding 329
Special Populations and Combined Antithrombotic Therapy 330
Laboratory Monitoring of Antithrombotic Therapy 331
Newer Antithrombotic Agents and Emerging Pharmacologic Considerations 333
Antithrombotic Therapy in Special Hematologic Populations 334
Systems-Level Safety Measures and Error Prevention 336
Communicating Periprocedural Plans and Patient Education 337
THE PLATELET CRISIS DECISION COMPASS — Periprocedural Antithrombotic Decision Arc 338
Summary and Key Concepts 338
CHAPTER 19: PLATELET TRANSFUSION MEDICINE: PRODUCTS, INDICATIONS, AND REFRACTORINESS 339
Platelet Products: Preparation, Storage, and Dosing 339
Special Platelet Products and Modifications 341
Prophylactic Platelet Transfusion Thresholds 342
THE PLATELET CRISIS DECISION COMPASS — Refractoriness Recognition Arc 344

Therapeutic Platelet Transfusion for Active Bleeding 344
Complications and Risks of Platelet Transfusion 345
Alloimmunization and Platelet Transfusion Refractoriness 346
THE PLATELET CRISIS DECISION COMPASS — Nonimmune Versus Alloimmune Refractoriness Arc 348
Management of the Alloimmunized, Refractory Patient 348
Blood Bank and Transfusion Service Logistics 349
Platelet Transfusion in Specific Procedural Contexts 351
Cost, Sustainability, and Judicious Platelet Utilization 352
Neonatal, Pediatric, and Massive Transfusion Considerations 353
Documentation, Monitoring, and Quality Metrics 354
Ethical Considerations in Scarce Compatible Product Allocation 355
Patient Communication and Informed Consent 355
THE PLATELET CRISIS DECISION COMPASS — Transfusion Refractoriness Diagnostic Arc 356
Summary and Key Concepts 356
CHAPTER 20: EMERGING AND INVESTIGATIONAL PLATELET-DIRECTED THERAPIES 358
Expanding Applications of Thrombopoietin Receptor Agonists 358
Novel Agents in Immune Thrombocytopenia and Autoimmune Platelet Destruction 359
THE PLATELET CRISIS DECISION COMPASS — Emerging Therapy Evaluation Arc 361
THE PLATELET CRISIS DECISION COMPASS — Investigational Access Arc 362
Gene Therapy and Gene Editing in Inherited Platelet Disorders 362
Novel Antithrombotic Strategies in Development 364
Ex Vivo Platelet Generation and Artificial Platelet Substitutes 365
Cellular and Antibody-Based Immunotherapy in Autoimmune Platelet Disorders 367
Regulatory Pathways and Health Technology Assessment 368
Biomarkers and Precision Medicine in Platelet Disorders 370
Preparing Clinical Practice for an Evolving Therapeutic Landscape 371
Critical Evaluation of Emerging Therapies 372
Synthesis: The Future of Platelet-Directed Clinical Practice 374
THE PLATELET CRISIS DECISION COMPASS — Emerging Therapy Evaluation and Closing Synthesis 375

Summary and Key Concepts 375
THE PLATELET CRISIS MASTER COMPASS 376
The Platelet Crisis Master Compass: Indexed Pattern Atlas 376
Part I: Foundational Platelet Biology 376
Part II: Clinical Evaluation and Diagnostic Approach 378
Part III: Thrombocytopenia — Immune, Drug-Induced, Consumptive, and Special-Population Disorders 380
Part IV: Inherited Platelet Disorders 383
Part V: Thrombocytosis, Pharmacology, Transfusion Medicine, and Emerging Therapies 384
Using the Master Compass in Practice 389
CONCLUSION 391

PREFACE

Platelet medicine occupies an unusual place in clinical hematology. The organelle itself is small, anucleate, and short-lived, yet the syndromes that arise when its number or function goes wrong are among the most consequential a hematologist will encounter. A falling platelet count on a morning laboratory panel can mean nothing at all, or it can mean that a patient will not survive the day without plasma exchange. The problem is that, at the moment the abnormal count first appears, these two possibilities frequently look identical. Thrombotic thrombocytopenic purpura, heparin-induced thrombocytopenia, disseminated intravascular coagulation, immune thrombocytopenia, and the thrombocytopenia of preeclampsia and HELLP syndrome can all present with a platelet count in the same range, on the same hospital day, in a patient with the same vague complaint of fatigue or bruising. Each of these conditions demands a different, time-sensitive action, and several of the correct actions are directly contraindicated in the other diagnoses. This handbook exists because that specific problem — differentiating look-alike platelet syndromes under time pressure, correctly, on the first attempt — is the single most consistently cited source of diagnostic anxiety among hematology and oncology fellows learning benign hematology.

The chapters that follow are organized to build outward from mechanism. The book begins with the biology of the megakaryocyte and the platelet itself — how the cell is produced, how it is built, how it senses injury and responds — because the clinical syndromes described in later chapters are, almost without exception, direct consequences of a specific breakdown somewhere in that biology. A reader who understands why a platelet aggregates the way it does will find the pharmacology of antiplatelet therapy intuitive rather than memorized, and a reader who understands the kinetics of platelet clearance will find the differential diagnosis of thrombocytopenia organized rather than exhausting. From there, the book moves through clinical and laboratory evaluation, then through the thrombocytopenic disorders in the order a consulting hematologist typically encounters them, then through the platelet function disorders and thrombocytoses, and finally through the therapeutics — antithrombotic pharmacology, reversal strategies, and platelet transfusion medicine — that translate diagnosis into action.

Running through every chapter is a single structural device built specifically to address the look-alike problem described above: **The Platelet Crisis Decision Compass**. At each major clinical decision point in the book, a Compass callout names the presenting picture exactly as it appears at the bedside, lists the specific look-alike syndromes that share that picture, states the definitive action the picture demands, flags the discriminating trap that causes experienced clinicians to miscall it, and closes with a single anchoring rule. Every chapter ends with a consolidated recap of that chapter's Compass instances, and the book closes with a dedicated Anchor Section, The Platelet Crisis Master Compass, that indexes every Compass instance in the book by presenting clinical and laboratory picture, cross-referenced back to its originating chapter. A reader on call, standing at a bedside with an unexplained platelet count, should be able to find the relevant picture in the Master Compass in under a minute.

This book contains no practice questions, board-style items, or self-assessment exercises of any kind. It is written as a clinical reference — one to be consulted during a consult, before a rotation, or while building a teaching point for a resident — rather than as an examination-preparation workbook. Every clinical case in the text is a narrative scenario with guided diagnostic and management reasoning, not a stem with lettered answer choices. The intent is that a hematology fellow, a practicing hematologist, or a transfusion medicine physician can open this book at any chapter and find authoritative, current, evidence-grounded guidance written in the same voice a thoughtful attending would use at the bedside.

Clinical practice in platelet medicine continues to evolve, particularly in the pharmacology of antithrombotic reversal, the classification of inherited platelet disorders, and the recognition of atypical thrombotic microangiopathies. Readers are encouraged to confirm specific drug doses, laboratory reference ranges, and guideline-directed thresholds against current institutional formularies and the most recent society guidelines at the time of use. It is hoped that the Platelet Crisis Decision Compass, built into every chapter of this book, will remain useful as that evidence base continues to move forward — because the underlying clinical problem it addresses, telling one falling platelet count apart from another under time pressure, is not going away.

CHAPTER 1: MEGAKARYOPOIESIS, THROMBOPOIESIS, AND PLATELET PRODUCTION

Learning Objectives

1. Describe the stages of megakaryocyte differentiation from the hematopoietic stem cell, including the transcription factors that commit a progenitor to the megakaryocytic lineage.
2. Explain the physiologic regulation of thrombopoietin, including the hepatic constitutive-synthesis model and the role of platelet and megakaryocyte mass in setting circulating thrombopoietin levels.
3. Describe the process of proplatelet formation and intravascular platelet release, including the contribution of pulmonary microcirculation to platelet biogenesis.
4. Distinguish central (production) causes of thrombocytopenia and thrombocytosis from peripheral (destruction, consumption, sequestration, and dilutional) causes using platelet kinetics.
5. Apply the corrected count increment to distinguish immune platelet transfusion refractoriness from non-immune consumptive refractoriness.
6. Recognize the clinical and morphologic features that suggest an inherited disorder of platelet production, using thrombocytopenia with absent radii syndrome as a model.

Chapter Outline

This chapter begins at the level of the hematopoietic stem cell and follows lineage commitment through megakaryocyte maturation, thrombopoietin regulation, proplatelet formation, and platelet release into the circulation. It then turns to platelet kinetics after release — lifespan, splenic sequestration, and clearance — before closing with an organizing framework for the disorders of platelet production that occupy later chapters. Two Platelet Crisis Decision Compass instances are embedded at the points in the chapter where foundational biology first intersects with a genuine bedside decision: the workup of isolated thrombocytosis, and the interpretation of a disappointing platelet count rise after transfusion.

Everything a clinician does with an abnormal platelet count, whether high or low, ultimately traces back to one of three variables: how many platelets are being made, how long they survive once made, and where in the body they are being held or destroyed. A hematologist who can locate an abnormal count on this three-variable map — production, lifespan, distribution — has already done most of the intellectual work of building a differential diagnosis, well before a single additional test has returned. This chapter builds that map in detail, because every later chapter in this book assumes the reader already has it.

Platelets are unusual among blood cells in that they are not cells in the conventional sense at all. They are anucleate cytoplasmic fragments, produced not by cell division but by the deliberate fragmentation of a single, enormous precursor cell, the megakaryocyte. This production strategy is unlike anything else in hematopoiesis, and understanding why it evolved this way, and what can go wrong at each step, is the foundation for the entire clinical discipline of platelet medicine. A production system built around a single, massive, terminally differentiated precursor cell is inherently more vulnerable to catastrophic failure than a system built around ongoing division of a self-renewing progenitor pool, which is one reason why disorders that damage the marrow broadly, such as chemotherapy, radiation, and infiltrative malignancy, so often produce thrombocytopenia earlier and more severely than they produce anemia or leukopenia; the megakaryocyte compartment simply has less redundancy to draw on.

Megakaryocyte Development and Differentiation

Hematopoietic Stem Cell Commitment and Lineage Determination

Megakaryocyte production begins with the same multipotent hematopoietic stem cell that gives rise to every other blood lineage. Lineage commitment toward the megakaryocyte-erythroid path is driven by a small set of transcription factors whose relative expression levels determine whether a common progenitor becomes a megakaryocyte or an erythroid precursor. GATA1 and its cofactor FOG1 are required for both lineages, but the balance shifts toward megakaryopoiesis when RUNX1 and FLI1 rise in relative expression, activating megakaryocyte-specific genes including those encoding glycoprotein IIb-IIIa and the thrombopoietin receptor MPL. NF-E2 acts further downstream, coordinating the terminal maturation program that produces platelet-specific granule proteins.

This transcriptional logic matters clinically because inherited mutations in these same factors produce recognizable syndromes rather than nonspecific cytopenia. A germline RUNX1 mutation produces familial platelet disorder with a predisposition to myeloid malignancy, in which mild thrombocytopenia and a qualitative platelet defect coexist with a lifetime risk of transformation to acute myeloid leukemia that is high enough to change how relatives of an affected patient are counseled and screened. A GATA1 mutation, depending on which functional domain is affected, can produce either a macrothrombocytopenia with anemia or a combined phenotype resembling a congenital dyserythropoietic anemia. Recognizing that a patient's thrombocytopenia traces to a transcription-factor lesion rather than an acquired process changes the entire subsequent evaluation, shifting it from a search for an acquired cause toward genetic testing and family counseling.

KEY POINT: A platelet count that has been mildly low since childhood, particularly with a family history of cytopenia or leukemia, should prompt consideration of an inherited transcription-factor disorder before an extensive acquired workup is pursued.

Progenitor Heterogeneity: Direct and Stepwise Pathways to Megakaryocyte Fate

The classical model of megakaryopoiesis, in which a multipotent stem cell passes sequentially through a common myeloid progenitor and then a bipotent megakaryocyte-erythroid progenitor before finally committing to the megakaryocyte lineage, has been substantially revised by lineage-tracing studies over the past decade. These studies have identified a distinct population of megakaryocyte-biased hematopoietic stem cells that can generate platelets directly, bypassing the classical progenitor hierarchy entirely, through what is now referred to as the direct pathway. This direct pathway appears to dominate during states of acute physiologic stress, including acute inflammation, infection, and acute blood loss, allowing the marrow to rapidly restore platelet production without waiting for the multi-step maturation sequence that characterizes steady-state, or stepwise, megakaryopoiesis.

The clinical significance of this dual-pathway model is still an active area of investigation, but it already offers a mechanistic explanation for an observation that has long been recognized empirically: the platelet count response to acute stress, such as major surgery or acute infection, is often disproportionately fast relative to the several-day maturation timeline expected from stepwise megakaryopoiesis alone. It also raises the possibility that megakaryocyte-biased stem cells could be selectively depleted or dysfunctional in some acquired marrow disorders even when erythroid and myeloid lineages remain grossly intact, a hypothesis that may eventually help explain isolated thrombocytopenia phenotypes in acquired bone marrow failure syndromes that do not fit cleanly into the classical central-versus-peripheral framework.

Megakaryocyte Maturation and Endomitosis

Once committed, the megakaryocyte progenitor undergoes a maturation process unlike that of any other hematopoietic cell: rather than dividing, it enlarges through repeated rounds of endomitosis, a truncated mitotic cycle in which the cell replicates its DNA and begins to separate chromosomes but fails to complete cytokinesis. The result is a single cell with a polyploid nucleus that can reach a DNA content of 64N or higher, occupying a cell body that grows to ten or more times the diameter of a typical marrow cell. This polyploidy is not incidental; it is the mechanism by which a single cell accumulates enough cytoplasmic mass, membrane, and organelle content to eventually supply thousands of platelets.

As ploidy increases, the megakaryocyte's cytoplasm becomes progressively organized into a demarcation membrane system, an elaborate, folded reservoir of membrane continuous with the plasma membrane that will later be reorganized into the boundaries of individual platelets. Alpha granules and dense granules are synthesized and trafficked into the maturing cytoplasm during this same window, so that by the time a megakaryocyte is ready to release platelets, the granule cargo that will drive platelet activation at a future site of vascular injury is already packaged and positioned. A megakaryocyte that is destroyed or fails to mature before this packaging is complete, as occurs in some marrow infiltrative processes, produces platelets that may be normal in number but deficient in granule content, a distinction that becomes clinically important when a patient has a normal platelet count but an unexplained bleeding tendency.

The Bone Marrow Megakaryocyte Niche

Megakaryocytes mature within a specialized marrow microenvironment organized around the sinusoidal vasculature. Unlike most hematopoietic progenitors, which mature deep within the marrow parenchyma near the endosteal surface, megakaryocytes migrate toward the vascular sinusoids as they mature, a process directed by a gradient of the chemokine CXCL12 acting on its receptor CXCR4, together with signaling through the sphingosine-1-phosphate pathway. This migration positions the mature megakaryocyte with its demarcation membrane system directly adjacent to the sinusoidal endothelium, so that proplatelet extensions can be released directly into the vascular lumen rather than into marrow stroma, where they would be unable to enter the circulation.

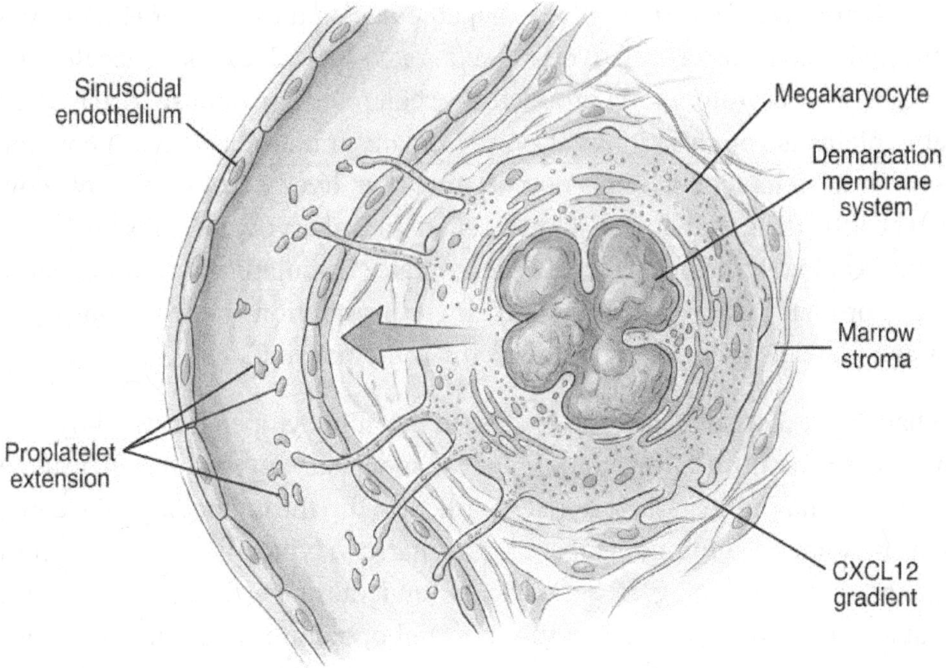

The niche also regulates megakaryocyte number through direct cell contact and locally produced cytokines, including stromal-derived thrombopoietin, interleukin-6, and interleukin-11, which act alongside circulating thrombopoietin discussed in the next section. Disruption of this niche, whether by marrow fibrosis, infiltrative malignancy, or radiation injury, impairs megakaryopoiesis independent of any defect in the megakaryocyte itself, which is why marrow biopsy, rather than platelet count alone, is often required to distinguish a niche-level production problem from a primary megakaryocyte disorder. Primary myelofibrosis provides a particularly instructive example of niche-level disruption: reticulin and collagen fibrosis deposited by reactive marrow fibroblasts, driven in large part by growth factors including platelet-derived growth factor and transforming growth factor beta released from the abnormal megakaryocytes themselves, progressively destroys the sinusoidal architecture on which normal megakaryocyte positioning and platelet release depend. Paradoxically, this process often begins against a background of megakaryocyte hyperplasia and even thrombocytosis, before eventually progressing to thrombocytopenia once fibrosis has advanced far enough to disrupt the niche architecture required for effective platelet release, illustrating that platelet count trajectory over time, not a single measurement, is often what best reflects the stage of an evolving niche-level process.

Thrombopoietin Physiology and Regulation

Thrombopoietin Synthesis and the Hepatic Set-Point Model

Thrombopoietin is synthesized constitutively by hepatocytes, and to a lesser extent by renal tubular cells and marrow stromal cells, at a relatively fixed rate that does not accelerate in response to thrombocytopenia the way erythropoietin production accelerates in response to anemia. This constitutive-synthesis model explains an observation that puzzles many trainees on first encounter: thrombopoietin levels rise when the platelet count falls, not because the liver senses the low count and increases production, but because there are fewer platelets and megakaryocytes present to bind and clear the thrombopoietin that is already being made at a steady rate. Circulating thrombopoietin is therefore best understood as a hormone whose level is set by consumption rather than by production, with megakaryocytes and platelets themselves acting as the principal sink.

This distinction has direct diagnostic consequences. In thrombocytopenia caused by a production failure, such as marrow aplasia or infiltration, there are few megakaryocytes present to consume circulating thrombopoietin, so thrombopoietin levels rise markedly. In thrombocytopenia caused by peripheral destruction, such as immune thrombocytopenia, the marrow typically contains a normal or increased number of megakaryocytes working to compensate, and these megakaryocytes continue to consume thrombopoietin at a near-normal rate, so measured thrombopoietin levels remain closer to normal despite the low platelet count. In practice, thrombopoietin level is rarely measured because the clinical and morphologic distinction between production failure and peripheral destruction can usually be made more quickly by marrow examination when needed, but the underlying physiology explains why marrow megakaryocyte number, not platelet count alone, is the variable that separates these two broad categories of thrombocytopenia.

The MPL Receptor and Downstream Signaling

Thrombopoietin acts through MPL, a homodimeric receptor expressed on hematopoietic stem cells, megakaryocyte progenitors, and mature megakaryocytes and platelets. Ligand binding activates the JAK2-STAT5 pathway along with the RAS-MAPK and PI3K-AKT pathways, driving progenitor proliferation, megakaryocyte maturation, and endomitosis. This same signaling axis is the direct target of the acquired JAK2 V617F mutation and analogous mutations in MPL and calreticulin that drive the myeloproliferative neoplasms discussed in Chapter 17; a mutation that renders MPL signaling constitutively active produces unregulated megakaryocyte proliferation independent of thrombopoietin level, which is the mechanistic basis for the clonal thrombocytosis that these mutations cause.

Loss-of-function mutations in MPL itself produce the opposite phenotype: congenital amegakaryocytic thrombocytopenia, in which megakaryocyte progenitors fail to respond to thrombopoietin at all, leading to severe thrombocytopenia from birth that typically progresses to trilineage marrow failure in later childhood as the stem cell compartment, which also depends on MPL signaling for self-renewal, becomes exhausted. This progression from isolated thrombocytopenia to full marrow failure is itself a diagnostic clue: any inherited thrombocytopenia syndrome in which MPL signaling is disrupted should prompt long-term surveillance for evolving pancytopenia, not just management of the presenting platelet count.

Feedback Regulation by Platelet and Megakaryocyte Mass

Because circulating thrombopoietin level reflects the balance between constitutive hepatic synthesis and consumption by the total megakaryocyte-platelet mass, the system behaves as a negative feedback loop even though production itself is not directly regulated. An expansion of platelet mass, whether from a rising count or from unusually large platelets, increases thrombopoietin clearance and lowers the circulating level, which in turn reduces the stimulus for further megakaryopoiesis. Conversely, a contraction in platelet mass raises circulating thrombopoietin and stimulates compensatory megakaryocyte proliferation and maturation. This is the physiologic basis for the platelet count rebound seen after resolution of an acute consumptive process, and it is also the physiologic rationale for thrombopoietin receptor agonist drugs, which bypass the endogenous ligand entirely and directly activate MPL to drive platelet production in conditions such as immune thrombocytopenia and certain forms of aplastic anemia, discussed further in later chapters.

THE PLATELET CRISIS DECISION COMPASS — Isolated Thrombocytosis on a Routine Panel

The Presentation: A platelet count above the upper reference limit, discovered incidentally on a routine or preoperative complete blood count, in a patient who is otherwise asymptomatic and has no prior hematologic history.

Mimic Signature: Reactive thrombocytosis from iron deficiency, acute or chronic inflammation, recent surgery, or splenectomy; a clonal myeloproliferative neoplasm, most often essential thrombocythemia, presenting at a subclinical stage; and spurious elevation from red cell or white cell fragments miscounted as platelets by automated analyzers.

The Decision: Review the peripheral smear to exclude a counting artifact, obtain a history and basic laboratory panel (ferritin, inflammatory markers, recent surgical or infectious history) to screen for a reactive cause, and if no reactive explanation is identified and the count remains persistently elevated on repeat testing, proceed to JAK2, CALR, and MPL mutation testing before reassuring the patient.

Trap Logic: The absence of symptoms is not evidence against a myeloproliferative neoplasm; early essential thrombocythemia is frequently asymptomatic, and the danger of dismissing an incidental thrombocytosis as benign is that clonal thrombocytosis carries a meaningful long-term risk of arterial and venous thrombosis that is not mitigated by reassurance.

Crisis Anchor: Persistent thrombocytosis without an identified reactive cause after a basic screening evaluation should proceed to molecular testing, not to a default diagnosis of reactive thrombocytosis by exclusion of history alone.

Platelet Formation and Release

Proplatelet Formation and Cytoskeletal Remodeling

Once a megakaryocyte has reached full maturity, it begins extending long, branching cytoplasmic processes called proplatelets, which are threaded through the demarcation membrane system and studded with periodic swellings that will ultimately become individual platelets. Proplatelet elongation is driven by a coordinated reorganization of the microtubule and actin cytoskeleton: bundled microtubules form the structural core of each proplatelet shaft, and molecular motors including dynein slide these microtubule bundles against one another to drive elongation, while localized actin polymerization at branch points generates the forked architecture characteristic of a mature proplatelet. This process converts the megakaryocyte's cytoplasm, over a period of several hours, from a compact polyploid cell body into an extensively branched network capable of yielding several thousand platelets from a single progenitor.

Mutations affecting this cytoskeletal machinery produce a recognizable group of inherited macrothrombocytopenias. MYH9-related disease, caused by mutations in the gene encoding non-muscle myosin heavy chain IIA, impairs the fission of proplatelet swellings into individual platelets, resulting in fewer, larger platelets than normal along with variable sensorineural hearing loss, nephropathy, and cataracts depending on the specific mutation. Similarly, mutations in the actin-regulatory protein Wiskott-Aldrich syndrome protein produce small, rather than large, platelets through a distinct cytoskeletal mechanism, illustrating that platelet size itself, easily measured as the mean platelet volume on a routine complete blood count, carries mechanistic information about which part of the production pathway has failed.

CLINICAL PEARL: Mean platelet volume is not a nuisance parameter to be ignored when the platelet count is abnormal. A markedly elevated mean platelet volume in the setting of thrombocytopenia points toward a production or peripheral-destruction process with compensatory release of large, young platelets, or toward an inherited macrothrombocytopenia, while a low mean platelet volume in thrombocytopenia is a recognized feature of Wiskott-Aldrich syndrome and related X-linked disorders.

Intravascular and Intrapulmonary Platelet Release

For decades, platelet release was taught as occurring exclusively within the bone marrow sinusoids, with proplatelets shedding their terminal swellings directly into the marrow vascular lumen. More recent evidence has substantially revised this picture: a large fraction of platelet release appears to occur not in the marrow itself but in the pulmonary microcirculation, where intact megakaryocytes and long proplatelet fragments that have entered the venous circulation become lodged in the narrow-caliber pulmonary capillary bed and continue to shed platelets as they transit or become trapped there. This finding reframes the lung not merely as a filter for megakaryocyte fragments but as an active site of terminal platelet biogenesis, and it may help explain the platelet count derangements observed in some pulmonary and cardiopulmonary bypass conditions, where disruption of this pulmonary microcirculatory bed measurably affects circulating platelet number.

Whatever the precise anatomic distribution of terminal release, the shared final step is membrane fission: individual platelet-sized fragments separate from the proplatelet shaft through a calcium-dependent, cytoskeleton-driven scission event, and each resulting platelet retains a portion of the parent megakaryocyte's cytoplasm, organelles, and granule content while remaining anucleate. A single megakaryocyte is estimated to yield on the order of one thousand to several thousand platelets over its productive lifespan, which is why a marrow that contains an apparently adequate number of megakaryocytes can still fail to sustain a normal platelet count if those megakaryocytes are dysplastic, poorly matured, or unable to complete proplatelet formation efficiently — a distinction between megakaryocyte number and megakaryocyte function that is central to interpreting a bone marrow biopsy in thrombocytopenia.

Determinants of Platelet Size and Granule Content

The size and granule content of a newly released platelet are determined largely during the megakaryocyte maturation phase discussed earlier in this chapter, before proplatelet formation even begins, because granule packaging occurs during cytoplasmic maturation and is simply partitioned among daughter platelets at the moment of fission rather than being synthesized anew in each platelet. This has a practical corollary: a process that shortens megakaryocyte maturation time, forcing premature proplatelet formation before granule packaging is complete, produces platelets that are structurally intact but functionally deficient, a pattern seen in some cases of accelerated compensatory thrombopoiesis and in certain marrow stress states. Recognizing this distinction, between a platelet that is present in normal number but poorly granulated and a platelet that is simply absent, is essential when a patient has an unexplained bleeding diathesis despite a normal platelet count, a scenario addressed in detail in Chapter 16.

Platelet size also correlates, on a population level, with platelet reactivity: larger, younger platelets released during compensatory thrombopoiesis tend to be enzymatically and functionally more active than older, smaller platelets nearing the end of their circulating lifespan, containing modestly higher densities of surface glycoprotein receptors and greater granule content per unit volume. This size-reactivity relationship is the physiologic rationale for the observation that a rapidly regenerating platelet population, such as that seen shortly after recovery from chemotherapy-induced thrombocytopenia or after splenectomy, can achieve adequate hemostasis at a lower absolute platelet count than would otherwise be expected, because the platelets present, though fewer, are disproportionately young and functionally competent.

Parameter	Neonate (Term)	Adult Reference Range	Clinical Note
Platelet count	150-450 x10^9/L (overlaps adult range by term)	150-450 x10^9/L	Preterm infants have lower physiologic nadirs and a higher baseline incidence of thrombocytopenia.

Mean platelet volume	Slightly lower than adult values at birth	7.5-11.5 fL (assay-dependent; confirm local reference range)	Rises over the first weeks of life as compensatory thrombopoiesis matures.
Platelet lifespan	Similar order of magnitude to adult (approximately 7-10 days)	Approximately 7-10 days	Estimates vary by labeling methodology; confirm assay-specific reference data when precise kinetics are clinically required.
Megakaryocyte ploidy	Lower average ploidy than adult marrow	Typically 16N-32N, up to 64N or higher	Neonatal megakaryocytes are smaller and lower-ploidy, yielding fewer platelets per cell, a contributor to neonatal thrombocytopenia risk.

Platelet Kinetics, Lifespan, and Clearance

Circulating Lifespan and Senescence Pathways

A healthy circulating platelet survives for approximately seven to ten days before being cleared, a lifespan far shorter than that of an erythrocyte and one that reflects the platelet's role as a rapidly renewable, disposable hemostatic effector rather than a long-lived structural cell. Clearance of aged platelets occurs predominantly through a desialylation-dependent mechanism: as a platelet ages, sialic acid residues are progressively removed from surface glycoproteins, exposing underlying galactose residues that are recognized by the hepatic Ashwell-Morell receptor, which mediates uptake and clearance by hepatocytes. This pathway operates continuously at low level to remove senescent platelets from the circulation and has been shown, in some circumstances, to also drive accelerated thrombopoietin production through a hepatic sensing mechanism linked to the same desialylation signal, providing a second, more rapid layer of feedback regulation on top of the platelet-mass-consumption model described earlier in this chapter.

Pathologic acceleration of this same desialylation pathway has been implicated in the thrombocytopenia associated with some bacterial and viral infections, in which pathogen-derived or host neuraminidase activity strips sialic acid from platelets prematurely, marking otherwise healthy young platelets for clearance well before their natural lifespan has elapsed. This mechanism is distinct from, and can coexist with, antibody-mediated immune destruction, and it is one of several reasons why sepsis-associated thrombocytopenia, discussed in Chapter 14, often has a multifactorial rather than single-mechanism explanation.

Splenic Sequestration and the Marginal Pool

At any given moment, approximately one-third of the body's total platelet mass resides not in the general circulation but within a slowly exchanging marginal pool sequestered in the splenic sinusoids and cords. This is a normal, physiologic distribution, not a pathologic one, and it means that a peripheral venous platelet count reflects only the circulating two-thirds of total platelet mass. Splenomegaly expands the splenic marginal pool disproportionately, so that a markedly enlarged spleen can sequester sixty to ninety percent of total platelet mass, producing a peripheral platelet count that appears substantially low even though total platelet production and total platelet mass in the body may be entirely normal.

Figure 1.3: Splenomegaly with Platelet Sequestration

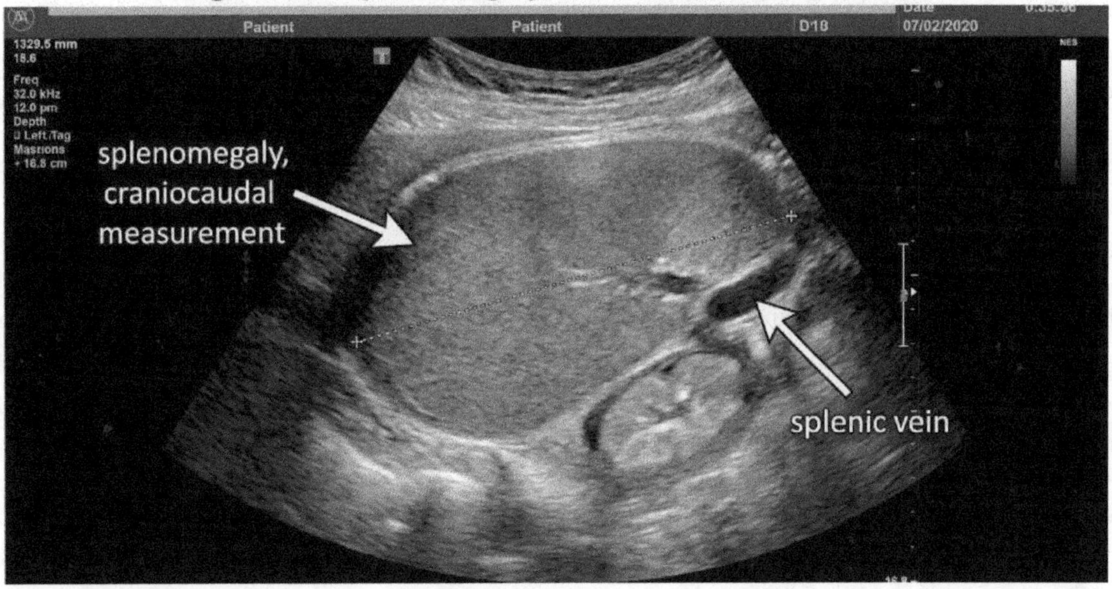

This distinction between true thrombocytopenia and splenic redistribution is one of the first branch points in the diagnostic approach to a low platelet count, addressed in detail in Chapter 8, and it explains why the physical examination finding of splenomegaly is weighted so heavily in that evaluation: a palpable spleen reframes an isolated low platelet count from a possible production or destruction problem into a probable distribution problem, fundamentally changing the subsequent workup.

Determinants of Steady-State Platelet Count

The steady-state circulating platelet count observed on any given complete blood count is therefore the net result of three independent variables operating simultaneously: the rate of platelet production by marrow megakaryocytes, the rate of platelet clearance through senescence and other destruction pathways, and the fraction of total platelet mass sequestered outside the peripheral circulation at that moment. An abnormal count can result from a derangement in any one of these variables in isolation, or from simultaneous derangements in more than one, which is why the clinical evaluation of thrombocytopenia, formalized in Chapter 8, is structured explicitly around identifying which of these three mechanisms, or which combination, is responsible in a given patient, rather than proceeding directly to a list of specific diseases.

THE PLATELET CRISIS DECISION COMPASS — A Disappointing Platelet Count Rise After Transfusion

The Presentation: A platelet transfusion is administered for thrombocytopenia, and the post-transfusion platelet count, measured at ten minutes to one hour or at eighteen to twenty-four hours, rises far less than the calculated corrected count increment predicts for the dose given and the patient's body surface area.

Mimic Signature: Non-immune consumptive refractoriness from sepsis, disseminated intravascular coagulation, active bleeding, or splenomegaly; immune refractoriness from HLA class I alloimmunization or, less commonly, human platelet antigen alloimmunization; and technical causes including inappropriately stored or ABO-incompatible product.

The Decision: Calculate the corrected count increment from the ten-minute to one-hour post-transfusion count; if low on a single occasion, evaluate first for a non-immune consumptive cause, since these are far more common than alloimmunization at first presentation; reserve HLA and platelet-specific antibody testing, and consideration of HLA-matched or crossmatched platelet products, for refractoriness that persists across two or more sequential, ABO-compatible, appropriately stored transfusions.

Trap Logic: Ordering an HLA antibody panel after a single refractory transfusion, before excluding sepsis, active bleeding, or splenomegaly, delays identification of the far more common and often more urgent non-immune cause and can commit a patient to an unnecessary search for HLA-matched platelet products.

Crisis Anchor: One low corrected count increment is a consumptive-cause screen; a pattern of low corrected count increments across multiple ABO-compatible transfusions is what should trigger an alloimmunization workup.

Megakaryopoiesis Across the Lifespan: Fetal, Neonatal, Pregnancy, and Aging Physiology

Fetal and Neonatal Megakaryopoiesis

Megakaryocytes present in the fetal liver and, later, the fetal and neonatal bone marrow differ systematically from their adult counterparts in ways that have direct clinical consequences. Fetal and neonatal megakaryocytes are smaller, achieve a lower maximum ploidy, and produce fewer platelets per cell than adult megakaryocytes, a pattern that persists into early infancy and gradually normalizes over the first months to years of life. This reduced per-cell platelet yield means that neonates, and particularly preterm neonates, operate with a narrower production reserve than older children and adults, so that a stressor that would be readily compensated for in an adult, such as a modest consumptive process or a brief period of marrow suppression, can produce more pronounced and more prolonged thrombocytopenia in a neonate. Preterm infants born before thirty-two weeks of gestation are disproportionately affected, both because their megakaryocytes are at an even earlier, lower-ploidy stage of developmental maturation and because they more frequently experience the placental insufficiency and perinatal stress states that independently suppress platelet production.

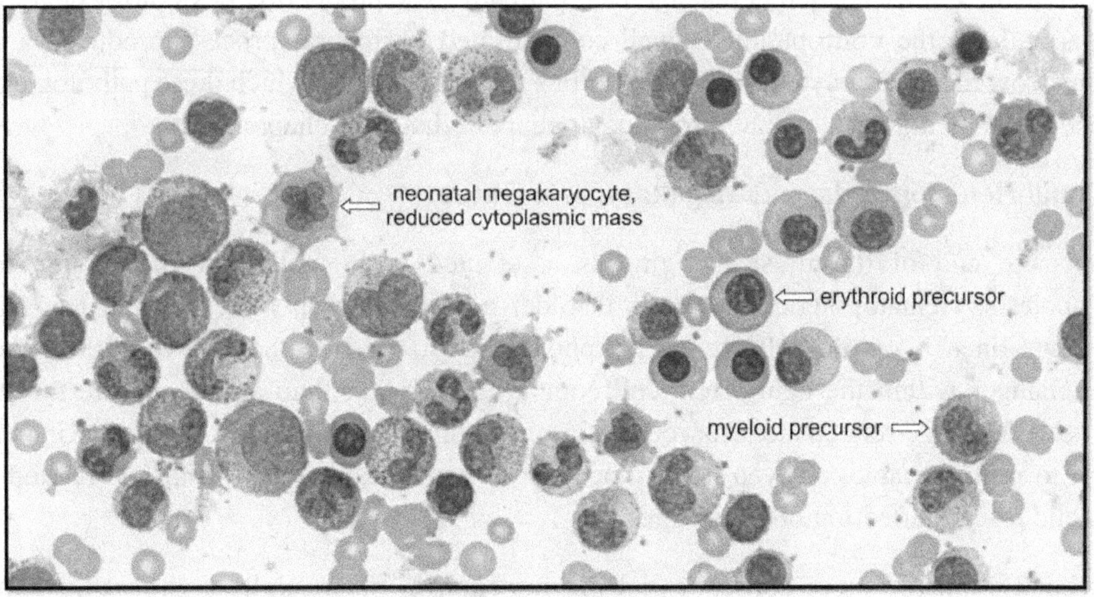

Figure 1.2: Neonatal Bone Marrow Megakaryocytes

This developmental physiology also explains why the platelet count reference range used for neonates, particularly preterm neonates, should not simply be borrowed from adult laboratory reporting without adjustment, and why a platelet count in the lower end of the adult reference range, which would prompt no evaluation in an adult, may already represent a meaningfully abnormal value relative to a gestational-age-adjusted neonatal norm. Clinical laboratories that serve neonatal intensive care populations increasingly report gestational-age-stratified reference intervals for exactly this reason, and clinicians interpreting a neonatal platelet count should confirm which reference standard, adult or age-adjusted, is being applied before concluding that a borderline count is normal.

Megakaryopoiesis and Platelet Turnover in Pregnancy

Pregnancy is associated with a well-described, physiologic decline in maternal platelet count, most pronounced in the third trimester, driven by a combination of hemodilution from expanded plasma volume and modestly increased platelet consumption related to the low-grade activation state of pregnancy and the uteroplacental circulation. This physiologic gestational thrombocytopenia typically keeps the platelet count above 100 x10^9/L and resolves spontaneously within one to two months of delivery, and it is the most common cause of thrombocytopenia identified during pregnancy, accounting for the substantial majority of cases. Megakaryopoiesis itself compensates for this increased peripheral turnover by increasing in a manner broadly analogous to the compensatory mechanisms described earlier in this chapter for other consumptive states, so that marrow megakaryocyte number in gestational thrombocytopenia is typically normal to increased rather than reduced.

The clinical importance of recognizing physiologic gestational thrombocytopenia lies chiefly in distinguishing it from the pathologic causes of thrombocytopenia in pregnancy addressed in Chapter 13, including pregnancy-associated immune thrombocytopenia, preeclampsia and HELLP syndrome, and pregnancy-associated thrombotic microangiopathy, each of which carries materially different maternal and fetal risk and requires a different management pathway. The production physiology developed in this chapter, particularly the concept that a well-compensated peripheral process produces a normal-to-increased marrow megakaryocyte response, underlies the reasoning by which these pathologic entities are distinguished from benign gestational thrombocytopenia in that later chapter.

Aging, Clonal Hematopoiesis, and Megakaryocyte Output

At the opposite end of the lifespan, aging is associated with subtle but measurable changes in megakaryopoiesis. Hematopoietic stem cells in older adults show an increased intrinsic bias toward megakaryocyte-lineage output relative to lymphoid output, a shift thought to reflect cell-intrinsic epigenetic changes within the aging stem cell compartment rather than any change in thrombopoietin signaling itself. This age-related megakaryocyte bias may help explain why platelet counts in healthy older adults tend to remain stable, or even trend modestly upward, despite an overall age-related decline in hematopoietic reserve affecting other lineages.

A separate and clinically more consequential phenomenon in older adults is clonal hematopoiesis of indeterminate potential, in which an acquired somatic mutation in a gene such as DNMT3A, TET2, ASXL1, or JAK2 confers a proliferative advantage to a single hematopoietic stem cell clone without yet meeting diagnostic criteria for a hematologic malignancy. When the mutation involves a gene directly coupled to megakaryocyte or myeloid proliferation, most notably JAK2, the resulting clone can manifest first as an otherwise unexplained thrombocytosis in an older adult, effectively representing a subclinical precursor to the myeloproliferative neoplasms discussed later in this book. This is one of several reasons why the Platelet Crisis Decision Compass presented earlier in this chapter for isolated thrombocytosis emphasizes molecular testing rather than reassurance by exclusion of symptoms alone, since a clinically silent JAK2-mutant clone can be present for years before any other hematologic abnormality becomes apparent.

KEY POINT: Reference ranges, compensatory capacity, and the pretest probability of specific diagnoses all shift meaningfully across the lifespan. A platelet count or a clinical picture that would be unremarkable in one age group, whether a preterm neonate, a pregnant patient in the third trimester, or an older adult with an incidental thrombocytosis, may carry an entirely different diagnostic weight in another.

Disorders of Platelet Production: an Overview and Roadmap

Quantitative Versus Qualitative Disorders of Production

Disorders of platelet production divide naturally into two categories that require different diagnostic approaches. Quantitative disorders reduce or increase the number of platelets released, without necessarily affecting the function of the platelets that are produced; these include the marrow failure syndromes, infiltrative processes, and the myeloproliferative neoplasms introduced earlier in this chapter. Qualitative disorders, by contrast, may leave the platelet count entirely normal while impairing the structural or functional integrity of each platelet produced, as occurs in MYH9-related disease, Wiskott-Aldrich syndrome, and the inherited platelet function disorders discussed in Chapter 16. A patient can therefore present with a bleeding tendency and a normal platelet count, a combination that is easy to dismiss incorrectly as functional or non-hematologic if the possibility of a qualitative production defect is not actively considered.

Central Versus Peripheral Causes: Locating the Lesion

Every disorder of platelet number discussed in this book can be located on the same three-variable map introduced earlier: a central (marrow production) defect, a peripheral destruction or consumption process, or an abnormal distribution between the circulating and sequestered pools. Bone marrow examination remains the single most direct way to distinguish a central production defect, in which megakaryocyte number is reduced or the megakaryocytes present are dysplastic, from a peripheral process, in which megakaryocyte number is typically normal or increased as the marrow compensates for ongoing peripheral loss. This central-versus-peripheral distinction, more than any single laboratory test, is what organizes the diagnostic algorithm presented in Chapter 8 and underlies the clinical reasoning in nearly every chapter that follows.

How This Book Is Organized Around the Production-to-Clearance Axis

Genetic Counseling and Family Screening in Inherited Production Disorders

When a thrombocytopenia is traced to a germline lesion in the megakaryopoiesis pathway, the clinical task extends beyond the affected patient to their family. Familial platelet disorder with predisposition to myeloid malignancy, caused by germline RUNX1 mutation and introduced earlier in this chapter, illustrates why this extension matters: first-degree relatives who share the mutation carry the same lifetime leukemia risk, estimated at roughly forty percent by some cohort series, regardless of whether they themselves have a clinically apparent bleeding history. Identification of a RUNX1 mutation in an index patient should therefore prompt an offer of cascade genetic testing to first-degree relatives, and mutation-positive relatives, even if asymptomatic, are generally recommended to undergo periodic surveillance blood counts and to have their case discussed with a center experienced in inherited bone marrow failure syndromes, since early identification of clonal evolution toward myelodysplastic syndrome or acute myeloid leukemia in this population can materially change transplantation timing and donor selection, including the exclusion of a mutation-positive sibling as a stem cell donor who might otherwise appear to be an ideal match.

Thrombocytopenia with absent radii syndrome, illustrated in the case that follows, raises a different counseling question, centered on recurrence risk for future pregnancies rather than malignancy surveillance. Because the syndrome requires both a chromosome 1q21.1 deletion and a hypomorphic RBM8A variant on the opposite allele, recurrence risk calculation depends on which parent carries which lesion: a parent who carries only the common, population-frequency hypomorphic RBM8A variant without the deletion is generally unaffected and has a modest recurrence risk driven by the population frequency of the deletion in a partner, whereas a parent who carries the 1q21.1 deletion itself, typically without radial anomalies if the deletion is inherited rather than de novo, faces a substantially higher recurrence risk with each pregnancy. Accurate counseling therefore requires parental testing for both the deletion and the RBM8A variant, not testing of the affected child alone, and should generally involve a clinical genetics consultation before a family proceeds with future pregnancy planning.

Megakaryocyte Rupture Versus Proplatelet Shedding: Resolving a Historical Debate

For much of the twentieth century, two competing models of platelet release coexisted in the hematology literature. One model held that mature megakaryocytes simply fragmented, or ruptured, within the marrow sinusoid, releasing platelet-sized cytoplasmic pieces directly. The other, favored by most investigators by the century's end and substantially confirmed by intravital microscopy studies performed directly within living marrow, described the proplatelet mechanism detailed earlier in this chapter, in which platelets are shed in an organized, cytoskeleton-directed fashion from the tips of elongating proplatelet processes rather than through indiscriminate cell rupture. The distinction is not merely historical trivia: the proplatelet model explains several features of platelet biology that a simple rupture model cannot, including the observation that proplatelet-derived platelets show a consistent, reproducible size distribution rather than the highly variable fragment sizes that indiscriminate cellular rupture would be expected to produce, and the observation that megakaryocyte nuclei are essentially never found free in the circulation despite the release of thousands of platelets per cell, which is explained by orderly proplatelet shedding but would be difficult to reconcile with a rupture mechanism.

Understanding platelet release as an organized, receptor- and cytoskeleton-directed process rather than passive fragmentation also clarifies why so many inherited platelet disorders selectively affect platelet size, number, or granule content without producing a global megakaryocyte failure: each of the inherited syndromes discussed throughout this chapter maps onto a specific, discrete step within the proplatelet formation and release pathway, from cytoskeletal elongation to membrane fission, rather than onto a nonspecific disruption of an unregulated rupture process. This mechanistic specificity is precisely what allows platelet size and morphology, easily assessed on a routine peripheral smear, to function as a diagnostic clue pointing toward a particular step in the production pathway, a theme that recurs throughout this book whenever an inherited platelet disorder is discussed.

EVIDENCE: Intravital imaging studies tracking megakaryocytes and proplatelets directly within living bone marrow and pulmonary microvasculature have been central to resolving the release-mechanism debate described above, and have further established that circulating megakaryocyte fragments and intact megakaryocytes reaching the lung continue to generate platelets there, reframing the lung as an active site of terminal thrombopoiesis rather than a passive filter.

The chapters that follow this one move systematically along the axis established here. Chapters 2 through 4 complete the biology of the mature platelet itself, covering its ultrastructure, receptor repertoire, and activation signaling. Chapters 5 through 7 build the clinical and laboratory toolkit for evaluating a suspected platelet disorder. Chapters 8 through 15 work through the thrombocytopenic disorders, generally proceeding from more central to more peripheral mechanisms. Chapters 16 and 17 address platelet function disorders and the thrombocytoses, respectively, returning conceptually to the production-side abnormalities introduced in this chapter but now at the level of established clinical disease. The final chapters address the therapeutics, including transfusion medicine, that translate this diagnostic framework into bedside action.

The following case illustrates how a disorder rooted entirely in the biology covered in this chapter, a failure of megakaryocyte production during fetal development, presents clinically and how the production-versus-peripheral framework guides its recognition.

CLINICAL CASE: A full-term female infant is noted at birth to have bilateral absence of the radii with intact thumbs, and a complete blood count obtained because of feeding difficulty and scattered petechiae reveals a platelet count of 22 x10^9/L with an otherwise normal white cell count and hemoglobin. The combination of a specific skeletal malformation and severe thrombocytopenia present from birth, rather than a nonspecific cytopenia alone, is the clinical signature that should immediately narrow the differential toward an inherited bone marrow failure or megakaryocyte-specific production syndrome rather than an acquired neonatal process such as alloimmune thrombocytopenia or sepsis-associated consumption, both of which are far more common overall but neither of which produces a limb malformation. Bilateral radial aplasia with preserved thumbs, combined with thrombocytopenia that is typically most severe in infancy and tends to improve somewhat with age, is the classic phenotype of thrombocytopenia with absent radii syndrome, caused by a deletion on chromosome 1q21.1 in combination with a hypomorphic RBM8A variant on the remaining allele. The mechanism is a partial, rather than complete, loss of RBM8A function, which impairs megakaryocyte maturation and proplatelet formation during a critical developmental window; complete biallelic loss of RBM8A is embryonic lethal, which is why every affected patient carries at least one hypomorphic allele rather than a full deletion on both chromosomes. Diagnosis is confirmed by chromosomal microarray demonstrating the 1q21.1 deletion together with targeted sequencing or a minor-allele-frequency assay for the RBM8A variant, since the variant alone is common in the general population and only becomes pathogenic in combination with deletion of the other allele. Management in infancy centers on platelet transfusion support during the period of most severe thrombocytopenia and orthopedic evaluation of the limb malformation, while longer-term surveillance addresses the tendency for the platelet count to rise gradually over the first several years of life as compensatory megakaryopoiesis, through mechanisms not yet fully defined, partially overcomes the underlying RBM8A deficiency. This case demonstrates a principle that recurs throughout the book: a production-level lesion, once correctly localized to a specific step in megakaryopoiesis, converts a nonspecific finding of thrombocytopenia into a precise, mechanistically explicable, and prognostically informative diagnosis. Longitudinal follow-up of this infant illustrates the second half of the principle: because the underlying defect is a partial rather than complete loss of RBM8A function, compensatory megakaryopoiesis through pathways that remain incompletely characterized typically raises the platelet count over the first several years of life, so that many affected children eventually reach a range that no longer requires regular transfusion support, even though the radial malformation and its orthopedic and functional consequences persist unchanged. Multidisciplinary follow-up accordingly shifts in emphasis over time, from hematology-led transfusion management and bleeding precautions in infancy toward orthopedic and occupational therapy-led functional management in later childhood, while periodic blood counts continue to track the expected gradual improvement and would prompt renewed hematologic evaluation if the trajectory instead reversed.

PATIENT EDUCATION: Families of an infant with thrombocytopenia with absent radii syndrome should be counseled that the platelet count is expected to improve gradually over the first several years of life even without a change in treatment, that bleeding precautions (avoiding intramuscular injections where oral or intravenous alternatives exist, using soft toothbrushes, and seeking urgent care for head trauma) apply throughout the period of most severe thrombocytopenia, and that cow's milk protein intolerance, a recognized and clinically significant association in this syndrome, should be considered if feeding difficulty or gastrointestinal symptoms persist beyond the neonatal period.

Figure 1.4 Bone Marrow Aspiration Technique for a Suspected Production Disorder

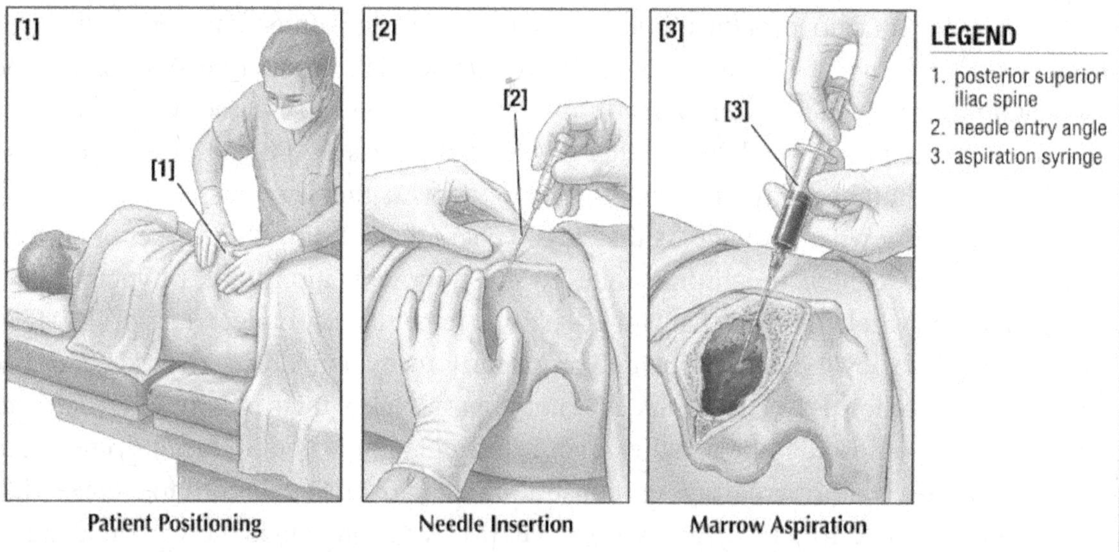

Bone marrow examination, illustrated above, remains the definitive tool for distinguishing central from peripheral thrombocytopenia whenever the distinction cannot be made confidently from history, physical examination, and basic laboratory testing alone, and its interpretation depends entirely on the megakaryocyte biology developed in this chapter: an aspirate or biopsy is examined specifically for megakaryocyte number, ploidy distribution, and morphology, each of which maps directly back to a specific stage of the maturation pathway described above.

Compass Recap: Isolated Thrombocytosis: An incidental thrombocytosis without an identified reactive cause after basic screening warrants JAK2, CALR, and MPL mutation testing before reassurance is offered; asymptomatic status does not exclude a clonal myeloproliferative process.

Compass Recap: Post-Transfusion Increment: A single low corrected count increment after platelet transfusion should first prompt evaluation for non-immune consumptive causes; alloimmunization workup is reserved for refractoriness that persists across multiple ABO-compatible transfusions.

Chapter Anchor: Every disorder of platelet number in this book can be located on the same three-variable map established in this chapter: production, lifespan and clearance, and distribution between circulating and sequestered pools. Locating a patient's abnormal count on this map before consulting a disease-specific chapter is the single habit of mind this book is built to reinforce.

Summary and Key Concepts

Megakaryocyte commitment and maturation are governed by a defined transcription factor program (GATA1, FOG1, RUNX1, FLI1, NF-E2); inherited mutations in these factors produce recognizable, often familial, thrombocytopenia syndromes with distinct prognostic implications.

Endomitosis produces the megakaryocyte's characteristic polyploidy, accumulating the cytoplasmic mass needed to support proplatelet formation and eventual release of thousands of platelets from a single cell.

Thrombopoietin is synthesized constitutively by the liver and cleared by megakaryocyte and platelet mass; circulating levels rise when platelet mass falls, making thrombopoietin level a marker of consumption rather than a directly regulated hormone.

Platelet release occurs through proplatelet formation and fission, with a substantial fraction of terminal release now understood to occur in the pulmonary microcirculation rather than exclusively within the bone marrow.

The steady-state platelet count reflects the balance of production, clearance (chiefly via desialylation and hepatic Ashwell-Morell receptor-mediated uptake), and distribution between the circulating and splenic marginal pools.

Locating an abnormal platelet count on the production-clearance-distribution map, and distinguishing central from peripheral mechanisms using bone marrow megakaryocyte number, organizes the entire diagnostic approach developed in the chapters that follow.

CHAPTER 2: PLATELET ULTRASTRUCTURE, GRANULES, AND RECEPTOR BIOLOGY

Learning Objectives

1. Describe the platelet plasma membrane and its specialized invaginations, the open canalicular system and the dense tubular system, and explain their distinct functional roles.
2. Identify the major platelet surface glycoprotein receptors, their ligands, and the inherited disorders that result from their absence or dysfunction.
3. Explain the cytoskeletal reorganization that underlies platelet shape change, and relate specific cytoskeletal defects to recognizable clinical syndromes.
4. Distinguish alpha granules, dense granules, and lysosomes by contents, and describe the clinical consequences of selective granule deficiency.
5. Interpret platelet electron microscopy and flow cytometry findings in the context of a suspected structural platelet disorder.
6. Explain how platelet Toll-like, Fc, and complement receptors couple platelet activation to innate immune and inflammatory processes beyond classical hemostasis.

Chapter Outline

This chapter dissects the mature, resting platelet from the outside in: the plasma membrane and its receptor repertoire, the specialized membrane invaginations that expand platelet surface area and enable rapid calcium signaling, the cytoskeleton that gives the resting platelet its discoid shape and drives its activation-associated transformation, and the three principal granule populations that store the mediators released during hemostasis. Two Platelet Crisis Decision Compass instances appear at the points where structural biology first produces a recognizable bedside problem: an unexpectedly prolonged bleeding time despite a normal platelet count, and a platelet function panel that suggests a storage pool disorder. The chapter closes with sections on platelet immune receptor biology, bioenergetics, and membrane remodeling with circulating age, three areas of platelet structural biology that receive comparatively little attention in traditional teaching but that connect directly to material developed in later chapters on sepsis-associated thrombocytopenia, transfusion medicine, and the interpretation of modern automated hematology analyzer parameters.

A resting platelet circulating in the bloodstream is a discoid structure roughly two to four micrometers in diameter, but this simple external shape conceals an extraordinarily organized internal architecture, purpose-built to convert a mechanical or chemical injury signal into a rapid, coordinated hemostatic response within seconds. Every element of that architecture described in this chapter exists to serve one of three functions: sensing injury through surface receptors, transmitting that signal through the cytoskeleton and internal membrane systems, and executing the response through regulated release of granule contents. Disorders of any one of these three functions produce a bleeding phenotype, and distinguishing which function has failed is the organizing task of platelet function disorder diagnosis, addressed in full in Chapter 16.

This three-function framework, sensing, transmission, and execution, deliberately parallels the three-variable production framework established in Chapter 1, and the two frameworks are meant to be used together in practice. A clinician first locates an abnormal platelet count on the production-clearance-distribution map from Chapter 1, and then, if the count itself is normal or if a functional bleeding phenotype persists despite a normal count, locates the abnormality on the sensing-transmission-execution map developed in this chapter. Used together, these two frameworks account for essentially the entire differential diagnosis of a platelet-related bleeding or thrombotic presentation before a single specialized platelet function test has been ordered, and both frameworks are revisited explicitly at the start of every disease-specific chapter that follows in this book.

Platelet Membrane Architecture and Surface Receptors

The Plasma Membrane and the Open Canalicular System

The platelet plasma membrane is a phospholipid bilayer whose composition is itself functionally important: phosphatidylserine and phosphatidylethanolamine, which are normally confined to the inner leaflet of the resting membrane by an ATP-dependent flippase, are externalized to the outer leaflet upon activation through the action of a scramblase, most notably TMEM16F. This externalized phosphatidylserine provides the anionic phospholipid surface required for assembly of the tenase and prothrombinase complexes of the coagulation cascade, directly coupling platelet activation to acceleration of thrombin generation, a link that makes the platelet not merely a mechanical plug but an active catalytic surface for coagulation. Loss-of-function mutations in TMEM16F produce Scott syndrome, a rare bleeding disorder in which platelet aggregation is entirely normal but the platelet surface fails to support efficient thrombin generation, illustrating that a normal platelet count and normal aggregation are not sufficient to guarantee normal hemostasis.

The plasma membrane is deeply invaginated into a branching network known as the open canalicular system, which threads throughout the platelet interior and communicates directly with the external environment. This system dramatically expands the platelet's effective surface area available for receptor-ligand interaction and provides a conduit through which granule contents, once released by fusion with the canalicular membrane, can reach the exterior without requiring the granule to migrate all the way to the peripheral plasma membrane. The open canalicular system also serves as a membrane reservoir: as a platelet spreads and forms filopodia during activation, membrane stored in the folded canalicular system unfurls to supply the substantial increase in surface area that spreading requires, without the platelet needing to synthesize new membrane on the rapid timescale that hemostasis demands.

The Dense Tubular System and Calcium Signaling

Distinct from the open canalicular system, the dense tubular system is a separate, closed membranous network derived from the megakaryocyte's smooth endoplasmic reticulum and functions as the platelet's principal intracellular calcium store, analogous to the sarcoplasmic reticulum of a muscle cell. Receptor activation triggers phospholipase C-mediated generation of inositol trisphosphate, which opens calcium release channels on the dense tubular system membrane and floods the cytoplasm with calcium, the central second messenger that drives shape change, granule secretion, and integrin activation. The dense tubular system also houses the enzymatic machinery for thromboxane A2 synthesis, including cyclooxygenase-1, the direct target of aspirin, positioning thromboxane generation immediately adjacent to the calcium signaling apparatus it helps amplify.

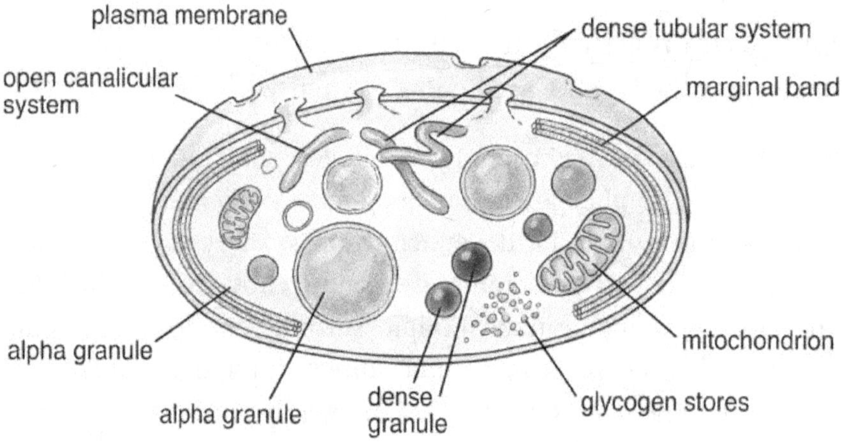

Figure 2.1: Platelet Ultrastructure in Cross-Section

Surface Glycoprotein Receptors: The Adhesion and Aggregation Repertoire

The platelet surface displays a defined repertoire of glycoprotein receptors, each coupling a specific extracellular ligand to an intracellular signaling or structural response. Glycoprotein Ib-IX-V, the platelet's von Willebrand factor receptor, mediates the initial, high-shear tethering of a platelet to exposed subendothelial matrix and is the receptor absent or dysfunctional in Bernard-Soulier syndrome, producing macrothrombocytopenia with markedly impaired primary hemostasis. Glycoprotein VI, together with the integrin alpha2beta1, mediates direct platelet adhesion to exposed collagen and initiates strong activating signals through an immunoreceptor tyrosine-based activation motif pathway analogous to that used by immune cell receptors. Glycoprotein IIb-IIIa, the integrin alphaIIbbeta3, is the most abundant platelet surface receptor and, once activated through inside-out signaling, binds fibrinogen and von Willebrand factor to mediate platelet-platelet aggregation; its absence or dysfunction produces Glanzmann thrombasthenia, a disorder addressed in detail in Chapter 16.

A second tier of surface receptors amplifies and sustains the initial adhesion signal. The P2Y12 receptor for adenosine diphosphate, released from dense granules upon activation, is the target of the thienopyridine and related antiplatelet drugs discussed in Chapter 18, and its activation is essential for stabilizing platelet aggregates under flow. The thromboxane A2 receptor and the protease-activated receptors PAR-1 and PAR-4, which respond to thrombin generated locally at the injury site, complete a set of amplification loops that convert an initial, reversible platelet tether into a stable, irreversible hemostatic plug. Each of these receptors represents both a physiologic amplification node and a pharmacologic target, and understanding their individual contributions is what allows a clinician to reason about which antiplatelet agent addresses which specific step in the activation cascade.

Receptor	Primary Ligand	Associated Inherited Disorder (Absence/Dysfunction)
Glycoprotein Ib-IX-V	von Willebrand factor	Bernard-Soulier syndrome
Glycoprotein VI / integrin alpha2beta1	Collagen	Rare collagen receptor deficiency (uncommon)
Integrin alphaIIbbeta3 (GPIIb-IIIa)	Fibrinogen, von Willebrand factor	Glanzmann thrombasthenia
P2Y12	Adenosine diphosphate	Congenital P2Y12 deficiency (rare)
TMEM16F (scramblase)	N/A (membrane phospholipid scrambling)	Scott syndrome

THE PLATELET CRISIS DECISION COMPASS — Prolonged Bleeding Time with a Normal Platelet Count

---

The Presentation: A patient with mucocutaneous bleeding symptoms and a normal platelet count on complete blood count, in whom a screening bleeding time or platelet function analyzer closure time returns prolonged.

Mimic Signature: Von Willebrand disease affecting glycoprotein Ib-IX-V-mediated adhesion; an inherited platelet receptor or granule disorder with normal platelet number, such as Glanzmann thrombasthenia, Bernard-Soulier syndrome, or a storage pool disorder; acquired platelet dysfunction from antiplatelet medication, uremia, or a paraprotein; and a preanalytic artifact from difficult venipuncture or sample handling.

The Decision: Confirm the abnormal screening result is reproducible on a repeat, well-collected sample; take a directed medication and supplement history; send von Willebrand factor antigen, activity, and factor VIII level as the highest-yield first-line evaluation given the relative prevalence of von Willebrand disease; and proceed to light transmission aggregometry and, where available, flow cytometric receptor quantification only if von Willebrand disease is excluded or the phenotype does not fit.

Trap Logic: Ordering aggregometry before excluding von Willebrand disease inverts the correct diagnostic sequence, since von Willebrand disease is far more prevalent than any inherited platelet receptor disorder and aggregometry itself can be secondarily abnormal in von Willebrand disease, producing a confusing result that delays the correct diagnosis.

Crisis Anchor: Von Willebrand factor testing precedes platelet function testing in the evaluation of mucocutaneous bleeding with a normal platelet count, not the reverse.

The Cytoskeleton and Platelet Shape Change

The Resting Marginal Microtubule Band

The discoid shape of a resting platelet is actively maintained, not passive, by a circumferential bundle of microtubules known as the marginal band, positioned just beneath the plasma membrane at the platelet's equator. This band is composed of a single microtubule coiled repeatedly around the platelet circumference and is stabilized by microtubule-associated proteins that resist depolymerization under the shear forces of normal circulation. Loss of marginal band integrity, whether through pharmacologic microtubule disruption or through mutation of the beta1-tubulin gene TUBB1, produces platelets that fail to maintain their discoid shape and often exhibit an abnormally rounded or oval morphology on peripheral smear, together with mild thrombocytopenia in some TUBB1 variants. The marginal band is also cold-sensitive: exposure to temperatures below approximately 4 degrees Celsius causes the band to depolymerize and reassemble abnormally upon rewarming, producing irreversible platelet activation and clearance, which is the direct structural explanation for why platelet concentrates intended for transfusion are stored at room temperature with continuous gentle agitation rather than refrigerated as red cell products are, a point that connects the structural biology introduced here to the platelet storage lesion discussed later in this chapter and to platelet transfusion practice covered fully in Chapter 19.

Actin Reorganization During Activation

Upon activation, the platelet undergoes a dramatic and rapid shape change, converting from a smooth discoid form to a spread, irregular form studded with filopodia and lamellipodia, driven by coordinated actin polymerization and depolymerization. The Arp2/3 complex nucleates branched actin networks that drive lamellipodial spreading, while formins drive the elongation of unbranched actin filaments into filopodial spikes, and this entire process is coordinated by Rho-family GTPases, principally Cdc42 and Rac1, acting downstream of the same calcium and diacylglycerol signals generated by receptor activation. This shape change dramatically increases the platelet's effective contact area with the injured vessel wall and with adjacent platelets, converting a point contact into a broad adhesive surface within seconds of activation.

Wiskott-Aldrich syndrome protein, mentioned in Chapter 1 as a determinant of platelet size, functions specifically as an activator of the Arp2/3 complex, and its absence in Wiskott-Aldrich syndrome and the related X-linked thrombocytopenia impairs actin branching during both megakaryocyte proplatelet formation and mature platelet activation, producing a combined defect in platelet production and platelet function that helps explain why bleeding symptoms in this condition are often disproportionate to the platelet count alone. MYH9-related disease, introduced in Chapter 1 for its effect on proplatelet fission, similarly affects the contractile actomyosin apparatus required for platelet spreading and clot retraction in the mature platelet, again illustrating how a single cytoskeletal gene defect can produce parallel abnormalities at both the production and functional level.

Clot Retraction and the Contractile Apparatus

In the final phase of platelet-mediated hemostasis, activated platelets bound to fibrin through integrin alphaIIbbeta3 generate contractile force through an actomyosin mechanism analogous to muscle contraction, pulling on the surrounding fibrin meshwork to physically retract and consolidate the clot. This clot retraction, historically assessed by simple visual observation of retracting whole blood clots in a test tube, requires functional integrin alphaIIbbeta3, an intact contractile cytoskeleton, and adequate platelet number, and its absence in the historical clot retraction assay was one of the earliest clinical clues to Glanzmann thrombasthenia, decades before glycoprotein-specific flow cytometry became available. Although largely superseded by more specific testing in modern practice, the underlying biology of clot retraction remains clinically relevant: it is thought to contribute to wound contraction and to the mechanical stability of a formed clot against premature dislodgement, and its impairment likely contributes to the bleeding phenotype seen in disorders of the contractile apparatus even when initial platelet plug formation is adequate. The same actomyosin contractile machinery that drives clot retraction also generates the mechanical forces that platelets exert on the surrounding fibrin network during the broader process of clot maturation, and impaired force generation has been associated in some studies with reduced clot stiffness, a mechanical property increasingly measured directly by viscoelastic assays such as thromboelastography and rotational thromboelastometry, discussed further as diagnostic tools in Chapter 7; a soft, poorly retracted clot on these assays in the presence of a normal platelet count and normal standard coagulation studies can be an important clue toward an underlying platelet contractile or receptor defect that would otherwise be missed.

Granule Biology: Alpha Granules, Dense Granules, and Lysosomes

Alpha Granules: Contents and Biogenesis

Alpha granules are the most numerous platelet granule, with fifty to eighty present in a typical platelet, and they carry an extraordinarily diverse cargo of proteins synthesized by the megakaryocyte and, in some cases, taken up from plasma by endocytosis. This cargo includes adhesive proteins such as von Willebrand factor and fibrinogen, growth factors including platelet-derived growth factor and transforming growth factor beta, angiogenic and antiangiogenic factors, coagulation factors including factor V, and membrane-bound receptors such as P-selectin that are inserted into the plasma membrane upon granule fusion and serve as a marker of platelet activation detectable by flow cytometry. Recent evidence indicates that alpha granule cargo is not uniformly distributed but is instead packaged into at least partially distinct granule subpopulations, so that a single activating stimulus can trigger differential release of pro-angiogenic versus anti-angiogenic cargo depending on the specific receptor engaged, a level of regulatory sophistication that helps explain platelet involvement in processes well beyond classical hemostasis, including wound healing, tumor angiogenesis, and immune modulation.

Gray platelet syndrome results from selective alpha granule deficiency, caused most commonly by mutation in NBEAL2, a gene required for alpha granule biogenesis within the megakaryocyte. Platelets in this disorder are large, appear pale or gray on Wright-stained peripheral smear because they lack the alpha granule content that normally imparts a granular appearance, and produce a moderate bleeding phenotype together with progressive marrow fibrosis in many patients, thought to result from chronic leakage of growth factors that should have been packaged into alpha granules but instead are released constitutively into the marrow microenvironment, driving the same fibrotic niche disruption discussed in Chapter 1 in the context of primary myelofibrosis.

Dense Granules: Contents and the Storage Pool Disorders

Dense granules, present in smaller numbers than alpha granules at three to eight per platelet, store a distinct set of small-molecule mediators rather than proteins: adenosine diphosphate and adenosine triphosphate at extraordinarily high concentration, serotonin taken up from plasma, calcium, and polyphosphate. Dense granule adenosine diphosphate release upon activation feeds directly into the P2Y12 amplification loop discussed earlier in this chapter, making dense granule content essential for normal secondary aggregation even when the initial adhesion and primary activation machinery is entirely intact. Hermansky-Pudlak syndrome and Chediak-Higashi syndrome, both disorders of lysosome-related organelle biogenesis that affect dense granules along with melanosomes and, in Chediak-Higashi syndrome, other lysosome-related structures throughout the body, produce dense granule deficiency together with oculocutaneous albinism, linking a bleeding phenotype to a pigmentation phenotype through a shared organelle biogenesis defect that is easy to overlook if the two findings are not considered together.

Figure 2.2: Platelet Ultrastructure by Transmission Electron Microscopy

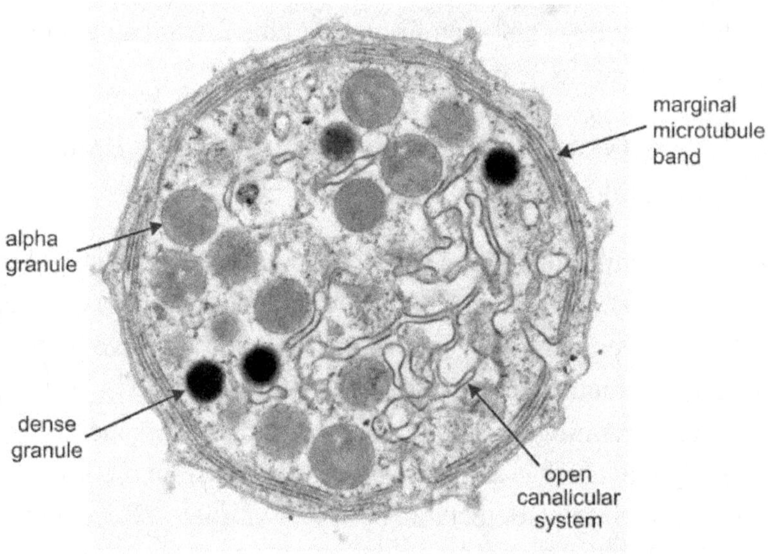

Lysosomes and Minor Granule Populations

A smaller population of lysosomal granules, containing acid hydrolases including cathepsins and glycosidases, is also present in platelets and is released, though generally more slowly and less completely than alpha or dense granule contents, upon strong platelet activation. The physiologic role of platelet lysosomal release remains less well defined than that of the other two granule populations, but proposed functions include extracellular matrix remodeling at the site of injury and modulation of the local inflammatory response. Because lysosomal markers overlap partially with those used to identify other granule populations by flow cytometry, isolated lysosomal granule disorders are rarely characterized as distinct clinical entities and are instead typically identified, when relevant, as part of a broader evaluation for a combined storage pool disorder.

Granule biogenesis for both alpha and dense granules depends on a shared, though partially divergent, intracellular trafficking machinery originating in the megakaryocyte's endosomal system, and mutations affecting shared trafficking components tend to produce combined rather than isolated granule deficiencies. VPS33B and its binding partner VIPAS39, for example, are required for normal alpha granule cargo trafficking, and biallelic mutation in either gene produces arthrogryposis-renal dysfunction-cholestasis syndrome, in which a gray-platelet-like alpha granule deficiency coexists with congenital joint contractures, renal tubular dysfunction, and neonatal cholestasis, a multisystem phenotype that reflects the broader role of this trafficking pathway outside the megakaryocyte lineage. Recognizing that a granule defect can be either an isolated hematologic finding or one manifestation of a shared, multisystem trafficking defect is essential when a patient presents with unexplained bleeding alongside findings in other organ systems, since the combination itself is diagnostically informative and should prompt a search for a shared underlying mechanism rather than being treated as coincidental.

THE PLATELET CRISIS DECISION COMPASS — A Platelet Function Panel Suggesting a Storage Pool Disorder

The Presentation: Light transmission aggregometry shows a normal primary wave of aggregation to multiple agonists but an absent or blunted secondary wave, particularly to adenosine diphosphate and epinephrine, with normal aggregation to ristocetin.

Mimic Signature: An inherited dense granule storage pool disorder (isolated or as part of Hermansky-Pudlak or Chediak-Higashi syndrome); acquired platelet dysfunction from recent aspirin, other nonsteroidal anti-inflammatory drug, or P2Y12 inhibitor exposure that can produce a similar aggregometry pattern; and uremia, which impairs granule release through mechanisms distinct from a structural storage pool defect.

The Decision: Confirm a genuine medication washout period before final interpretation, since recent antiplatelet exposure is a far more common cause of this pattern than an inherited disorder; if the pattern persists after an adequate washout, proceed to dense granule quantification by whole-mount electron microscopy or mepacrine uptake flow cytometry, and examine for associated oculocutaneous albinism suggesting Hermansky-Pudlak or Chediak-Higashi syndrome.

Trap Logic: Diagnosing an inherited storage pool disorder from a single aggregometry tracing obtained without confirming an adequate medication washout risks a false inherited-disorder label that follows the patient for life and can affect future perioperative and obstetric management unnecessarily.

Crisis Anchor: A blunted secondary aggregation wave is confirmed as a genuine storage pool disorder only after medication-related and uremic causes have been excluded and, ideally, after direct granule content quantification supports the diagnosis.

Platelet Receptors in Immune Surveillance and Inflammation

Toll-Like Receptors and Pathogen Sensing

Beyond the classical adhesion and aggregation receptors described earlier in this chapter, platelets express a functional repertoire of Toll-like receptors, most notably TLR2 and TLR4, that allow direct platelet sensing of bacterial and other pathogen-associated molecular patterns independent of classical hemostatic activation. Engagement of TLR4 by bacterial lipopolysaccharide, for example, triggers platelet degranulation, enhanced platelet-leukocyte aggregate formation, and release of neutrophil extracellular trap-promoting signals, positioning the platelet as an active participant in the innate immune response to systemic infection rather than a passive bystander. This immune-sensing function has direct relevance to the thrombocytopenia of sepsis discussed in Chapter 14, where pathogen-driven platelet activation through these same receptors contributes to accelerated platelet consumption independent of the disseminated intravascular coagulation that classically dominates teaching on that topic.

The clinical corollary of this pathogen-sensing function is that platelet activation markers, including surface P-selectin expression and platelet-leukocyte aggregate frequency, rise measurably during systemic infection even before overt coagulopathy develops, and some centers use these markers experimentally as early indicators of evolving sepsis-associated coagulopathy, although this remains a research rather than a standard clinical application at present. Understanding that platelets can be activated through pathogen-sensing receptors entirely independent of vascular injury also explains why an infected patient can develop clinically significant platelet activation and consumption in the complete absence of any mechanical or endothelial injury, a mechanism worth keeping distinct from the injury-triggered activation pathway that dominates the rest of this chapter.

Fc Receptors and Platelet Involvement in Antibody-Mediated Processes

Platelets express FcgammaRIIA, the only activating Fc receptor for immunoglobulin G present on human platelets, and this single receptor has outsized clinical importance because it is the mechanistic entry point for several of the most consequential acquired platelet disorders addressed later in this book. In heparin-induced thrombocytopenia, discussed in Chapter 11, immune complexes formed between heparin, platelet factor 4, and IgG antibody engage FcgammaRIIA to drive pathologic platelet activation and a paradoxical prothrombotic state despite a falling platelet count, a mechanism that is essential to understand because it explains why heparin-induced thrombocytopenia causes thrombosis rather than bleeding despite its name. In immune thrombocytopenia, discussed in Chapter 9, antibody-coated platelets are instead recognized and phagocytosed by Fc receptor-bearing macrophages in the spleen and liver, a distinct FcgammaRdependent clearance mechanism operating on macrophages rather than on the platelet's own FcgammaRIIA. The shared involvement of Fc receptor biology across these otherwise mechanistically distinct disorders is one reason this book returns repeatedly to antibody-receptor interactions as a unifying theme across the acquired thrombocytopenic disorders in Part III.

Complement Receptors and Platelet-Complement Crosstalk

Platelets also express receptors for complement components, including C1q and complement receptors that engage opsonized surfaces, and activated platelets can themselves serve as a surface for complement activation through both the classical and alternative pathways. This platelet-complement crosstalk is bidirectional: complement activation products, including C5a, can further activate platelets, while platelet activation can accelerate local complement deposition, creating an amplification loop that is increasingly recognized as clinically important in the thrombotic microangiopathies discussed in Chapter 12, particularly atypical hemolytic uremic syndrome, in which dysregulated alternative complement pathway activation on endothelial and platelet surfaces is the primary pathogenic mechanism rather than a secondary bystander phenomenon. Recognizing platelets as active participants in, rather than passive targets of, complement-mediated microvascular injury has directly informed the development of complement-targeted therapeutics used in that disorder.

Platelet Metabolism, Mitochondria, and Energy Supply for Activation

Mitochondrial Biology in an Anucleate Cell

Despite lacking a nucleus, each platelet retains several mitochondria inherited directly from the parent megakaryocyte's cytoplasm at the moment of proplatelet fission, and these mitochondria remain fully functional throughout the platelet's circulating lifespan, since platelets, unlike most anucleate cells, retain the capacity for oxidative phosphorylation. This mitochondrial retention is not incidental; activation, shape change, and secretion are energetically demanding processes that occur on a timescale of seconds and require a rapidly mobilizable adenosine triphosphate supply that glycolysis alone, though present and active in platelets, cannot fully provide under all circumstances. Platelet mitochondrial DNA content and function have additionally become a subject of interest as a biomarker in their own right, since circulating mitochondrial DNA released from activated or damaged platelets can act as a damage-associated molecular pattern that engages innate immune signaling, linking platelet bioenergetics to platelet immune and inflammatory functions well beyond classical hemostasis.

Glycolysis, Oxidative Phosphorylation, and the Metabolic Switch During Activation

Resting platelets rely predominantly on oxidative phosphorylation to meet baseline energy demands, but activation triggers a rapid shift toward aerobic glycolysis, a metabolic pattern in which glucose is converted to lactate even in the presence of adequate oxygen, broadly analogous to the Warburg effect described in proliferating tumor cells. This glycolytic shift provides a faster, if less efficient, route to adenosine triphosphate generation and simultaneously supplies glycolytic intermediates that feed into the pentose phosphate pathway, supporting the nicotinamide adenine dinucleotide phosphate-dependent oxidative burst and lipid membrane remodeling that accompany shape change and granule secretion. The speed of this metabolic switch, occurring within seconds of receptor engagement, is itself made possible by the pre-positioned mitochondria and glycolytic enzyme pools inherited from the megakaryocyte, since an anucleate platelet cannot transcribe new metabolic enzymes in response to activation the way a nucleated cell could.

Platelet Bioenergetics in Storage and Disease

Platelet metabolic function is not merely a laboratory curiosity; it has direct relevance to platelet product quality in transfusion medicine, addressed further in Chapter 19. Platelets stored ex vivo for transfusion undergo a progressive metabolic decline termed the platelet storage lesion, characterized by falling adenosine triphosphate content, accumulating lactate from ongoing glycolysis without adequate clearance, declining pH, and progressive, low-level activation with granule release and morphologic change from discoid toward spherical form. This storage lesion is the principal factor limiting the shelf life of platelet concentrates and is the reason platelet products, unlike red cell products, are stored at room temperature with continuous agitation rather than refrigerated, since cold storage accelerates a distinct but related activation and clearance pathway. Inherited primary mitochondrial disorders, in which oxidative phosphorylation is impaired throughout the body, can also produce a mild platelet function defect as one component of a broader multisystem phenotype, illustrating that the same metabolic machinery discussed in this section, when genetically compromised, has hemostatic consequences that a clinician evaluating an unexplained bleeding tendency in the context of a known or suspected mitochondrial disease should keep in mind.

Storage Parameter	Fresh Platelet Concentrate (Day 0-1)	End of Standard Shelf Life (Day 5-7)	Clinical Significance
Adenosine triphosphate content	Near baseline	Progressively declining	Falling ATP reflects the metabolic storage lesion and correlates with declining post-transfusion viability.
pH	7.2-7.4 (assay-dependent; confirm local standard)	Trends downward as lactate accumulates	A pH below the product's validated release threshold is a criterion for discard.
Lactate	Low	Progressively rising	Reflects sustained aerobic glycolysis without adequate clearance in the closed storage bag.
Platelet morphology (discoid score)	Predominantly discoid	Shift toward spherical, activated morphology	Loss of discoid form on visual or automated swirl assessment is used as

			a bedside quality indicator before release for transfusion.

This same bioenergetic decline is the reason platelet concentrates carry a shelf life measured in days rather than the weeks-to-months window available for red cell products, and it is also the reason platelet inventory management, discussed further in Chapter 19, is a persistent operational challenge for blood banks: unlike red cells, which can be frozen for long-term storage, platelets cannot currently be cryopreserved in a manner that preserves adequate function for routine clinical use at scale, so supply is continuously constrained by the same metabolic fragility that gives the platelet its rapid, energetically demanding hemostatic responsiveness in vivo.

Platelet Membrane Remodeling With Circulating Age

Receptor Density Changes During Platelet Aging

A newly released platelet is not functionally identical to one nearing the end of its seven-to-ten-day circulating lifespan discussed in Chapter 1, and surface receptor density is one of the parameters that changes measurably across that interval. Glycoprotein Ib-IX-V surface density, in particular, declines gradually as a platelet ages, a change linked to the same desialylation process that ultimately targets the platelet for hepatic clearance through the Ashwell-Morell receptor pathway, so that receptor loss and clearance marking appear to be mechanistically coupled rather than coincidental parallel processes. Integrin alphaIIbbeta3 density, by contrast, appears comparatively more stable across the platelet lifespan, though its activation state, rather than its total surface density, is what varies most with platelet age, with older platelets generally showing a reduced capacity for full integrin activation in response to a standard agonist stimulus compared with young platelets.

Reticulated Platelets and the Immature Platelet Fraction

The youngest platelets released from the marrow retain small residual amounts of megakaryocyte-derived messenger RNA for a brief period after entering the circulation, a feature exploited clinically through thiazole orange or oxazine-based staining, which binds residual RNA and identifies these newly released cells as reticulated platelets, directly analogous to the reticulocyte concept in red cell biology. Modern automated hematology analyzers report this same population as the immature platelet fraction, a parameter now widely available alongside the routine complete blood count on many platforms and increasingly incorporated into the diagnostic evaluation of thrombocytopenia discussed in Chapter 8. Because reticulated platelets and the immature platelet fraction directly reflect the rate of recent platelet release from the marrow, they function as a real-time surrogate for marrow megakaryocyte production activity without requiring a bone marrow biopsy, closing the loop back to the production-versus-peripheral framework established in Chapter 1.

Clinical Use of the Immature Platelet Fraction

An elevated immature platelet fraction in the setting of thrombocytopenia indicates that the marrow is actively releasing young platelets at an increased rate, a pattern consistent with a peripheral destruction or consumption process in which the marrow is compensating appropriately, such as immune thrombocytopenia or a resolving consumptive process. A low or inappropriately normal immature platelet fraction in the setting of thrombocytopenia, by contrast, suggests that the marrow is not mounting an adequate compensatory response, pointing toward a central production defect such as marrow aplasia, infiltration, or a myelosuppressive drug effect. This distinction can often be made within minutes from an automated analyzer result, well before a bone marrow biopsy could be scheduled and performed, and an increasing number of centers use a low immature platelet fraction as one of the factors supporting an earlier decision to proceed to marrow examination in an undifferentiated thrombocytopenia, rather than waiting through a longer trial of empiric management.

EVIDENCE: Comparative studies of the immature platelet fraction against bone marrow megakaryocyte assessment have generally shown good correlation between a low immature platelet fraction and reduced marrow megakaryocyte mass, supporting its use as a rapid, noninvasive adjunct, though not yet a replacement, for direct marrow examination when the central-versus-peripheral distinction is clinically urgent, such as in a critically ill patient in whom empiric management cannot safely await a scheduled biopsy.

Structural Basis of Inherited Platelet Disorders: an Integrative Roadmap

Mapping Structure to Syndrome

Every inherited platelet disorder addressed in this book maps onto a specific structural element introduced in this chapter: a surface receptor, a cytoskeletal component, or a granule population. This mapping is not merely an organizing convenience; it is the basis for a rational, mechanism-first approach to evaluating a patient with a suspected inherited platelet disorder, in which the pattern of laboratory abnormalities, aggregometry response, and associated clinical features (macrothrombocytopenia, albinism, hearing loss, nephropathy, and others introduced throughout this chapter) are used to localize the defect to a specific structural compartment before genetic testing is pursued, rather than proceeding directly to broad genetic panel testing without a working hypothesis.

This structural framework also clarifies why platelet count alone is an unreliable screen for platelet disorders as a category: receptor disorders such as Glanzmann thrombasthenia and granule disorders such as most storage pool disorders typically leave the platelet count entirely normal, while cytoskeletal disorders such as MYH9-related disease and Wiskott-Aldrich syndrome typically do not. A clinician evaluating unexplained mucocutaneous bleeding should therefore never allow a normal platelet count to end the evaluation prematurely; the structural elements described in this chapter, not the platelet count, are where a true functional platelet disorder is most often found.

It is also worth emphasizing that acquired disease frequently exploits the same structural vulnerabilities described throughout this chapter as inherited disease, so that the receptor, cytoskeletal, and granule framework developed here is not merely a scaffold for rare congenital syndromes but a lens applicable to the far more common acquired platelet disorders addressed in later chapters. Uremic platelet dysfunction, for example, impairs granule secretion and integrin activation through accumulation of guanidino compounds and altered nitric oxide signaling, producing a functional phenotype that overlaps substantially with the inherited granule and receptor disorders discussed above despite arising from an entirely acquired, reversible metabolic derangement. Myelodysplastic and myeloproliferative disease can likewise produce dysplastic megakaryocytes that generate platelets with reduced granule content or receptor density, an acquired parallel to the inherited production and structural disorders covered in this chapter and the preceding one. Recognizing this shared structural vocabulary across inherited and acquired disease is part of what allows a clinician to reason efficiently from an unfamiliar clinical presentation back to a specific, testable hypothesis about which structural compartment has failed, rather than requiring a distinct diagnostic framework for every individual disease encountered in clinical practice.

CLINICAL PEARL: A normal platelet count excludes a quantitative disorder but says nothing about receptor, cytoskeletal, or granule integrity. Persistent mucocutaneous bleeding with a normal platelet count should proceed to von Willebrand factor testing and, if indicated, platelet function testing, not to reassurance.

Diagnostic Algorithm: From Clinical Phenotype to Structural Compartment

The structural framework developed across this chapter can be converted into a stepwise evaluation sequence for a patient with suspected inherited platelet dysfunction, moving from the least to the most specialized testing in a manner intended to reach a structural localization efficiently and without unnecessary testing.

1. Confirm the platelet count and review peripheral smear morphology directly, noting platelet size, granularity, and the presence of any red or white cell clues to a syndromic diagnosis; this step alone begins to separate cytoskeletal disorders, which frequently alter platelet size, from receptor and granule disorders, which typically do not.
2. Take a directed medication history covering aspirin, other nonsteroidal anti-inflammatory drugs, P2Y12 inhibitors, and other agents with recognized antiplatelet effect, and confirm an adequate washout period, generally seven to ten days for irreversible cyclooxygenase and P2Y12 inhibitors, before proceeding further, since an unrecognized medication effect is the single most common cause of an abnormal platelet function evaluation.
3. Send von Willebrand factor antigen, activity, and factor VIII level as first-line testing whenever the presenting phenotype is mucocutaneous bleeding, given the substantially higher population prevalence of von Willebrand disease relative to any single inherited platelet receptor or granule disorder.
4. If von Willebrand disease is excluded or the phenotype does not fit, proceed to light transmission aggregometry using a standard agonist panel (adenosine diphosphate, epinephrine, collagen, arachidonic acid, and ristocetin), interpreting the pattern against the receptor and granule biology developed in this chapter: absent aggregation to all agonists except ristocetin localizes to integrin

alphaIIbbeta3; absent ristocetin-induced agglutination with preserved response to other agonists localizes to glycoprotein Ib-IX-V; and an isolated blunted secondary wave localizes to a granule secretion defect.

5. Confirm a receptor-level abnormality suggested by aggregometry using flow cytometric quantification of the relevant glycoprotein, and confirm a suspected granule defect using electron microscopy or a granule-specific uptake assay, before committing to genetic testing, so that genetic panel selection can be targeted to the implicated gene or gene family rather than sent as an unfocused broad panel.
6. Screen for associated syndromic features at each step along the way, including hearing loss, nephropathy, and cataracts suggesting MYH9-related disease; oculocutaneous albinism suggesting Hermansky-Pudlak or Chediak-Higashi syndrome; and eczema, recurrent infection, and small platelet size suggesting Wiskott-Aldrich syndrome, since identification of a syndromic association can substantially narrow genetic testing before it is even ordered.

CAUTION: Aggregometry is technically demanding and highly sensitive to preanalytic variables, including time from collection, sample temperature, and platelet count itself, since severe thrombocytopenia can produce an artifactually abnormal aggregometry tracing unrelated to any structural platelet defect. Results should always be interpreted by a laboratory experienced in platelet function testing, and an unexpected or internally inconsistent pattern should prompt repeat testing before a structural diagnosis is finalized.

Combined Structural Defects: Syndromes Spanning More Than One Compartment

Not every inherited platelet disorder confines itself neatly to a single structural compartment, and recognizing the syndromes that span more than one is important both for accurate diagnosis and for anticipating the full clinical phenotype. Wiskott-Aldrich syndrome protein, discussed earlier in this chapter for its role in cytoskeletal actin branching during mature platelet activation, is also required for normal proplatelet formation during megakaryopoiesis, so that its absence produces a combined defect spanning both the production biology covered in Chapter 1 and the cytoskeletal biology covered in this chapter, manifesting clinically as small platelets present in reduced number with additionally impaired function. MYH9-related disease similarly spans compartments, impairing both proplatelet fission during production and the contractile actomyosin apparatus required for mature platelet clot retraction and spreading.

This pattern of overlapping structural involvement is not coincidental; the megakaryocyte and the platelets it produces share the same cytoskeletal and trafficking machinery across the production and mature-cell phases of the lineage, so a gene defect affecting a core structural component, such as a cytoskeletal motor protein or a shared vesicular trafficking factor, will generally manifest at both stages simultaneously rather than at only one. A clinician who identifies an abnormality in platelet size or number should therefore always also assess platelet function directly, rather than assuming that a quantitative abnormality and a qualitative abnormality are mutually exclusive findings that point to separate, unrelated diagnoses.

Figure 2.3: Flow Cytometric Assessment of Platelet Surface Glycoproteins

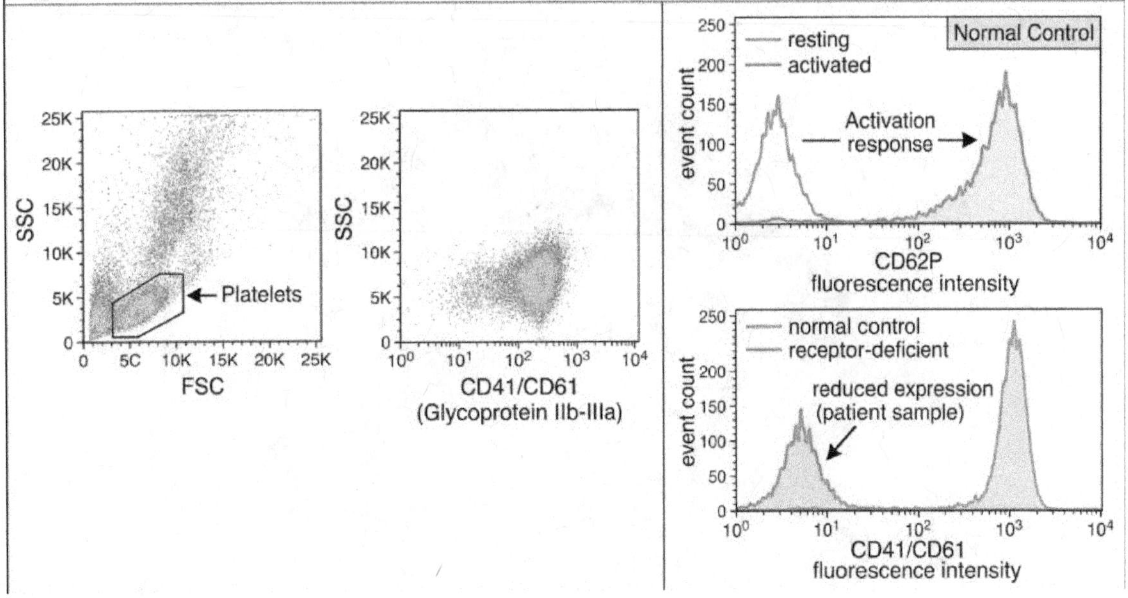

CLINICAL CASE: A 19-year-old man of consanguineous parentage presents for evaluation of lifelong easy bruising, recurrent epistaxis requiring cautery on two occasions, and heavy bleeding after a dental extraction that required repacking. His platelet count is 260 x10^9/L and peripheral smear morphology is unremarkable. Coagulation studies, including prothrombin time and activated partial thromboplastin time, are normal, and von Willebrand factor antigen, activity, and factor VIII level are all within normal limits, excluding von Willebrand disease as the explanation for his bleeding phenotype and, per the Compass instance earlier in this chapter, appropriately directing the workup toward platelet-specific testing. Light transmission aggregometry shows absent aggregation in response to adenosine diphosphate, epinephrine, collagen, and arachidonic acid, but preserved aggregation in response to ristocetin, a pattern that localizes the defect specifically to the fibrinogen-binding integrin alphaIIbbeta3 rather than to the ristocetin-dependent glycoprotein Ib-IX-V receptor, since ristocetin-induced agglutination does not require alphaIIbbeta3 activation in the same way that agonist-induced aggregation does. Flow cytometry confirms markedly reduced surface expression of CD41 and CD61, the components of integrin alphaIIbbeta3, and genetic testing identifies a homozygous loss-of-function mutation in ITGA2B, confirming Glanzmann thrombasthenia. Management centers on avoidance of antiplatelet and anticoagulant medications, use of antifibrinolytic agents for mucosal bleeding and dental procedures, and reservation of platelet transfusion for major bleeding or surgery given the risk of alloimmunization against the very receptor the patient lacks, which can render future platelet transfusions ineffective; recombinant activated factor VII is used in refractory cases specifically because it can generate thrombin, and therefore support hemostasis, through a pathway that bypasses the defective integrin entirely. This case demonstrates the full diagnostic logic developed in this chapter: a normal platelet count and normal von Willebrand factor testing redirected the evaluation toward platelet receptor biology, and the specific aggregometry pattern, differentiating a fibrinogen receptor defect from a von Willebrand factor receptor defect, localized the diagnosis before genetic confirmation was even obtained.

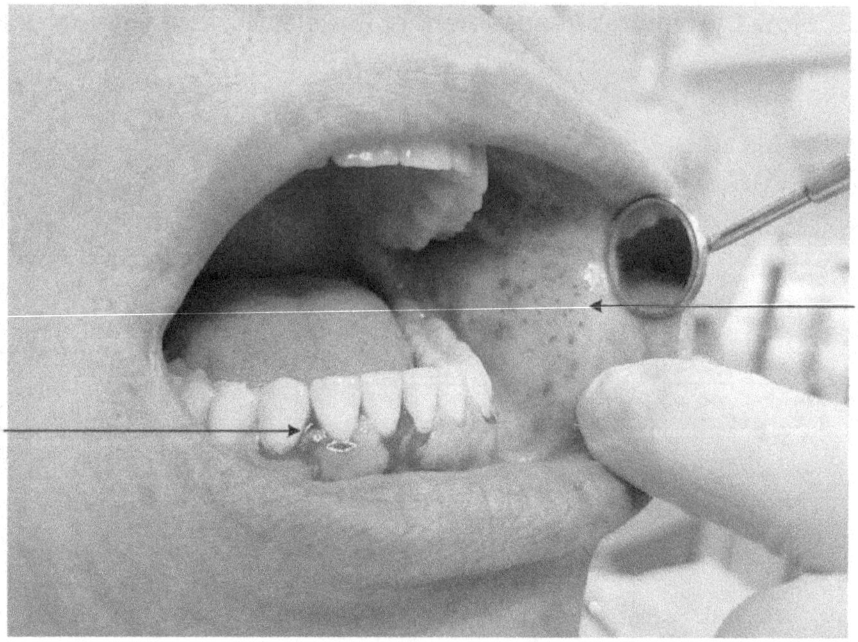

Alloimmunization Risk and Family Counseling in Glanzmann Thrombasthenia

The alloimmunization risk mentioned in the case above deserves elaboration because it fundamentally shapes long-term management. A patient whose platelets entirely lack surface integrin alphaIIbbeta3, as in severe Glanzmann thrombasthenia, has never been immunologically tolerized to this protein and can mount a robust alloantibody response against alphaIIbbeta3 on transfused donor platelets after even a single exposure, particularly in the context of pregnancy or repeated transfusion. Once such alloantibodies develop, subsequent platelet transfusions can be rendered rapidly and completely ineffective, and in a pregnant patient, maternal alloantibodies against alphaIIbbeta3 can cross the placenta and cause severe fetal or neonatal alloimmune thrombocytopenia in a manner mechanistically related to, but distinct from, the human platelet antigen alloimmunization discussed in Chapter 13. For this reason, platelet transfusion in Glanzmann thrombasthenia is reserved for major hemorrhage or surgery unresponsive to antifibrinolytic and recombinant factor VIIa therapy, and every transfusion decision, particularly in a patient of reproductive age, should be made jointly with a hematologist experienced in this disorder, with the transfusion history clearly documented for future reference given the lifelong implications of an established alloimmune response.

Because Glanzmann thrombasthenia follows autosomal recessive inheritance, genetic counseling for the family in this case addresses both recurrence risk for future children, generally one in four for parents who are each heterozygous carriers, and the possibility of identifying carrier status in siblings who may themselves be considered as future platelet or, in severe refractory cases, hematopoietic stem cell transplant donors; heterozygous carriers are generally asymptomatic and are not excluded as transplant donors on the basis of carrier status alone in the way that a RUNX1 mutation carrier would be excluded in the familial platelet disorder scenario discussed in Chapter 1, since Glanzmann thrombasthenia carries no analogous malignancy predisposition.

Compass Recap: Prolonged Bleeding Time, Normal Count: Von Willebrand factor testing precedes platelet function testing when mucocutaneous bleeding occurs with a normal platelet count, given the relative prevalence of von Willebrand disease.

Compass Recap: Storage Pool Pattern on Aggregometry: A blunted secondary aggregation wave is attributed to an inherited storage pool disorder only after medication-related and uremic causes have been excluded through an adequate washout and clinical correlation.

Chapter Anchor: Every inherited platelet disorder in this book localizes to one of three structural compartments introduced in this chapter: surface receptor, cytoskeleton, or granule population. A normal platelet count rules out a quantitative disorder, never a structural one.

Summary and Key Concepts

The platelet plasma membrane, open canalicular system, and dense tubular system together enable rapid surface-area expansion, calcium signaling, and thromboxane generation during activation.

Glycoprotein Ib-IX-V, glycoprotein VI/integrin alpha2beta1, and integrin alphaIIbbeta3 mediate sequential adhesion and aggregation steps; their absence produces Bernard-Soulier syndrome and Glanzmann thrombasthenia respectively for the von Willebrand factor and fibrinogen receptors.

Activation-driven cytoskeletal reorganization, coordinated by Rho-family GTPases acting on actin and stabilized by the marginal microtubule band at rest, drives platelet shape change, spreading, and clot retraction.

Alpha granules, dense granules, and lysosomes store functionally distinct cargo; selective deficiency of any one population produces a recognizable syndrome, including gray platelet syndrome (alpha granules) and Hermansky-Pudlak or Chediak-Higashi syndrome (dense granules, with associated albinism).

Mucocutaneous bleeding with a normal platelet count and normal von Willebrand factor testing should proceed to platelet function testing, since receptor and granule disorders typically leave the platelet count entirely normal.

Aggregometry response patterns localize structural platelet defects to a specific receptor or granule compartment before genetic testing is pursued, converting a nonspecific bleeding history into a mechanistically precise diagnosis.

Platelet Toll-like, Fc, and complement receptors extend platelet function into innate immunity and inflammation, mechanistically linking sepsis-associated thrombocytopenia, heparin-induced thrombocytopenia, and atypical hemolytic uremic syndrome to the structural biology developed in this chapter.

CHAPTER 3: PLATELET ACTIVATION, SIGNALING, AND AGGREGATION MECHANISMS

Learning Objectives

1. Describe the sequential steps of platelet adhesion, activation, and aggregation at a site of vascular injury, from initial tethering through stable thrombus formation.
2. Explain the intracellular signaling cascades triggered by collagen, thrombin, adenosine diphosphate, and thromboxane A2, and identify the point in each cascade targeted by a major antiplatelet drug class.
3. Describe inside-out and outside-in signaling through integrin alphaIIbbeta3 and their respective roles in platelet aggregation and clot stabilization.
4. Explain the role of platelets in thrombin generation and coagulation cascade amplification through phosphatidylserine externalization and procoagulant platelet formation.
5. Describe platelet-leukocyte crosstalk, including P-selectin-mediated aggregate formation and platelet-induced neutrophil extracellular trap generation, and relate this immunothrombotic pathway to sepsis-associated thrombocytopenia.
6. Distinguish primary from secondary hemostasis and relate this distinction to the interpretation of screening coagulation and platelet function tests.
7. Recognize the clinical presentations of pharmacologically induced platelet hyperreactivity and hyporeactivity and apply this knowledge to periprocedural risk assessment.
8. Compare the mechanisms of arterial, venous, and microvascular thrombosis and relate each to its corresponding first-line antithrombotic treatment strategy.

Chapter Outline

This chapter follows the platelet through the complete arc of hemostatic activation: initial tethering and adhesion to injured vessel wall, the intracellular signaling cascades that convert receptor engagement into shape change and secretion, the aggregation process that links individual activated platelets into a growing thrombus, and the procoagulant function that couples platelet activation directly to thrombin generation. Two Platelet Crisis Decision Compass instances address the points where this activation biology intersects most urgently with bedside decision-making: interpreting an unexpected bleeding complication in a patient on dual antiplatelet therapy, and recognizing early laboratory and clinical signs of platelet-driven microvascular thrombosis.

The preceding two chapters established what a platelet is built from and what its structural components are capable of; this chapter explains how those components are actually deployed, in real time, at the site of a bleeding vessel. Nearly every antiplatelet drug in clinical use, and nearly every acquired platelet function disorder discussed later in this book, is best understood as an interruption at one specific point along the activation cascade described here, which is why this chapter functions as the pharmacologic and mechanistic foundation for Chapter 18 as much as it does for the disease chapters that precede it.

This chapter also introduces a distinction that recurs throughout the remainder of this book: not every vascular bed activates platelets the same way, and not every thrombotic disease process is mechanistically identical simply because it involves platelets. Arterial, venous, and microvascular thrombosis each depend on different combinations of the mechanisms developed in this chapter, and correctly identifying which mechanism, or combination of mechanisms, predominates in a given patient is what determines whether antiplatelet therapy, anticoagulation, plasma exchange, or some combination of these approaches is the mechanistically correct treatment, a theme this chapter closes by making explicit before the disease-specific chapters that follow put it into practice.

Initial Adhesion and Tethering at the Site of Injury

Von Willebrand Factor-Mediated Tethering Under Shear

When the vascular endothelium is disrupted, the subendothelial matrix, including collagen, is exposed to flowing blood. Under the high shear conditions present in arterioles and small arteries, platelets cannot adhere directly and stably to exposed collagen on first contact, because the force of flowing blood would simply sweep them away before a stable bond could form. Von Willebrand factor, an enormous multimeric glycoprotein synthesized by endothelial cells and megakaryocytes, solves this problem: it unfolds under high shear stress to expose binding sites for both collagen and the platelet receptor glycoprotein Ib-IX-V, forming a rapid, high-on-rate but also high-off-rate bond that allows a platelet to tether transiently to the injured vessel wall and roll along its surface rather than being swept past entirely. This rolling behavior converts a flowing platelet into a surface-associated one long enough for slower, higher-affinity adhesion receptors to engage.

The shear-dependence of this mechanism has an important corollary: von Willebrand factor-mediated tethering is most critical in the high-shear microvasculature and small arterioles, which is why von Willebrand disease characteristically produces mucocutaneous bleeding, arising from small superficial vessels with high shear rates, rather than the deep soft tissue and joint bleeding characteristic of the coagulation factor deficiencies discussed in relation to secondary hemostasis later in this chapter. This same shear-dependent unfolding mechanism is also directly exploited by ristocetin in the laboratory: ristocetin artificially induces the same von Willebrand factor conformational change that high shear stress produces physiologically, which is why ristocetin-induced platelet agglutination, discussed in Chapter 2, functions as a laboratory surrogate for a process that would otherwise require high-shear flow conditions to reproduce.

Firm Adhesion Through Glycoprotein VI and Integrin alpha2beta1

Once transient tethering has slowed the platelet sufficiently, glycoprotein VI engages exposed collagen directly and generates a strong activating signal through its associated Fc receptor gamma-chain, employing an immunoreceptor tyrosine-based activation motif signaling module that recruits and activates the tyrosine kinase Syk, ultimately triggering phospholipase C-gamma2 activation and the downstream calcium and diacylglycerol signaling that drives the remainder of the activation cascade described in this chapter. Integrin alpha2beta1 engages collagen with substantially higher affinity than glycoprotein VI but transmits a comparatively weaker independent activating signal, functioning primarily to consolidate firm, stable adhesion once glycoprotein VI signaling has already triggered the initial activation response, illustrating a common pattern in platelet biology in which one receptor initiates signaling while a second, higher-affinity receptor stabilizes the resulting adhesion.

Figure 3.1: Sequential Platelet Adhesion Under Shear

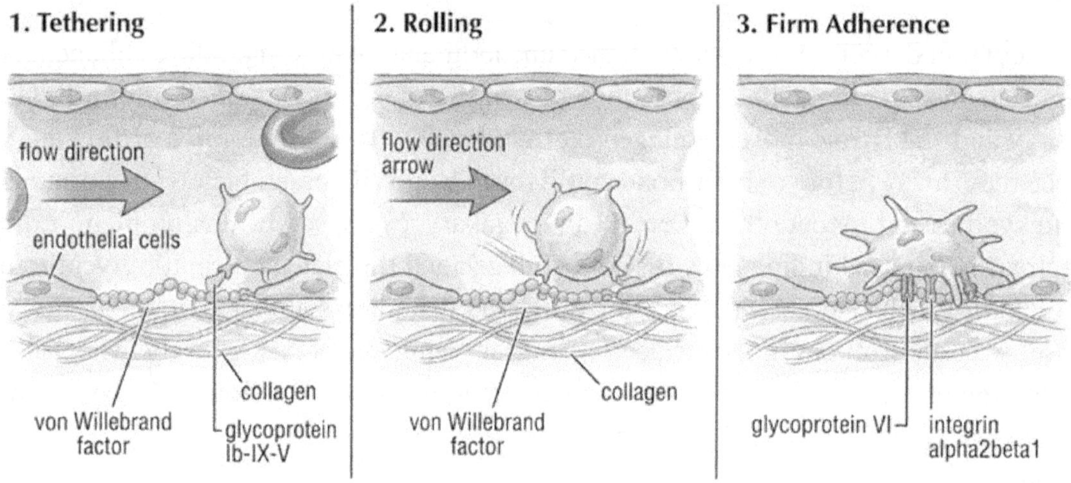

Intracellular Signaling Cascades and Amplification

Calcium Mobilization and the Phospholipase C Pathway

Receptor engagement by collagen, thrombin, or other agonists converges on activation of phospholipase C, which hydrolyzes membrane phosphatidylinositol 4,5-bisphosphate into inositol trisphosphate and diacylglycerol. Inositol trisphosphate diffuses to the dense tubular system introduced in Chapter 2 and opens calcium release channels, flooding the platelet cytoplasm with calcium and triggering downstream effects including cytoskeletal reorganization, granule secretion, and integrin activation. Diacylglycerol, acting in parallel, activates protein kinase C isoforms that phosphorylate targets throughout the activation cascade, including proteins that regulate integrin alphaIIbbeta3 affinity. This calcium-diacylglycerol signaling module is the shared downstream convergence point for essentially every activating platelet receptor discussed in this book, which is why disorders and drugs that interrupt this common pathway, rather than a single upstream receptor, tend to produce the most profound global platelet dysfunction.

Thromboxane A2 Generation and Cyclooxygenase Signaling

Activated platelets liberate arachidonic acid from membrane phospholipids through phospholipase A2 activity, and cyclooxygenase-1, located in the dense tubular system as noted in Chapter 2, converts this arachidonic acid to prostaglandin H2, which thromboxane synthase then converts to thromboxane A2. Thromboxane A2 is released from the activated platelet and acts both on the same platelet in an autocrine fashion and on neighboring platelets in a paracrine fashion, engaging the thromboxane receptor to further amplify calcium signaling and recruit additional platelets into the growing aggregate. This amplification loop is the direct target of aspirin, which irreversibly acetylates a serine residue within the cyclooxygenase-1 active site, permanently disabling thromboxane generation for the remaining lifespan of each affected platelet, since an anucleate platelet cannot synthesize new cyclooxygenase-1 protein to replace the inhibited enzyme; this is the mechanistic reason aspirin's antiplatelet effect persists for the full seven-to-ten-day circulating platelet lifespan despite the drug itself having a plasma half-life of only about twenty minutes.

KEY POINT: Aspirin's clinical duration of action reflects platelet lifespan, not drug pharmacokinetics. A patient who has taken a single aspirin dose has irreversibly inhibited cyclooxygenase-1 in every platelet exposed at that moment, and full functional recovery requires replacement of the affected platelet population over the subsequent seven to ten days, which is the basis for standard preoperative aspirin discontinuation windows.

A partial exception to this all-or-nothing lifespan logic is provided by megakaryocytes actively undergoing proplatelet formation at the moment of aspirin exposure, discussed in Chapter 1: because cyclooxygenase-1 protein synthesized after aspirin has cleared from the plasma is not itself acetylated, platelets released from megakaryocytes that were still maturing when the aspirin dose was cleared can retain normal thromboxane-generating capacity, meaning that the platelet population's aggregate recovery from aspirin effect is not a simple, uniform seven-to-ten-day step function but a gradual repopulation curve tracking new platelet release, an important nuance when interpreting platelet function testing performed at an intermediate time point after aspirin discontinuation rather than at the fully recovered endpoint.

Adenosine Diphosphate Feedback Through P2Y1 and P2Y12

Adenosine diphosphate released from dense granules upon activation, as introduced in Chapter 2, engages two distinct receptors that together sustain and stabilize the aggregation response. P2Y1, coupled to Gq, triggers a rapid but transient calcium mobilization and initiates shape change, while P2Y12, coupled to Gi, inhibits adenylyl cyclase, lowering cyclic adenosine monophosphate and thereby removing a braking signal that would otherwise limit integrin activation; the combined engagement of both receptors is required for full, sustained platelet aggregation, and loss of either receptor alone produces a measurable, though generally milder, aggregation defect. P2Y12 is the specific target of the thienopyridine drugs clopidogrel and prasugrel, which require hepatic metabolic activation to an active thiol metabolite that irreversibly binds the receptor, and the direct-acting reversible P2Y12 inhibitor ticagrelor, which binds the receptor without requiring metabolic activation and dissociates over time, producing a shorter and more readily reversible antiplatelet effect than the thienopyridines.

Platelet Activation Across Arterial, Venous, and Microvascular Contexts

Arterial (Platelet-Rich) Thrombosis

The high-shear, platelet-driven activation cascade developed throughout this chapter is most directly relevant to arterial thrombosis, which characteristically forms at sites of atherosclerotic plaque rupture or erosion, exposing subendothelial collagen and tissue factor to high-velocity, high-shear arterial flow. Arterial thrombi are accordingly platelet-rich, sometimes described as white thrombi, reflecting their predominant platelet and fibrin composition with relatively few entrapped red cells, and this platelet-dominant composition is the direct rationale for antiplatelet therapy, rather than anticoagulation, as the primary pharmacologic strategy for both secondary prevention and acute management of arterial thrombotic events such as myocardial infarction and ischemic stroke.

The core-shell architecture discussed earlier in this chapter is most extensively characterized in arterial thrombosis models, and the shear-dependent adhesion mechanisms, including von Willebrand factor-mediated tethering and shear-induced aggregation, are correspondingly most clinically relevant in this high-shear arterial context. This is also the setting in which the antiplatelet drug map summarized in this chapter's table finds its principal clinical application, since arterial thrombotic events are the primary indication for the aspirin, P2Y12 inhibitor, and integrin antagonist therapies discussed throughout this chapter.

Venous (Fibrin-Rich) Thrombosis

Venous thrombosis arises through a mechanistically distinct process, typically initiated not by high-shear exposure of subendothelial collagen but by localized stasis, endothelial activation without frank denudation, and tissue factor exposure in a low-shear environment, classically at venous valve pockets where blood flow is naturally sluggish. Venous thrombi are accordingly fibrin- and red-cell-rich, sometimes described as red thrombi, with platelets present but generally less central to thrombus initiation than in the arterial setting, reflecting the comparatively minor role of shear-dependent platelet adhesion mechanisms under low-flow venous conditions. This mechanistic distinction is the primary rationale for anticoagulation, rather than antiplatelet therapy, as the mainstay treatment for venous thromboembolism, although platelets are not entirely absent from venous thrombus pathophysiology and are increasingly recognized as contributing to venous thrombus propagation through mechanisms that overlap partially with the immunothrombosis pathway discussed earlier in this chapter.

This arterial-venous distinction is directly relevant to a platelet disorder textbook because it clarifies which patients are, and are not, expected to benefit mechanistically from platelet-directed therapy: a patient with predominantly venous thrombotic disease, such as isolated deep vein thrombosis without an arterial component, derives little direct mechanistic benefit from antiplatelet therapy, whereas a patient with predominantly arterial disease derives comparatively little benefit from anticoagulation alone unless a specific additional indication for anticoagulation, such as atrial fibrillation, is also present. This distinction becomes clinically important in the thrombocytosis and myeloproliferative neoplasm chapters later in this book, where thrombotic risk spans both arterial and venous beds and management must account for both platelet-directed and coagulation-directed prevention strategies simultaneously.

Microvascular Thrombosis

Microvascular thrombosis, the pathologic process underlying the thrombotic microangiopathies introduced earlier in this chapter and covered in full in Chapter 12, represents a third, distinct pattern, characterized by platelet-rich microthrombi forming diffusely throughout small vessels rather than at a single, localized site of injury. Unlike arterial thrombosis, which requires a discrete initiating lesion such as plaque rupture, microvascular thrombosis in disorders such as thrombotic thrombocytopenic purpura arises from a systemic failure of the restraining mechanisms discussed earlier in this chapter, particularly ADAMTS13-mediated von Willebrand factor cleavage, allowing spontaneous, disseminated platelet-von Willebrand factor interaction to occur throughout the microvasculature simultaneously rather than at a single injured site.

Recognizing microvascular thrombosis as mechanistically distinct from both arterial and venous macrovascular thrombosis is essential for correct management: unlike arterial thrombosis, which is treated with antiplatelet therapy, and unlike venous thrombosis, which is treated with anticoagulation, thrombotic microangiopathy is treated by removing or neutralizing the specific restraining-mechanism failure responsible, such as through plasma exchange in thrombotic thrombocytopenic purpura, and platelet transfusion is generally avoided in this setting because it can provide additional substrate for ongoing pathologic microvascular aggregation rather than correcting the underlying problem, a principle addressed in detail with the full Compass instance dedicated to this exact scenario in Chapter 12.

Aggregation, Integrin Activation, and Thrombus Growth

Inside-Out Signaling and Integrin alphaIIbbeta3 Activation

In its resting conformation, integrin alphaIIbbeta3 has low affinity for its ligands fibrinogen and von Willebrand factor, despite being present in high copy number on the resting platelet surface as discussed in Chapter 2; without this low-affinity resting state, circulating platelets would aggregate spontaneously in the absence of injury, an obviously catastrophic outcome. The calcium and diacylglycerol signaling cascades described above converge on activation of the small guanosine triphosphatase Rap1, which recruits and activates talin and kindlin, two cytoplasmic proteins that bind the integrin's cytoplasmic tail and mechanically trigger a conformational change that propagates across the membrane to convert the extracellular ligand-binding head domain from a low-affinity, bent conformation to a high-affinity, extended conformation. This process, termed inside-out signaling because it originates from intracellular signals and produces an extracellular conformational consequence, is the final common step by which every upstream activating pathway discussed in this chapter culminates in the platelet's capacity to bind fibrinogen and aggregate.

Fibrinogen-Independent Aggregation Pathways

Although fibrinogen is the dominant integrin alphaIIbbeta3 ligand supporting platelet aggregation under most physiologic conditions, it is not the only one, and this redundancy has both physiologic and clinical significance. Von Willebrand factor itself can serve as an alternative alphaIIbbeta3 ligand, particularly under high shear conditions where its unfolded conformation exposes an integrin-binding site in addition to the glycoprotein Ib-IX-V binding site discussed earlier in this chapter, and fibronectin can contribute a similar bridging function under certain conditions. This redundancy explains the clinically important observation that patients with afibrinogenemia, a rare inherited disorder of absent circulating fibrinogen, typically have a milder bleeding phenotype than patients with Glanzmann thrombasthenia despite both conditions superficially involving loss of aggregation-supporting capacity, because afibrinogenemic patients retain the alternative von Willebrand factor and fibronectin-mediated aggregation pathways operating through the same, structurally intact alphaIIbbeta3 receptor, while Glanzmann thrombasthenia eliminates the receptor itself and therefore all ligand-dependent aggregation pathways simultaneously.

This fibrinogen-independent capacity also has practical relevance to the interpretation of aggregometry in a patient with a suspected but atypical bleeding disorder: a patient with a documented severe fibrinogen deficiency who nonetheless shows some residual aggregation response on laboratory testing is demonstrating exactly this redundant pathway rather than an inconsistency in the diagnosis, and this observation should not be used to argue against a fibrinogen deficiency diagnosis that is otherwise well supported by a low measured fibrinogen level and a consistent clinical bleeding history.

Outside-In Signaling and Clot Stabilization

Once integrin alphaIIbbeta3 has bound fibrinogen or von Willebrand factor, ligand engagement itself triggers a second, reciprocal signaling wave, termed outside-in signaling, that reinforces platelet spreading, promotes further granule secretion, and drives the clot retraction process discussed in Chapter 2. This outside-in signal is essential for converting the initial, mechanically fragile platelet aggregate into a stable, retracted thrombus capable of withstanding the shear forces of ongoing blood flow, and its disruption, even when initial inside-out activation and aggregation proceed normally, can produce a thrombus that forms but subsequently disaggregates prematurely, a phenomenon documented with certain integrin antagonist drugs and one of the reasons dual-pathway inhibition, blocking both an upstream receptor and providing an integrin antagonist, is sometimes used in high-risk percutaneous coronary intervention despite the additional bleeding risk this combination carries.

THE PLATELET CRISIS DECISION COMPASS — Bleeding on Dual Antiplatelet Therapy

The Presentation: A patient established on dual antiplatelet therapy, typically aspirin plus a P2Y12 inhibitor after coronary stenting, develops a bleeding complication ranging from minor mucocutaneous bleeding to a major gastrointestinal or intracranial hemorrhage.

Mimic Signature: Expected pharmacologic bleeding risk from appropriately prescribed dual antiplatelet therapy; an unrecognized additional bleeding risk factor such as concurrent anticoagulation, an underlying structural lesion (peptic ulcer, arteriovenous malformation), or renal impairment amplifying drug effect; and a superimposed, previously unrecognized platelet or coagulation disorder unmasked by the pharmacologic stress of dual therapy.

The Decision: Localize the bleeding source and assess severity first; for major or life-threatening bleeding, involve cardiology before any antiplatelet discontinuation decision given the competing risk of stent thrombosis, particularly within the first weeks after stent placement; platelet transfusion is generally reserved for major bleeding or urgent procedures, since it does not reverse the drugs already bound to circulating platelets but does supply additional, unaffected platelets to the hemostatic pool.

Trap Logic: Reflexively and unilaterally discontinuing dual antiplatelet therapy for a bleeding complication, without cardiology input on stent thrombosis timing, can convert a manageable bleeding problem into a fatal stent thrombosis, particularly within the first month after placement of a coronary stent.

Crisis Anchor: Antiplatelet therapy is modified only after weighing bleeding severity against stent thrombosis risk together with the prescribing cardiologist; it is never stopped unilaterally on hematology's initiative alone outside of immediately life-threatening hemorrhage.

Platelet Aggregate Architecture: the Core-Shell Model of Thrombus Structure

Heterogeneity Within a Single Growing Thrombus

Intravital microscopy studies imaging thrombus formation directly in living microvasculature have substantially revised the classical picture of a hemostatic plug as a uniform mass of identically activated platelets. A growing thrombus instead displays clear architectural heterogeneity, organized into a densely packed, highly activated core immediately adjacent to the site of injury, surrounded by a looser, less fully activated shell of platelets at the thrombus periphery. Core platelets are exposed to the highest local concentrations of thrombin, collagen, and thromboxane A2, and consequently display full integrin alphaIIbbeta3 activation, extensive phosphatidylserine externalization consistent with the procoagulant phenotype discussed later in this chapter, and minimal ongoing movement once incorporated into the thrombus. Shell platelets, by contrast, experience a diluted agonist concentration further from the injury site and remain more loosely attached, more readily activated and deactivated, and capable of detaching and reattaching dynamically as the thrombus continues to grow and remodel.

Functional Significance of Core-Shell Organization

This architectural distinction is not merely descriptive; it has direct functional consequences for both normal hemostasis and antiplatelet pharmacology. The stable, fully activated core is thought to provide the mechanical foundation that seals the injured vessel wall, while the more dynamic shell is thought to allow the thrombus to adapt its size and shape to changing flow conditions without becoming so rigid that it fails catastrophically under shear stress. Antiplatelet drugs appear to act preferentially on shell platelets, which depend more heavily on the amplification signaling (thromboxane A2, adenosine diphosphate feedback) that these drugs target, while core platelets, having already received a maximal, unamplified thrombin and collagen stimulus directly at the injury site, are comparatively more resistant to pharmacologic inhibition. This differential drug sensitivity is one proposed explanation for why complete platelet inhibition is difficult to achieve pharmacologically even with combination antiplatelet therapy, and why some degree of hemostatic capacity, sufficient to prevent catastrophic bleeding, typically persists even in patients on aggressive antiplatelet regimens.

Clinical Relevance to Rebleeding and Thrombus Instability

Core-shell heterogeneity also offers a mechanistic framework for understanding why some hemostatic plugs are more prone to premature dissolution and rebleeding than others. A thrombus with an inadequately formed or undersized core, whether from insufficient local thrombin generation, an underlying platelet function defect, or pharmacologic inhibition of core-stabilizing signals, may rely disproportionately on its shell for mechanical integrity, and shell-dominant thrombi are structurally less stable under the sustained shear stress of ongoing blood flow. This concept has practical relevance in the evaluation of a patient with recurrent bleeding from an apparently well-treated site, such as a gastrointestinal ulcer that has been endoscopically managed but continues to rebleed, in whom an underlying platelet function abnormality affecting core stability, rather than a purely mechanical or vascular explanation, should be considered as a contributing factor.

Negative Regulation: Keeping Platelet Activation Contained

Endothelial Prostacyclin and Nitric Oxide

Platelet activation must be confined to the immediate site of vascular injury, since unrestrained activation throughout the circulation would produce diffuse, life-threatening thrombosis. Intact endothelium adjacent to an injury site actively restrains platelet activation through continuous synthesis of prostacyclin and nitric oxide, both of which raise cyclic nucleotide levels, cyclic adenosine monophosphate for prostacyclin acting through its receptor and cyclic guanosine monophosphate for nitric oxide acting through soluble guanylyl cyclase, within nearby platelets. Elevated cyclic nucleotide levels activate protein kinase A and protein kinase G, which phosphorylate and inhibit key nodes in the activation cascade described earlier in this chapter, including proteins involved in inside-out integrin activation, effectively raising the activation threshold for platelets passing over or adjacent to healthy, intact endothelium. This continuous restraining signal is why platelet activation normally occurs only where the endothelium has actually been breached, exposing subendothelial collagen and von Willebrand factor while simultaneously removing the local source of inhibitory prostacyclin and nitric oxide.

CD39, CD73, and Purinergic Signal Termination

A second, complementary restraining mechanism operates through the ectonucleotidases CD39 and CD73, expressed on endothelial cells and, to a lesser degree, on platelets themselves. CD39 rapidly hydrolyzes extracellular adenosine triphosphate and adenosine diphosphate, the latter being the direct P2Y1 and P2Y12 agonist discussed earlier in this chapter, converting it first to adenosine monophosphate and then, through CD73, to adenosine, which itself engages platelet adenosine receptors to further raise cyclic adenosine monophosphate and reinforce the inhibitory signal described above. This enzymatic degradation pathway limits the spatial and temporal spread of adenosine diphosphate-driven platelet recruitment away from the immediate injury site, preventing a locally appropriate hemostatic response from propagating into inappropriate, diffuse platelet activation throughout adjacent, uninjured vasculature.

ADAMTS13 and Restraint of Von Willebrand Factor-Mediated Aggregation

A distinct but equally important restraining mechanism operates on von Willebrand factor itself rather than on platelet-intrinsic signaling. Newly secreted, ultra-large von Willebrand factor multimers are considerably more adhesive and more prone to spontaneous platelet-tethering than the smaller multimers that predominate in normal plasma, and the plasma metalloprotease ADAMTS13 continuously cleaves these ultra-large multimers down to a less thrombogenic size under the shear conditions present in flowing blood. This restraining mechanism is entirely distinct from the cyclic nucleotide and purinergic pathways described above, targeting the adhesive substrate rather than the platelet's own signaling machinery, and its failure, whether from severe congenital ADAMTS13 deficiency or from an acquired autoantibody against the enzyme, removes this restraint entirely, allowing ultra-large von Willebrand factor multimers to persist and drive spontaneous, disseminated platelet aggregation throughout the microvasculature. This is the central pathogenic mechanism of thrombotic thrombocytopenic purpura, addressed in full mechanistic and clinical detail in Chapter 12, and its inclusion here, alongside the endothelial and purinergic restraining mechanisms, completes the picture of platelet activation as a tightly regulated process with multiple, mechanistically distinct layers of negative control, any one of which can fail to produce a distinct clinical syndrome of pathologic platelet activation.

KEY POINT: Platelet activation is normally restrained by at least three independent mechanisms operating at different levels: endothelial cyclic nucleotide signaling acting on the platelet directly, ectonucleotidase-mediated degradation of extracellular adenosine diphosphate, and ADAMTS13-mediated cleavage of the adhesive substrate itself. Failure of any one of these mechanisms, rather than a single unified pathway, can produce pathologic platelet activation, which is why the thrombotic microangiopathies discussed in Chapter 12 are mechanistically heterogeneous despite sharing a common clinical presentation.

Platelet-Leukocyte Interactions and Immunothrombosis

P-Selectin, PSGL-1, and Leukocyte Recruitment

Activated platelets do not interact solely with one another; alpha granule fusion, discussed in Chapter 2, inserts P-selectin into the platelet plasma membrane, where it engages P-selectin glycoprotein ligand-1, expressed constitutively on circulating neutrophils and monocytes. This interaction tethers leukocytes to the surface of an activated platelet or a growing platelet aggregate, recruiting them directly into the developing hemostatic response at the site of vascular injury. Platelet-leukocyte aggregate formation is detectable by flow cytometry and is increasingly used as a sensitive marker of in vivo platelet activation, often positive earlier and more reliably in low-level activation states than P-selectin surface expression measured on platelets alone, since the aggregate readout integrates activation signal from a larger effective platelet population passing through the leukocyte-rich circulation.

This platelet-leukocyte tethering is not a passive bystander phenomenon; it actively recruits leukocyte tissue factor and proteolytic machinery to the site of injury, further amplifying local coagulation activation, and it positions platelets to directly influence leukocyte behavior, including promoting neutrophil degranulation and the extracellular trap formation discussed in the following subsection. The clinical relevance of this crosstalk extends well beyond acute injury hemostasis: circulating platelet-monocyte aggregates are elevated in a range of inflammatory and cardiovascular conditions and have been studied as a biomarker of ongoing vascular inflammation, reflecting the same platelet activation biology developed throughout this chapter operating in a chronic, low-level, disease-associated rather than acute-injury context.

Platelet-Induced Neutrophil Extracellular Trap Formation

Activated platelets, whether through direct P-selectin-PSGL-1 contact or through secreted mediators including platelet-derived high mobility group box 1 protein, can trigger neutrophils to undergo NETosis, a specialized form of neutrophil death in which decondensed chromatin studded with antimicrobial proteins is extruded into the extracellular space, forming a web-like structure termed a neutrophil extracellular trap. These structures were originally described as an antimicrobial defense mechanism, physically ensnaring and concentrating antimicrobial peptides against invading pathogens, but the same chromatin scaffold provides a potent, negatively charged surface that further activates the intrinsic coagulation pathway and traps additional platelets and red cells, directly contributing to thrombus growth and stability at the site of injury.

This platelet-neutrophil extracellular trap axis, now commonly referred to under the umbrella term immunothrombosis, is of particular clinical relevance in sepsis, where excessive and dysregulated neutrophil extracellular trap formation is thought to contribute both to microvascular thrombosis and to the platelet consumption that produces sepsis-associated thrombocytopenia, addressed in Chapter 14, operating alongside and in addition to the direct pathogen-sensing mechanisms discussed in Chapter 2 and the disseminated intravascular coagulation mechanisms discussed in the same later chapter. Recognizing immunothrombosis as a distinct, platelet-initiated pathway helps explain why some patients with severe sepsis develop a thrombotic microvascular picture that does not fit neatly into either a classical disseminated intravascular coagulation or classical thrombotic microangiopathy framework, instead representing a third, immune-driven mechanism operating in parallel.

Therapeutic Implications of Immunothrombosis

Recognition of the platelet-leukocyte-coagulation axis described above has motivated interest in therapeutic strategies that target immunothrombosis specifically, rather than platelet activation or coagulation alone, including agents that disrupt P-selectin-PSGL-1 interaction and approaches aimed at degrading or preventing extracellular trap formation, though none of these approaches has yet become standard clinical practice for the platelet-related disorders discussed in this book. For the practicing clinician, the more immediately actionable implication is diagnostic rather than therapeutic: a critically ill patient with thrombocytopenia, evidence of microvascular dysfunction, and a clinical picture that does not fit cleanly into disseminated intravascular coagulation or a classical thrombotic microangiopathy should prompt consideration of an immunothrombotic process driven predominantly by overwhelming infection or severe inflammation, a distinction elaborated further in the differential diagnosis developed in Chapter 14.

Shear-Dependent Regulation of Platelet Aggregation

Shear-Induced Platelet Aggregation Independent of Soluble Agonists

Beyond its role in von Willebrand factor unfolding discussed earlier in this chapter, sufficiently high, pathologic shear stress can itself directly trigger platelet aggregation even in the complete absence of soluble agonists such as thrombin, collagen, or adenosine diphosphate, a phenomenon termed shear-induced platelet aggregation. This pathway depends on glycoprotein Ib-IX-V engagement of von Willebrand factor under very high shear rates, of the magnitude generated by severe arterial stenosis, malfunctioning prosthetic heart valves, or mechanical circulatory support devices, and triggers platelet activation through a signaling pathway that partially overlaps with, but is not identical to, the agonist-driven pathways described earlier in this chapter, involving calcium influx through mechanosensitive channels in addition to the classical phospholipase C-mediated calcium release.

Shear-induced platelet aggregation has direct clinical relevance to two distinct, clinically important phenomena. First, it contributes to arterial thrombosis at sites of severe atherosclerotic stenosis, where local shear rates can rise dramatically as blood is forced through a narrowed lumen, adding a mechanical trigger for platelet activation on top of any exposed atherosclerotic plaque material. Second, and less intuitively, extreme pathologic shear, as generated by continuous-flow ventricular assist devices and extracorporeal membrane oxygenation circuits, can paradoxically cause bleeding rather than thrombosis, through a mechanism addressed in the following subsection.

Acquired Von Willebrand Syndrome From Mechanical Shear

Extreme, sustained pathologic shear stress, as generated continuously by a mechanical circulatory support device, causes progressive proteolytic degradation of high-molecular-weight von Willebrand factor multimers, the same multimers that are most critical for effective platelet tethering under physiologic shear as described earlier in this chapter. This degradation occurs because sustained high shear keeps von Willebrand factor persistently unfolded, exposing it to ongoing proteolysis by ADAMTS13, discussed above in the context of thrombotic thrombocytopenic purpura, but here operating in the opposite clinical direction: excessive multimer cleavage depletes the specific multimer population most needed for effective hemostasis, producing an acquired bleeding phenotype termed acquired von Willebrand syndrome.

Acquired von Willebrand syndrome from mechanical shear is a well-recognized and clinically important complication in patients supported by continuous-flow ventricular assist devices and extracorporeal membrane oxygenation, producing a mucocutaneous and gastrointestinal bleeding tendency that can be substantial despite a normal platelet count, and it is diagnosed by demonstrating a disproportionate loss of high-molecular-weight von Willebrand factor multimers on multimer analysis relative to overall von Willebrand factor antigen level, a pattern distinct from the multimer patterns seen in the inherited subtypes of von Willebrand disease. Recognizing this acquired, device-related mechanism is essential in any patient supported by mechanical circulatory support who develops unexplained bleeding, since standard inherited bleeding disorder testing and management algorithms do not directly address a shear-driven acquired defect that will persist for as long as the device remains in place and that has direct implications for device selection, anticoagulation intensity, and bleeding management in this population.

CAUTION: A patient supported by a ventricular assist device or extracorporeal membrane oxygenation who develops unexplained mucocutaneous or gastrointestinal bleeding should be evaluated for acquired von Willebrand syndrome via multimer analysis, not assumed to have a bleeding complication attributable solely to concurrent anticoagulation; the two causes often coexist and require different management approaches.

Acquired von Willebrand syndrome from mechanical shear also illustrates a broader principle developed across this chapter: any process, whether pharmacologic, mechanical, or disease-driven, that meaningfully perturbs one of the specific molecular mechanisms detailed in this chapter, whether a receptor, a signaling node, or a restraining pathway, produces a predictable, mechanistically explicable clinical phenotype rather than a generic, undifferentiated bleeding or thrombotic tendency. A clinician who has internalized the receptor and signaling map developed in this chapter is therefore equipped to reason toward a specific mechanistic hypothesis for a novel or unusual platelet-related presentation, including one not explicitly named in this book, rather than relying solely on pattern recognition of previously described syndromes.

Platelets and Coagulation: The Procoagulant Platelet

Phosphatidylserine Externalization and the Tenase-Prothrombinase Surface

As introduced in Chapter 2, strong and sustained platelet activation, particularly the combined stimulation produced by collagen and thrombin acting together, drives a subpopulation of activated platelets to externalize phosphatidylserine through TMEM16F scramblase activity, converting the platelet surface into an anionic phospholipid-rich catalytic platform. This procoagulant platelet surface dramatically accelerates the assembly and catalytic efficiency of the intrinsic tenase complex, composed of factors IXa and VIIIa, and the prothrombinase complex, composed of factors Xa and Va, increasing local thrombin generation by several orders of magnitude compared with the same reactions occurring in the absence of an activated platelet surface. This direct coupling of platelet activation to coagulation factor complex assembly is why primary and secondary hemostasis, though often taught as separate, sequential processes, are in reality tightly integrated and mutually reinforcing in vivo: platelet activation accelerates thrombin generation, and thrombin generated locally further activates additional platelets through protease-activated receptors, creating a self-amplifying loop at the site of injury.

Protease-Activated Receptors and Thrombin Feedback

Human platelets express protease-activated receptors PAR-1 and PAR-4, both of which are activated by thrombin cleavage of an extracellular receptor domain that exposes a new, tethered ligand sequence capable of self-activating the same receptor. PAR-1 has substantially higher affinity for thrombin than PAR-4 and mediates the platelet's response to low concentrations of thrombin generated early in the hemostatic response, while PAR-4 requires higher thrombin concentrations and contributes predominantly once thrombin generation has been substantially amplified by the procoagulant platelet mechanism described above. This affinity difference explains the clinical rationale for PAR-1 antagonist drugs, such as vorapaxar, which selectively blunt the platelet's early, high-sensitivity response to thrombin while leaving PAR-4-mediated responses to high local thrombin concentrations comparatively intact, an attempt to reduce thrombotic risk while limiting the bleeding penalty that comes with more complete inhibition of thrombin-driven platelet activation.

Distinguishing Primary From Secondary Hemostasis at the Bedside

Despite the mechanistic integration described above, the traditional clinical distinction between primary hemostasis, referring to platelet plug formation, and secondary hemostasis, referring to the coagulation cascade and fibrin formation, retains real diagnostic value, because disorders that predominantly affect one component tend to produce recognizably different bleeding patterns. Primary hemostatic disorders, including thrombocytopenia and the platelet function disorders discussed throughout this book, characteristically produce immediate, mucocutaneous bleeding: petechiae, purpura, epistaxis, and prolonged bleeding from minor cuts. Secondary hemostatic disorders, including hemophilia and other coagulation factor deficiencies, characteristically produce delayed, deep bleeding into joints, muscles, and soft tissue, often hours after an inciting injury, because an initially adequate platelet plug forms normally but fails to be stabilized by an adequate fibrin mesh. Recognizing which bleeding pattern a patient describes is often the single fastest way to direct initial laboratory testing toward platelet-specific evaluation, as emphasized throughout this book, versus coagulation factor testing, which lies outside this book's scope but is addressed in companion texts on hemostasis and thrombosis.

This bedside distinction, while clinically valuable, is not absolute, and several conditions violate the classical pattern in ways that are important to recognize. Severe thrombocytopenia can occasionally produce deep bleeding resembling a coagulation factor deficiency pattern once the platelet count falls low enough to compromise the procoagulant platelet mechanism discussed later in this chapter, and von Willebrand disease, despite being classified as a primary hemostatic disorder because of its platelet-adhesion mechanism, can also produce a secondary reduction in factor VIII level, since von Willebrand factor serves as the plasma carrier protein that stabilizes circulating factor VIII, occasionally producing bleeding with features that overlap with a mild factor VIII deficiency. These exceptions do not invalidate the primary-secondary framework as a first-pass clinical tool, but they are a reminder that the framework organizes an initial diagnostic approach rather than serving as a rigid, universally exclusive classification.

THE PLATELET CRISIS DECISION COMPASS — Early Recognition of Platelet-Driven Microvascular Thrombosis

---

The Presentation: A patient develops new thrombocytopenia together with early signs suggesting diffuse microvascular platelet consumption: unexplained neurologic symptoms, evolving renal dysfunction, or a rapidly falling platelet count without an obvious bleeding source or overt disseminated intravascular coagulation picture.

Mimic Signature: Thrombotic thrombocytopenic purpura and other thrombotic microangiopathies, in which platelet activation and aggregation drive microvascular occlusion; disseminated intravascular coagulation, in which coagulation activation dominates but platelet consumption also occurs; and severe sepsis with combined platelet activation through the Toll-like receptor pathways discussed in Chapter 2.

The Decision: Obtain an immediate peripheral smear to assess for schistocytes, since this single, rapidly available test is the highest-yield initial discriminator between a primarily platelet-driven microangiopathic process and disseminated intravascular coagulation or sepsis-associated thrombocytopenia without microangiopathy; do not wait for a full coagulation panel before requesting this smear review.

Trap Logic: Waiting for a comprehensive coagulation and hemolysis laboratory panel before requesting an urgent peripheral smear delays recognition of a thrombotic microangiopathy, in which the correct intervention, addressed fully in Chapter 12, is time-critical and should not be deferred pending laboratory confirmation once clinical suspicion is high.

Crisis Anchor: An urgent peripheral smear for schistocytes is obtained the moment a thrombotic microangiopathy is suspected, in parallel with, not after, the remainder of the diagnostic workup.

Drug Class	Example Agents	Molecular Target	Mechanism Summary
Cyclooxygenase-1 inhibitor	Aspirin	Cyclooxygenase-1	Irreversible acetylation blocks thromboxane A2 synthesis for the platelet's remaining lifespan.
Thienopyridine P2Y12 inhibitor	Clopidogrel, prasugrel	P2Y12 receptor	Active metabolite irreversibly binds P2Y12, blocking adenosine diphosphate-mediated amplification.
Direct-acting P2Y12 inhibitor	Ticagrelor	P2Y12 receptor	Reversible binding without hepatic activation requirement; shorter, more readily reversible effect.
PAR-1 antagonist	Vorapaxar	Protease-activated receptor 1	Selectively blunts early, high-sensitivity thrombin-driven activation while sparing PAR-4 responses.
Integrin alphaIIbbeta3 antagonist	Abciximab, eptifibatide, tirofiban	Integrin alphaIIbbeta3	Directly blocks the final common aggregation receptor; reserved for high-risk percutaneous intervention.

CLINICAL CASE: A 58-year-old man with a drug-eluting coronary stent placed three weeks earlier for an acute coronary syndrome, maintained on aspirin and ticagrelor, presents with melena and a hemoglobin drop from 13.8 to 9.1 g/dL over twenty-four hours. He is hemodynamically stable. Upper endoscopy identifies a bleeding gastric ulcer, which is treated endoscopically. The admitting team's initial instinct is to discontinue both antiplatelet agents immediately given the ongoing bleeding, but the consulting hematologist, applying the Compass instance addressed earlier in this chapter, instead contacts the treating cardiologist before any medication change, given the well-established, substantially elevated risk of stent thrombosis within the first month after drug-eluting stent placement, a period during which the stent struts remain incompletely endothelialized and therefore intrinsically thrombogenic independent of the patient's antiplatelet regimen. The joint decision reached is to continue aspirin, which the patient's endoscopically controlled ulcer bleeding does not require discontinuing, while temporarily holding ticagrelor for a defined, short interval with a plan for early resumption once endoscopic hemostasis is confirmed durable, rather than stopping both agents indefinitely. This mechanistically informed, multidisciplinary approach reflects the pharmacology developed throughout this chapter: aspirin's cyclooxygenase-1 inhibition and ticagrelor's P2Y12 inhibition act on distinct points in the activation cascade, so a decision to modify one agent while retaining the other is a rational, mechanism-based approach to partially reducing bleeding risk while preserving substantial residual antithrombotic protection against stent thrombosis, rather than an all-or-nothing choice between full dual therapy and no antiplatelet coverage at all. At the two-week follow-up visit, the patient remains free of further melena, a repeat hemoglobin has stabilized, and ticagrelor is resumed at the cardiology team's direction, restoring full dual antiplatelet coverage roughly ten days after the bleeding event, a timeline chosen to balance the diminishing but still meaningful residual stent thrombosis risk against adequate confirmation of durable endoscopic hemostasis; the patient is additionally started on a proton pump inhibitor for ongoing gastric mucosal protection given the anticipated resumption of dual antiplatelet therapy, illustrating that mitigating future bleeding risk, not merely treating the acute event, is an integral part of the long-term management plan in a patient who will remain on antiplatelet therapy indefinitely.

THE PLATELET CRISIS DECISION COMPASS — Activation, Signaling, and the Antiplatelet Drug Map

---

Compass Recap: Bleeding on Dual Antiplatelet Therapy: Antiplatelet therapy is modified jointly with the prescribing cardiologist, weighing bleeding severity against stent thrombosis risk, never discontinued unilaterally outside immediately life-threatening hemorrhage.

Compass Recap: Early Microvascular Thrombosis Recognition: An urgent peripheral smear for schistocytes is obtained the moment a thrombotic microangiopathy is suspected, in parallel with the rest of the workup, not after it.

Chapter Anchor: Every major antiplatelet drug class targets a specific, named point in the activation cascade developed in this chapter: cyclooxygenase-1 (aspirin), P2Y12 (thienopyridines, ticagrelor), PAR-1 (vorapaxar), and integrin alphaIIbbeta3 (parenteral antagonists). Knowing which point a given drug targets is what allows a clinician to reason about combined antiplatelet regimens rather than treating them as an undifferentiated bleeding risk.

Summary and Key Concepts

Platelet adhesion under high shear begins with von Willebrand factor-mediated tethering through glycoprotein Ib-IX-V, followed by firm adhesion through glycoprotein VI and integrin alpha2beta1 engagement of exposed collagen.

Calcium mobilization through phospholipase C, thromboxane A2 generation through cyclooxygenase-1, and adenosine diphosphate feedback through P2Y1 and P2Y12 together form the core amplification signaling shared across virtually every platelet agonist.

Inside-out signaling converts integrin alphaIIbbeta3 to a high-affinity conformation to enable aggregation; outside-in signaling, triggered by ligand engagement, stabilizes the resulting thrombus and drives clot retraction.

Strong platelet activation drives phosphatidylserine externalization, creating a procoagulant platelet surface that dramatically accelerates tenase and prothrombinase assembly and directly couples platelet activation to thrombin generation.

Primary hemostatic disorders characteristically produce immediate mucocutaneous bleeding, while secondary hemostatic (coagulation factor) disorders characteristically produce delayed, deep soft-tissue and joint bleeding, a distinction that guides initial diagnostic direction at the bedside.

Every major antiplatelet drug class targets a specific, named point in the activation cascade, and antiplatelet therapy decisions around a bleeding complication should weigh drug-specific thrombotic risk (such as stent thrombosis timing) rather than being treated as a uniform bleeding-risk category.

Arterial, venous, and microvascular thrombosis are mechanistically distinct processes drawing on different combinations of the pathways developed in this chapter, and correctly identifying which predominates in a given patient determines whether antiplatelet therapy, anticoagulation, or plasma exchange is the mechanistically appropriate treatment.

Negative regulatory mechanisms, including endothelial prostacyclin and nitric oxide signaling, CD39/CD73-mediated adenosine diphosphate degradation, and ADAMTS13-mediated von Willebrand factor cleavage, normally confine platelet activation to the site of injury; failure of any one mechanism produces a distinct pathologic activation syndrome.

CHAPTER 4: PRIMARY HEMOSTASIS AND PLATELET-VESSEL WALL INTERACTIONS

Learning Objectives

1. Describe the sequence of events comprising primary hemostasis, from vasoconstriction through stable platelet plug formation.
2. Explain the role of the endothelium as an active regulator of hemostasis rather than a passive vessel lining.
3. Describe the structural and functional differences between large-vessel and microvascular hemostasis and relate these differences to distinct bleeding phenotypes.
4. Explain the physiology of the bleeding time and its modern replacements, and identify their limitations as clinical screening tools.
5. Describe the vascular contributions to bleeding disorders, including connective tissue and vasculitic causes, and distinguish these from platelet-intrinsic disorders.
6. Apply the concept of hemostatic reserve to periprocedural risk assessment in a patient with a mild, borderline platelet abnormality.

Chapter Outline

This chapter completes Part I of this book by placing the platelet within its vascular context, examining how the vessel wall itself actively participates in, rather than passively hosts, the hemostatic response. It covers the sequence of primary hemostasis, the endothelium's dual role as both hemostatic activator and restrainer, the distinct hemostatic demands of large vessels versus the microvasculature, and the vascular (non-platelet) causes of a primary hemostatic bleeding phenotype that must be considered whenever a platelet-focused evaluation returns unrevealing. Two Platelet Crisis Decision Compass instances address the evaluation of unexplained easy bruising with normal platelet studies, and the periprocedural risk assessment of a patient with a mild, borderline platelet count.

Every mechanism introduced in the preceding three chapters, megakaryocyte production, platelet structure, and platelet activation signaling, operates within and upon a vessel wall that is itself an active participant rather than an inert conduit. This chapter closes Part I by integrating those platelet-intrinsic mechanisms with vascular biology, establishing the complete primary hemostatic system before Part II turns to how that system is evaluated clinically and in the laboratory.

This chapter closes Part I of the book, and the two chapters that follow it, opening Part II, turn from mechanism to method: how a clinician takes a bleeding history capable of distinguishing the patterns introduced in this chapter, and how the laboratory translates the biology developed across Chapters 1 through 4 into a reproducible diagnostic evaluation. Everything developed in this chapter, the vascular contribution to primary hemostasis, the distinction between large-vessel and microvascular bleeding, and the concept of hemostatic reserve, functions as the direct conceptual bridge between the mechanistic chapters that precede it and the clinical evaluation chapters that follow.

The Sequence of Primary Hemostasis

Placing Vascular Biology Within This Book's Overall Framework

Chapter 1 introduced the production-clearance-distribution framework for locating an abnormal platelet count, and Chapter 2 introduced the sensing-transmission-execution framework for locating a structural platelet defect. This chapter adds a third organizing lens, the vascular context in which platelet biology operates, and the three lenses together, production and kinetics, structural and signaling integrity, and vascular context, are intended to be applied jointly whenever a platelet-related clinical problem is encountered in the remainder of this book, since most genuinely difficult diagnostic problems in platelet medicine involve some interaction between two or more of these three domains rather than a defect confined entirely within one.

Vasoconstriction as the Initial Response

The earliest response to vascular injury is a brief, localized vasoconstriction, mediated by direct smooth muscle contraction in response to injury itself, by locally released endothelin, and by thromboxane A2 and serotonin released from the earliest activated platelets, the biology of which was developed in Chapter 3. This vasoconstrictive response is transient, typically lasting only seconds to a few minutes, but it serves an important early function: reducing local blood flow and pressure at the injury site, which reduces the shear forces that a nascent, still-fragile platelet plug must withstand during the earliest and most vulnerable phase of its formation.

Vasoconstriction is most pronounced and most clinically significant in muscular arteries and arterioles, which possess a substantial smooth muscle layer capable of generating meaningful luminal narrowing, and is correspondingly less prominent in the thin-walled venules and capillaries that make up the microvasculature, a distinction that becomes relevant later in this chapter when large-vessel and microvascular hemostasis are compared directly. Clinically, this initial vasoconstrictive phase is rarely assessed directly, but its absence or impairment, as can occur in some connective tissue disorders affecting vascular smooth muscle, contributes to the bleeding phenotype of those disorders independent of any platelet-intrinsic abnormality.

Platelet Plug Formation: Integrating Chapters 1 Through 3

The platelet plug itself forms through the sequential adhesion, activation, and aggregation processes detailed in Chapter 3: initial tethering via von Willebrand factor and glycoprotein Ib-IX-V, firm adhesion via glycoprotein VI and integrin alpha2beta1, activation-driven shape change and granule release, and aggregation via inside-out activated integrin alphaIIbbeta3 binding fibrinogen and von Willebrand factor. This chapter does not repeat that mechanistic detail but instead emphasizes its integration with the vascular events on either side of it: the vasoconstriction that precedes it and reduces the mechanical demand placed upon it, and the coupling to secondary hemostasis that follows it and stabilizes it, mediated by the procoagulant platelet surface discussed in Chapter 3.

The adequacy of platelet plug formation depends not only on platelet number and function but on the local vascular environment in which it occurs, including the degree of vessel wall injury, local blood flow and shear rate, and the availability of an intact, functional endothelium immediately adjacent to the injury site to provide the restraining signals discussed in Chapter 3 that confine the growing plug appropriately rather than allowing it to propagate uncontrolled into adjacent, uninjured vessel.

Stabilization and the Transition to Secondary Hemostasis

The platelet plug formed through the mechanisms above is mechanically adequate to arrest bleeding from small vessels within minutes, but it remains inherently unstable until it is reinforced by fibrin generated through the coagulation cascade, itself accelerated directly by the procoagulant platelet surface discussed in Chapter 3. This transition from an unstable platelet plug to a stable, fibrin-reinforced clot typically occurs over several minutes following the initial injury, and it is during this transitional window that a patient with an isolated platelet disorder but normal coagulation factor levels remains at highest risk of early rebleeding, since the platelet plug, while present, has not yet been mechanically consolidated by fibrin.

This integration of primary and secondary hemostasis is the physiologic basis for combination therapy in some clinical bleeding scenarios, such as the simultaneous use of platelet transfusion and antifibrinolytic or coagulation factor support in a patient with combined defects, and it also explains why a patient with an isolated, severe platelet disorder can still achieve durable hemostasis for major bleeding once an adequate platelet count or function is restored, since the coagulation cascade itself, assuming it is intact, will proceed to stabilize whatever platelet plug is present.

The Endothelium as an Active Hemostatic Regulator

The Glycocalyx as a First-Line Antithrombotic Surface

Covering the luminal surface of intact endothelium is the endothelial glycocalyx, a dense, gel-like layer composed of proteoglycans, glycoproteins, and bound plasma proteins that extends several hundred nanometers to a micrometer into the vessel lumen, forming a physical barrier that normally prevents direct contact between circulating platelets and the underlying endothelial surface. Beyond this purely physical shielding function, the glycocalyx binds and concentrates antithrombin, heparin cofactor II, and other endogenous anticoagulant proteins at the vessel wall surface, effectively creating a continuous, locally concentrated anticoagulant zone along the entire length of otherwise healthy vasculature.

Glycocalyx degradation, which occurs in sepsis, hyperglycemia, and following ischemia-reperfusion injury, through the action of enzymes including heparanase and matrix metalloproteinases released during systemic inflammation, removes this protective layer and directly exposes the underlying prothrombotic endothelial cell surface and its adhesion molecules to circulating platelets, providing yet another mechanistic layer, distinct from but complementary to the direct endothelial activation discussed throughout this section, by which systemic illness converts vasculature that has not been mechanically injured into a surface capable of supporting pathologic platelet adhesion and activation. This glycocalyx-degradation mechanism is increasingly recognized as a contributor to the diffuse microvascular dysfunction observed in sepsis and critical illness, addressed further in Chapter 14, adding a distinct vascular contribution to the sepsis-associated thrombocytopenia and coagulopathy discussed in that chapter alongside the platelet-intrinsic and immunothrombotic mechanisms introduced in Chapters 2 and 3.

Constitutive Antithrombotic Endothelial Function

Intact, unactivated endothelium is not a passive barrier but an actively antithrombotic surface, continuously synthesizing the prostacyclin and nitric oxide discussed in Chapter 3, expressing thrombomodulin that redirects thrombin toward activation of protein C rather than fibrin generation, and displaying heparan sulfate proteoglycans that accelerate antithrombin activity. This constitutive antithrombotic phenotype ensures that platelets and coagulation factors passing over healthy endothelium remain quiescent, and it is the loss of this phenotype, rather than merely the physical exposure of subendothelial collagen, that fully explains why endothelial injury is so potently prothrombotic: injury simultaneously removes a restraining signal and exposes an activating one.

This dual mechanism, loss of restraint plus exposure of activating substrate, is a recurring theme worth making explicit here because it applies well beyond acute mechanical injury: any process that converts endothelium from its resting antithrombotic phenotype to an activated, prothrombotic phenotype, including inflammation, hypoxia, and the sepsis-associated processes discussed in Chapter 14, can trigger a comparable hemostatic activation even without frank endothelial denudation, since inflammatory endothelial activation independently suppresses the constitutive antithrombotic program described above.

Regulated Von Willebrand Factor Release From Weibel-Palade Bodies

Endothelial cells store preformed von Willebrand factor, along with P-selectin and several other mediators, in specialized storage organelles termed Weibel-Palade bodies, allowing rapid, regulated release in response to injury or specific agonists such as thrombin and histamine, without requiring new protein synthesis. This regulated release mechanism, directly analogous to the alpha granule release from platelets discussed in Chapter 2, ensures that a surge of highly adhesive von Willebrand factor is available within seconds of injury, immediately supporting the platelet tethering mechanism discussed in Chapter 3 at the precise moment and location it is needed.

Desmopressin, a synthetic vasopressin analog used clinically in mild von Willebrand disease and some inherited platelet function disorders, acts specifically by triggering Weibel-Palade body release from residual, functional endothelium, transiently raising circulating von Willebrand factor and factor VIII levels several-fold above baseline; understanding this endothelial storage-and-release mechanism explains both why desmopressin can be clinically useful in appropriately selected patients and why it is ineffective in patients whose endothelium cannot synthesize or store von Willebrand factor normally, such as those with severe type 3 von Willebrand disease, in whom no meaningful releasable pool exists regardless of the stimulus applied.

Endothelial Dysfunction as a Contributor to Bleeding and Thrombotic Risk

Chronic endothelial dysfunction, arising from conditions including diabetes, chronic kidney disease, and long-standing hypertension, produces a persistently altered balance between the antithrombotic and prothrombotic endothelial functions described above, generally shifting the balance toward a prothrombotic phenotype through reduced nitric oxide bioavailability and increased expression of adhesion molecules and tissue factor. This chronic endothelial contribution to thrombotic risk operates independently of, but frequently in addition to, the platelet-intrinsic abnormalities discussed throughout this book, and it is one of several reasons that thrombotic risk in a patient with a platelet disorder, such as essential thrombocythemia discussed in Chapter 17, cannot be assessed by platelet count or platelet-specific testing alone without also considering the patient's broader vascular risk profile.

Endothelial dysfunction is also increasingly recognized as bidirectionally linked to platelet activation itself, rather than existing as an entirely independent risk factor: chronically activated platelets release mediators, including CD40 ligand and additional inflammatory cytokines carried in alpha granules, that further impair endothelial nitric oxide production, creating a self-reinforcing cycle in which platelet activation worsens endothelial dysfunction and endothelial dysfunction in turn lowers the threshold for further platelet activation. This bidirectional relationship is one reason that antiplatelet therapy in chronic cardiovascular disease may confer benefit partly through interrupting this reinforcing cycle at the platelet end, in addition to its more directly appreciated effect of reducing acute thrombus formation at a ruptured plaque.

KEY POINT: The endothelium is not a passive backdrop against which platelet biology unfolds; it is an active participant that can independently shift the hemostatic balance in either direction. A full assessment of thrombotic or bleeding risk in a patient with a platelet disorder should always include consideration of the vascular, and not only the platelet-intrinsic, contribution.

Large-Vessel Versus Microvascular Hemostasis

Structural Differences and Their Hemostatic Consequences

Large arteries and veins possess a substantial smooth muscle media and adventitia capable of contributing meaningful vasoconstrictive force and mechanical tamponade to an injury, along with a comparatively lower surface-area-to-volume ratio of exposed subendothelial matrix relative to the total vessel lumen for any given injury size. Capillaries and postcapillary venules, by contrast, are composed of a single endothelial layer with minimal or absent smooth muscle support, relying almost entirely on platelet plug formation, with comparatively little contribution from vasoconstriction or mechanical tamponade, to achieve hemostasis after injury.

This structural difference directly explains why primary hemostatic disorders, including thrombocytopenia and platelet function disorders, characteristically produce bleeding from the smallest, most numerous, and most mechanically vulnerable vessels, manifesting as petechiae, purpura, and mucosal bleeding, rather than bleeding from larger vessels, which retain substantial mechanical and vasoconstrictive hemostatic reserve even when platelet-mediated plug formation is significantly impaired. A patient with severe thrombocytopenia is therefore at much greater risk from an unrecognized capillary-level bleed, such as intracranial microhemorrhage, than from a comparable injury to a larger vessel, which retains alternative hemostatic mechanisms largely independent of platelet function.

Retinal and cerebral microvasculature deserve particular emphasis within this framework because both are capillary-dominant vascular beds situated within confined, non-distensible anatomic spaces, so that even a small-volume microvascular hemorrhage, entirely consistent with the mechanistic vulnerability described above, can produce disproportionate clinical consequences, vision loss from retinal hemorrhage or neurologic deficit from intracranial hemorrhage, that would be inconsequential if the same hemorrhage volume occurred in a more distensible tissue bed such as subcutaneous fat. This combination of capillary-dominant structural vulnerability and confined anatomic space is the specific reason severe thrombocytopenia is treated as a genuine medical emergency warranting urgent correction, addressed in the diagnostic and management chapters that follow, rather than merely an abnormal laboratory value to be corrected electively.

Mucosal Surfaces as a Special Microvascular Case

Mucosal surfaces, including the gingiva, nasal mucosa, and gastrointestinal tract, combine the structural vulnerability of the microvasculature described above with additional factors that further predispose to clinically apparent bleeding in the setting of a primary hemostatic disorder: high local fibrinolytic activity, particularly in the oral cavity where salivary plasminogen activator continuously promotes clot dissolution, and frequent mechanical trauma from normal function such as chewing and tooth brushing. This combination explains why mucosal bleeding, particularly gingival bleeding and epistaxis, is often the earliest and most sensitive clinical indicator of a primary hemostatic disorder, appearing before more dramatic bleeding manifestations and often before the patient recognizes the pattern as abnormal rather than as ordinary minor trauma.

This same high local fibrinolytic activity is the pharmacologic rationale for antifibrinolytic agents such as tranexamic acid in the management of mucosal bleeding across nearly every disorder discussed in this book, from inherited platelet function disorders to immune thrombocytopenia to periprocedural bleeding prevention for dental extraction, since locally counteracting the high fibrinolytic environment of the oral cavity directly addresses one of the two structural vulnerabilities described in this subsection, complementing rather than replacing platelet-directed therapy.

Implications for Interpreting a Bleeding History

Understanding the structural basis for the large-vessel-versus-microvascular distinction allows a clinician to interpret a bleeding history with greater diagnostic precision than pattern recognition alone: a patient reporting primarily mucosal and cutaneous bleeding, with normal hemostasis after larger surgical incisions, is describing a pattern fully consistent with a primary hemostatic (platelet or von Willebrand factor) disorder, while a patient reporting normal mucosal hemostasis but delayed, deep bleeding after surgical incision is describing a pattern that points away from a platelet-intrinsic disorder and toward the coagulation factor deficiencies that lie outside this book's scope.

This structural framework also explains an occasionally counterintuitive clinical observation: a patient with even quite severe thrombocytopenia can sometimes tolerate a major surgical procedure with a large-vessel component reasonably well, provided platelet counts are appropriately supported perioperatively, while the same patient may experience disproportionate bleeding from a seemingly minor mucosal procedure such as a dental extraction performed without adequate platelet or antifibrinolytic support, precisely because the mucosal microvasculature depends so heavily on the platelet-mediated mechanism that is compromised in that patient.

Vascular Contributions to Bleeding: Beyond the Platelet

Connective Tissue Disorders and Vessel Wall Fragility

Inherited connective tissue disorders, including Ehlers-Danlos syndrome, particularly the vascular subtype, and osteogenesis imperfecta, can produce a clinically significant bleeding phenotype through structural fragility of the vessel wall itself, independent of any platelet or coagulation abnormality, since normal platelet plug formation and fibrin stabilization cannot compensate for a vessel wall that tears or ruptures more easily than normal under ordinary mechanical stress. These patients typically present with easy bruising, and in severe cases spontaneous vessel rupture, in the setting of entirely normal platelet count, platelet function testing, and coagulation studies, a combination that should prompt consideration of a vascular rather than hemostatic cause once the standard hematologic evaluation has been unrevealing.

Recognizing this category is clinically important both to avoid an exhaustive and ultimately unrevealing hematologic evaluation and because the management implications differ substantially: a connective tissue-related bleeding phenotype is not improved by platelet transfusion, desmopressin, or antifibrinolytic therapy in the way a platelet-intrinsic disorder might be, and management instead centers on mechanical precautions, genetic counseling, and, in the vascular subtype of Ehlers-Danlos syndrome specifically, surveillance for the arterial and organ rupture risk that defines the more severe end of that disorder's spectrum.

Vasculitis and Acquired Vascular Purpura

Acquired vasculitic and vasculopathic processes, including immunoglobulin A vasculitis, cutaneous small-vessel vasculitis, and the vasculopathy of long-standing corticosteroid use or aging (senile purpura), can produce cutaneous purpura that closely mimics the appearance of platelet-mediated purpura but arises from vessel wall inflammation or structural fragility rather than platelet dysfunction. Distinguishing these entities from a platelet disorder relies on a combination of the distribution and morphology of the lesions, which in vasculitis are often palpable rather than flat, reflecting the underlying vessel wall inflammation, together with a normal platelet count and platelet function evaluation and, when needed, skin biopsy demonstrating leukocytoclastic vasculitis or another specific histopathologic pattern rather than the simple extravasation seen in platelet-mediated purpura.

This distinction matters clinically because vasculitic purpura frequently signals an underlying systemic process, such as an autoimmune disease, malignancy, or drug reaction, requiring its own dedicated evaluation and treatment entirely separate from the platelet-focused algorithms developed throughout the remainder of this book, and because immunosuppressive or anti-inflammatory therapy, rather than platelet-directed therapy, is the appropriate management once a vasculitic cause is confirmed.

Vitamin C Deficiency and Scurvy: a Vascular Collagen Disorder

Vitamin C is an essential cofactor for prolyl and lysyl hydroxylase, enzymes required for normal collagen cross-linking, and its deficiency, producing the clinical syndrome of scurvy, causes vessel wall fragility through defective collagen support of small vessels, producing perifollicular hemorrhage, corkscrew hair, and gingival bleeding through a mechanism entirely independent of platelet number or function. Scurvy has seen a resurgence in modern clinical practice among patients with restrictive diets, alcohol use disorder, and certain gastrointestinal malabsorptive conditions, and it should be considered in any patient presenting with a bleeding phenotype and characteristic perifollicular or gingival findings whose platelet count and standard coagulation studies are normal, particularly when accompanied by a dietary history suggesting inadequate vitamin C intake, since this is a readily and inexpensively treatable cause of bleeding that is easy to overlook if not specifically considered.

Diagnosis of scurvy is generally made clinically, supported by a plasma or leukocyte vitamin C level when available and by the characteristic combination of perifollicular hemorrhage with corkscrew hairs, gingival changes, and a compatible dietary history, and response to vitamin C repletion, typically evident within one to two weeks, can itself serve as confirmatory evidence in an ambiguous case. Because scurvy is readily treatable and because an exhaustive, unrevealing hematologic workup can otherwise consume considerable time and resources, dietary history focused specifically on fruit and vegetable intake deserves a routine place in the evaluation of unexplained purpura, particularly in patients with recognized risk factors including alcohol use disorder, restrictive eating patterns, food insecurity, or malabsorptive gastrointestinal disease.

THE PLATELET CRISIS DECISION COMPASS — Unexplained Easy Bruising with Normal Platelet Studies

---

The Presentation: A patient reports easy bruising or recurrent petechiae, but platelet count, peripheral smear, von Willebrand factor testing, and platelet function testing are all normal.

Mimic Signature: A connective tissue disorder such as vascular Ehlers-Danlos syndrome; an acquired vasculitic or vasculopathic process; vitamin C deficiency (scurvy); normal physiologic bruising in a patient (particularly a child or older adult) who is simply more attentive to or more susceptible to minor bruising; and factitious or non-accidental injury in appropriate clinical contexts.

The Decision: Re-examine the lesion morphology and distribution directly, looking specifically for palpable purpura suggesting vasculitis, perifollicular distribution suggesting scurvy, or a distribution and pattern inconsistent with reported trauma; take a dietary and social history; and consider skin biopsy or dermatology and, where the history raises concern, appropriate safeguarding evaluation, rather than repeating platelet-focused testing that has already returned normal.

Trap Logic: Repeating platelet count, aggregometry, and von Willebrand factor testing multiple times in a patient whose initial evaluation was normal and adequately performed delays recognition of a vascular, nutritional, or non-hematologic explanation and can create the false impression that a hematologic cause simply has not yet been found.

Crisis Anchor: A normal, adequately performed platelet and von Willebrand factor evaluation should redirect, not repeat, the workup toward vascular, nutritional, and non-hematologic causes of a bruising or purpuric phenotype.

The Bleeding Time and Its Modern Replacements

The Historical Bleeding Time Test

The bleeding time, historically performed by making a standardized incision on the volar forearm and timing cessation of bleeding, was for decades the principal bedside screening test for primary hemostatic function, integrating vascular, platelet, and von Willebrand factor contributions into a single measured endpoint. The test proved poorly standardized between operators, insensitive to mild platelet defects, and poorly predictive of surgical bleeding risk in prospective studies, leading to its near-complete abandonment in modern clinical practice in favor of the platelet function analyzer and targeted laboratory testing discussed in Chapter 7.

Despite its abandonment, understanding the conceptual basis of the bleeding time remains useful, because it illustrates a principle that persists in modern practice: primary hemostatic function is most directly and physiologically assessed by observing an actual, standardized hemostatic challenge under conditions of physiologic shear, rather than by an isolated in vitro biochemical measurement, and every modern replacement for the bleeding time, discussed in Chapter 7, represents an attempt to reproduce this same physiologic, shear-dependent assessment in a more standardized, reproducible laboratory format.

The Platelet Function Analyzer as a Modern Surrogate

The platelet function analyzer, discussed in detail in Chapter 7, replaced the bleeding time by measuring the time required for citrated whole blood, aspirated under controlled high shear through a small aperture coated with collagen and either epinephrine or adenosine diphosphate, to occlude that aperture through platelet plug formation, producing a standardized closure time that is far more reproducible between operators than the historical bleeding time. This assay reproduces the shear-dependent, von Willebrand factor-mediated adhesion mechanism developed in Chapter 3 within a controlled in vitro system, which is why closure time is prolonged in both von Willebrand disease and significant platelet function disorders, but its clinical use and interpretation are addressed fully in Chapter 7 rather than here.

Limitations Shared by Bleeding Time and Its Replacements

Both the historical bleeding time and its modern replacements share an important conceptual limitation worth establishing here before Chapter 7 addresses laboratory testing in full detail: none of these tests directly measures in vivo hemostatic adequacy at a real anatomic bleeding site, and each instead measures a standardized surrogate process under artificial, though physiologically informed, conditions. A normal result on any of these tests substantially lowers, but does not entirely eliminate, the probability of a clinically significant primary hemostatic disorder, and an abnormal result requires further, more specific testing before a diagnosis is finalized, a principle that recurs throughout the diagnostic chapters of this book and that tempers overreliance on any single screening assay.

This limitation is precisely why current preoperative guidelines from major hematology and anesthesiology societies generally recommend against routine bleeding time or platelet function analyzer screening in an asymptomatic patient with no personal or family bleeding history, reserving these tests for patients whose bleeding history, physical examination, or specific procedure risk profile raises genuine concern; a structured bleeding history, addressed in detail in Chapter 5, has repeatedly been shown to outperform indiscriminate laboratory screening in predicting clinically significant perioperative bleeding, reversing what was once common practice of routine bleeding time testing before elective surgery regardless of clinical suspicion.

Platelet-Vessel Wall Interaction in Special Clinical Contexts

Diabetes, Atherosclerosis, and Chronic Endothelial Activation

Chronic hyperglycemia produces advanced glycation end products that accumulate on vessel wall collagen and other structural proteins, altering their conformation in ways that increase platelet adhesiveness and reduce nitric oxide bioavailability, layering an additional prothrombotic mechanism on top of the direct platelet hyperreactivity that has also been documented in diabetes, thought to relate to altered calcium handling and increased thromboxane generation at baseline. This combination of vascular and platelet-intrinsic prothrombotic changes is one contributor to the excess cardiovascular risk seen in diabetes, and it is part of the rationale, alongside purely atherosclerotic burden, for antiplatelet therapy in diabetic patients with established cardiovascular disease.

Atherosclerotic plaque itself represents a chronic, localized disruption of normal vessel wall biology, with plaque endothelium typically displaying reduced antithrombotic capacity even before frank rupture occurs, and plaque core material, rich in tissue factor and other prothrombotic substrates, poised to trigger the full activation cascade developed in Chapter 3 immediately upon rupture or erosion. This chronic vascular vulnerability is the structural basis for acute coronary syndromes and ischemic stroke, and it explains why arterial thrombotic risk in a patient with underlying atherosclerosis reflects both plaque burden, a vascular variable, and platelet reactivity, a hematologic variable, neither of which alone fully predicts an individual patient's risk.

Pregnancy-Associated Vascular Adaptation

Normal pregnancy is accompanied by substantial uteroplacental and systemic vascular remodeling, including trophoblast-mediated remodeling of the maternal spiral arteries to create a low-resistance, high-flow uteroplacental circulation, alongside a systemic shift toward a modestly prothrombotic hemostatic balance that likely serves to limit hemorrhage at delivery. This vascular adaptation depends on coordinated endothelial and, to a lesser degree, platelet participation, and its failure, as occurs in preeclampsia, produces widespread endothelial dysfunction with the specific downstream hematologic consequences, including the thrombocytopenia of preeclampsia and HELLP syndrome, addressed in full in Chapter 13.

The vascular biology developed in this chapter, particularly the concept of endothelial activation removing constitutive antithrombotic restraint while simultaneously exposing prothrombotic substrate, applies directly to preeclampsia, in which widespread maternal endothelial dysfunction, triggered by circulating antiangiogenic factors released from an abnormally implanted placenta, produces exactly this pattern of restraint loss and activation across the maternal vasculature, providing the mechanistic link between an abnormality of placental vascular development and the seemingly distant hematologic finding of maternal thrombocytopenia discussed in the later chapter.

Vascular Aging and Age-Related Bleeding Susceptibility

Vascular aging produces progressive loss of dermal collagen and subcutaneous supportive tissue around small vessels, a process substantially accelerated by chronic sun exposure and long-term corticosteroid use, that leaves small vessels relatively unsupported and prone to rupture with minimal mechanical stress, producing the common clinical entity of senile purpura, characterized by irregular ecchymoses typically on the dorsal forearms and hands. This age-related vascular fragility occurs independent of platelet count or function and should be distinguished, using the same lesion morphology and distribution principles introduced earlier in this chapter, from a genuine platelet or coagulation disorder before an older patient is subjected to unnecessary hematologic evaluation.

Distinguishing senile purpura from a pathologic bleeding disorder relies on the characteristic distribution, sparing the trunk and favoring sun-exposed extremities, the typically well, otherwise asymptomatic patient, and the absence of the mucosal bleeding, petechiae in other locations, or systemic symptoms that would suggest a true hematologic process; when these distinguishing features are present, reassurance and mechanical protection of vulnerable skin are appropriate, and extensive laboratory evaluation can reasonably be deferred.

Platelets Beyond Hemostasis: Wound Healing and Tissue Repair

Platelet-Derived Growth Factors in Wound Healing

Beyond their acute hemostatic role, platelets released at a site of tissue injury continue to participate actively in the subsequent wound healing process, releasing platelet-derived growth factor, transforming growth factor beta, and vascular endothelial growth factor from alpha granules, the biology of which was introduced in Chapter 2, to recruit and activate fibroblasts, promote angiogenesis, and coordinate the transition from the acute inflammatory phase of wound healing to the proliferative and remodeling phases that follow. This sustained biological role, extending well beyond the minutes-to-hours timescale of acute hemostasis, is the physiologic basis for platelet-rich plasma preparations used clinically in some orthopedic, dermatologic, and dental applications, which concentrate autologous platelet growth factor content and apply it directly to a healing tissue site.

This wound-healing function also has clinical relevance to patients with chronic thrombocytopenia or platelet function disorders, in whom impaired wound healing, not merely impaired acute hemostasis, can complicate recovery from surgery or traumatic injury, an often underappreciated consideration in the long-term management of patients with chronic platelet disorders addressed throughout the thrombocytopenic disorder chapters of this book, and one additional reason that achieving an adequate platelet count and function around a planned surgical procedure matters beyond the immediate perioperative bleeding risk alone.

Platelets in Angiogenesis: Dual Pro- and Antiangiogenic Roles

As introduced in Chapter 2 in the context of differential alpha granule cargo packaging, platelets carry both pro-angiogenic factors, including vascular endothelial growth factor and platelet-derived growth factor, and antiangiogenic factors, including endostatin and platelet factor 4, within at least partially distinct granule subpopulations, allowing platelets to either promote or restrain new blood vessel formation depending the specific activating stimulus and local tissue context. This dual capacity positions platelets as active participants in tumor angiogenesis as well as physiologic wound healing, and it is an area of active oncologic research given the observation that tumor-associated platelet activation can promote tumor vascularization and metastatic spread through mechanisms that overlap partially with the immunothrombosis pathway discussed in Chapter 3.

Clinically, this dual angiogenic role helps explain the relationship between thrombocytosis and malignancy discussed in Chapter 17, where reactive thrombocytosis is not merely a passive marker of underlying cancer but may actively participate in tumor progression through the angiogenic and immune-modulatory mechanisms outlined here, an evolving area of research that has begun to influence how markedly elevated platelet counts are interpreted as a potential paraneoplastic signal in appropriate clinical contexts.

Clinical Implications for Chronic Wound Management

The wound-healing and angiogenic functions of platelets described in this section have direct relevance to the management of chronic, non-healing wounds, including diabetic foot ulcers and venous stasis ulcers, in which local platelet-derived growth factor deficiency at the wound bed, whether from impaired local platelet activation or from a systemic platelet disorder, may contribute to delayed healing; this is the rationale underlying topical recombinant platelet-derived growth factor and platelet-rich plasma therapies used in selected chronic wound care settings. For the hematologist managing a patient with a chronic platelet disorder, recognizing that impaired wound healing, alongside impaired acute hemostasis, is a potential downstream consequence of that disorder supports a lower threshold for proactive surgical and wound care planning in this population.

Hemostatic Reserve and Periprocedural Risk Assessment

The Concept of Hemostatic Reserve

Hemostatic reserve refers to the margin between a patient's baseline hemostatic capacity and the minimum capacity required to prevent clinically significant bleeding under a given level of hemostatic challenge, and it is a more clinically useful concept than any single laboratory value in isolation, because it explicitly incorporates the magnitude of the anticipated challenge alongside the patient's baseline status. A platelet count that provides ample hemostatic reserve for daily activities may provide inadequate reserve for a major surgical procedure, while the same count might be entirely adequate for a minor procedure performed with meticulous local hemostatic technique, illustrating that periprocedural risk assessment cannot be reduced to a single universal platelet count threshold applicable across all clinical contexts.

This reserve concept also explains why the platelet count thresholds used for different procedures, addressed with specific numeric guidance in Chapter 19 in the context of prophylactic platelet transfusion, vary so substantially by procedure type, ranging from thresholds adequate for routine venipuncture to substantially higher thresholds required for neurosurgical or ophthalmologic procedures, where even a small hemorrhage in a confined anatomic space can produce catastrophic, irreversible consequences disproportionate to the bleeding volume itself.

Integrating Multiple Sources of Hemostatic Compromise

Periprocedural risk assessment must integrate every source of hemostatic compromise simultaneously rather than evaluating platelet count in isolation: concurrent anticoagulant or antiplatelet medication, discussed extensively in Chapter 3 and Chapter 18, renal or hepatic dysfunction affecting both platelet function and coagulation factor synthesis, and any qualitative platelet abnormality that may coexist with an otherwise reassuring platelet count, as emphasized throughout Chapter 2. A patient with a borderline platelet count who is also taking aspirin, or who has renal impairment producing uremic platelet dysfunction as discussed in Chapter 2, carries meaningfully less hemostatic reserve than the platelet count alone would suggest, and periprocedural planning should account for this combined burden explicitly rather than assessing each factor independently.

This integrative approach to hemostatic reserve is the conceptual foundation for the periprocedural management guidance provided throughout the disease-specific chapters of this book, each of which addresses procedure-specific platelet thresholds and bridging strategies relevant to that particular disorder, building on the general framework established in this chapter rather than repeating it from first principles in every subsequent discussion.

THE PLATELET CRISIS DECISION COMPASS — Periprocedural Assessment of a Mild, Borderline Platelet Count

The Presentation: A patient with a platelet count in the borderline range, generally 50 to 100 x10^9/L, is scheduled for an elective procedure, and the proceduralist requests hematology input on whether the procedure can proceed safely.

Mimic Signature: A patient with adequate hemostatic reserve for a low-bleeding-risk procedure despite the borderline count; a patient with inadequate reserve once concurrent antiplatelet or anticoagulant therapy, renal or hepatic dysfunction, or an unrecognized qualitative platelet defect is factored in; and a patient in whom the count itself is spuriously low due to a preanalytic artifact such as pseudothrombocytopenia, addressed further in Chapter 6.

The Decision: Confirm the count is accurate (repeat testing, review smear for clumping), classify the planned procedure's bleeding risk category, and integrate all concurrent hemostatic risk factors before recommending a threshold-based decision; low-bleeding-risk procedures often proceed safely at counts that would be inadequate for a high-bleeding-risk or closed-space procedure, and the recommendation should be procedure-specific rather than based on a single universal number.

Trap Logic: Applying a single, universal platelet count threshold to every procedure regardless of bleeding risk category either exposes a patient to unnecessary bleeding risk for a high-risk procedure or subjects a patient to unnecessary delay and platelet transfusion for a low-risk procedure that did not require it.

Crisis Anchor: Periprocedural platelet threshold recommendations are procedure-specific and account for concurrent hemostatic risk factors, never a single universal number applied uniformly across all procedure types.

Bleeding Risk Category	Example Procedures	General Platelet Count Consideration	Key Additional Factors
Minimal risk	Venipuncture, peripheral intravenous access, routine dental cleaning	Generally safe well below 50 x10^9/L absent other risk factors	Local pressure usually sufficient; concurrent coagulopathy still relevant.
Low risk	Central venous catheter placement	Often proceeds around 20-50	Ultrasound guidance and experienced

	(ultrasound-guided), bone marrow biopsy, routine dental extraction	x10^9/L depending on institutional protocol and technique	operator reduce risk; confirm local protocol.
Moderate risk	Major abdominal or orthopedic surgery, liver biopsy	Higher thresholds generally applied; confirm against current institutional and specialty guidance	Concurrent antiplatelet or anticoagulant therapy meaningfully raises effective risk.
High risk (closed space)	Neurosurgical procedures, ophthalmologic surgery	Highest thresholds generally applied given catastrophic consequence of even minor bleeding	Confined anatomic space means even small hemorrhage volume can be irreversible.

CAUTION: The platelet count thresholds referenced in the table above are general teaching illustrations, not fixed prescriptive numbers; actual thresholds vary by institution, specific procedure, operator experience, and concurrent patient risk factors, and current institutional and specialty-society guidance should always be confirmed before a final periprocedural recommendation is made.

CLINICAL CASE: A 71-year-old woman with stage 4 chronic kidney disease and a platelet count of 88 x10^9/L, stable over the preceding six months and attributed to her underlying kidney disease without a clear alternative explanation on prior workup, is referred for hematology clearance before an elective total knee arthroplasty. Her medications include low-dose aspirin for coronary artery disease, and her estimated glomerular filtration rate is 22 mL/min/1.73m2. Applying the hemostatic reserve framework developed in this chapter, the consulting hematologist recognizes that the borderline platelet count alone, viewed in isolation, might be considered marginally acceptable for a major orthopedic procedure by some published thresholds, but the patient's combined risk burden, uremic platelet dysfunction from advanced chronic kidney disease as introduced in Chapter 2, concurrent aspirin therapy, and a large-vessel, closed-space surgical field with substantial expected blood loss, together meaningfully reduce her actual hemostatic reserve below what the isolated count would suggest. The recommendation is to hold aspirin for the standard preoperative window with cardiology confirmation that this is safe given her cardiac history, to consider a short course of desmopressin perioperatively to transiently improve uremic platelet function through the endothelial Weibel-Palade body release mechanism discussed earlier in this chapter, and to ensure platelet concentrates are readily available intraoperatively rather than administered prophylactically in advance, reserving transfusion for actual excessive bleeding given that prophylactic transfusion in uremic thrombocytopathy provides only transient benefit as transfused platelets rapidly acquire the same uremic dysfunction once exposed to the patient's circulating uremic milieu. This case demonstrates the central lesson of this chapter: hemostatic risk is a composite, procedure-specific assessment integrating platelet count, platelet function, vascular factors, and medication history together, never a single number evaluated in isolation. The surgery proceeds without prophylactic platelet transfusion, aspirin is held for five days preoperatively with cardiology confirmation and resumed on postoperative day two once surgical hemostasis is confirmed adequate, a single dose of desmopressin is administered on the morning of surgery, and estimated intraoperative blood loss is within the expected range for the procedure without need for platelet transfusion; the patient is discharged on postoperative day three with an unremarkable hemoglobin trend, illustrating that a well-integrated, multifactorial periprocedural plan, rather than an isolated platelet count threshold or a reflexive prophylactic transfusion, achieved an uneventful surgical outcome despite a hemostatic profile that, viewed through any single variable alone, might have appeared more concerning than it proved to be in practice.

THE PLATELET CRISIS DECISION COMPASS — Vascular Integration and Hemostatic Reserve

Compass Recap: Bruising with Normal Platelet Studies: A normal, adequately performed platelet and von Willebrand factor evaluation redirects the workup toward vascular, nutritional, and non-hematologic causes rather than prompting repeat platelet-focused testing.

Compass Recap: Borderline Periprocedural Platelet Count: Periprocedural platelet thresholds are procedure-specific and integrate concurrent hemostatic risk factors; no single universal count threshold applies across all procedure types.

Chapter Anchor: Primary hemostasis is a vascular-platelet system, not a platelet-only system. Bleeding evaluation and periprocedural risk assessment that considers platelet count in isolation, without the vascular, medication, and organ-function context developed in this chapter, will systematically misjudge both bleeding and thrombotic risk.

Summary and Key Concepts

Primary hemostasis proceeds from transient vasoconstriction through platelet plug formation to fibrin-mediated stabilization, integrating the platelet biology of Chapters 1 through 3 with active vascular participation.

The endothelium is a dynamic hemostatic regulator, constitutively antithrombotic at rest and capable of rapid, regulated von Willebrand factor release from Weibel-Palade bodies, the basis for desmopressin's clinical effect.

Large vessels retain substantial vasoconstrictive and mechanical hemostatic reserve independent of platelet function, while capillaries and mucosal surfaces depend almost entirely on platelet plug formation, explaining the characteristic mucocutaneous distribution of primary hemostatic bleeding.

Connective tissue disorders, vasculitis, and vitamin C deficiency can each produce a bleeding or purpuric phenotype through vascular rather than platelet mechanisms and should be considered when platelet-focused testing is unrevealing.

The bleeding time has been replaced by the platelet function analyzer and targeted testing (Chapter 7), but both share the limitation of measuring a standardized surrogate rather than true in vivo hemostatic adequacy.

Periprocedural bleeding risk reflects hemostatic reserve, a composite of platelet count, platelet function, concurrent medications, organ dysfunction, and procedure-specific bleeding risk category, never a single platelet count threshold applied universally.

CHAPTER 5: CLINICAL APPROACH TO THE PATIENT WITH SUSPECTED PLATELET DISORDER

Learning Objectives

1. Take a structured bleeding history capable of distinguishing a genuine hemostatic disorder from normal variation in bruising and bleeding tendency.
2. Apply a validated bleeding assessment tool to quantify and standardize bleeding history.
3. Recognize physical examination findings that localize a bleeding tendency to a primary hemostatic (platelet or vascular) rather than secondary hemostatic (coagulation factor) cause.
4. Distinguish incidental thrombocytopenia discovered on routine testing from thrombocytopenia presenting with clinical bleeding, and adjust urgency accordingly.
5. Construct an efficient, stepwise initial evaluation for a patient with a newly identified platelet count abnormality.
6. Recognize when a platelet-related presentation constitutes a medical emergency requiring immediate action rather than routine outpatient evaluation.

Chapter Outline

This chapter opens Part II of the book and translates the biology developed in Part I into a structured clinical approach. It addresses the bleeding history and its standardized quantification, the physical examination findings that localize a bleeding tendency, the distinction between incidental and symptomatic thrombocytopenia, and the construction of an efficient initial evaluation pathway. Two Platelet Crisis Decision Compass instances address the recognition of a bleeding history that warrants urgent same-day evaluation, and the interpretation of a markedly low platelet count discovered incidentally in an asymptomatic patient.

The chapters that follow this one, covering laboratory evaluation and platelet function testing, are only as useful as the clinical framework that directs their use. A test ordered without a clear clinical hypothesis, or a bleeding history taken without a structured approach, produces a large volume of information that is difficult to interpret and act upon efficiently. This chapter provides that structured clinical framework, establishing the questions a clinician should ask, the examination findings that matter most, and the triage logic that separates a routine outpatient evaluation from a same-day hematologic emergency.

The Structured Bleeding History

Distinguishing Abnormal From Normal Bleeding Tendency

Nearly every person has bruised, bled from a minor cut, or noticed occasional gingival bleeding with brushing at some point, and the central challenge of the bleeding history is distinguishing this universal, physiologic experience from a genuine underlying hemostatic disorder. A structured approach directs attention toward features that discriminate pathologic from physiologic bleeding: spontaneous bleeding without an identifiable trigger, bleeding disproportionate to the inciting trauma, bleeding from multiple, unrelated anatomic sites, bleeding that required medical intervention such as cautery, packing, or transfusion, and a consistent pattern present since childhood or a clear acquired change from a previously normal baseline.

Equally important is directly asking about hemostatic challenges the patient may not have volunteered: prior surgical or dental procedures, including simple dental extractions, and their bleeding course; obstetric history in women, including postpartum hemorrhage; and any prior instance of unexpectedly prolonged bleeding after a minor procedure such as a skin biopsy or venipuncture. A patient who has undergone a major surgical procedure or childbirth without excessive bleeding has, in effect, already passed a substantial physiologic hemostatic challenge, and this history carries considerable diagnostic weight in judging the likelihood of a clinically significant underlying disorder.

Family History and Inheritance Patterns

A family history of bleeding, particularly in a pattern consistent with a specific inheritance mode, substantially raises the pretest probability of an inherited platelet or von Willebrand disorder among the conditions discussed throughout Part I of this book. Von Willebrand disease and most inherited platelet function disorders typically follow autosomal inheritance and can therefore appear in either sex across multiple generations, while a small number of platelet disorders, including Wiskott-Aldrich syndrome discussed in Chapter 2, follow X-linked inheritance and predominantly affect males, with carrier females occasionally showing a milder phenotype.

A negative family history does not exclude an inherited disorder, since de novo mutation, variable expressivity, and simple underrecognition of mild bleeding symptoms in relatives are all common, but a positive family history, particularly one following a recognizable pattern, should prompt directed evaluation even when the index patient's own bleeding history is comparatively mild, since family members are sometimes the first to recognize a pattern that any single affected individual might otherwise attribute to unrelated causes or dismiss as unremarkable.

Medication and Supplement History

A complete medication history, including over-the-counter analgesics, herbal supplements, and any recent new prescription, is essential before a bleeding history is interpreted as reflecting an underlying hematologic disorder, since the antiplatelet and anticoagulant mechanisms developed in Chapter 3 and addressed pharmacologically in Chapter 18 are collectively among the most common causes of an acquired bleeding tendency encountered in clinical practice. Patients frequently do not consider over-the-counter aspirin, nonsteroidal anti-inflammatory drugs, or supplements such as fish oil and certain herbal preparations with recognized antiplatelet activity as medications worth reporting, so directed questioning about these specific categories, rather than an open-ended request to list medications, substantially improves the yield of this portion of the history.

This medication history should also specifically probe recent changes, since a bleeding symptom that began shortly after starting a new medication, even one not classically recognized as having antiplatelet effect, raises the possibility of an idiosyncratic drug-induced platelet disorder, addressed in detail in Chapter 10, a category of thrombocytopenia that is substantially underrecognized in clinical practice precisely because the causative medication is often not among the drugs a clinician would immediately suspect.

Standardized Bleeding Assessment Tools

The Rationale for Structured Quantification

An unstructured bleeding history is subject to substantial interobserver variability and recall bias, and structured bleeding assessment tools were developed specifically to address this limitation by quantifying bleeding symptoms across a defined set of anatomic sites and severity categories, producing a numeric bleeding score that can be compared against validated normal reference ranges. The most widely used instrument in current practice, the International Society on Thrombosis and Haemostasis Bleeding Assessment Tool, assigns a graded score to bleeding symptoms across categories including epistaxis, cutaneous bleeding, minor wounds, oral cavity bleeding, gastrointestinal bleeding, menorrhagia, postpartum hemorrhage, surgical bleeding, and muscle or joint bleeding, producing a composite score validated against the likelihood of an underlying inherited bleeding disorder, most extensively studied in von Willebrand disease.

A normal score on a validated bleeding assessment tool carries substantial negative predictive value for a clinically significant inherited bleeding disorder and can reasonably support a decision to defer extensive laboratory evaluation in a patient with a low pretest probability based on other clinical features, while an elevated score supports proceeding to the laboratory evaluation detailed in Chapters 6 and 7. This structured approach represents a direct, modern substitute for the physiologic bleeding challenge that the historical bleeding time, discussed in Chapter 4, once attempted to provide through direct provocation, achieving comparable or superior diagnostic value through careful history alone.

Interpreting Menstrual Bleeding as a Sensitive Indicator

Heavy menstrual bleeding deserves particular emphasis within the structured bleeding history because it is among the most sensitive indicators of an underlying primary hemostatic disorder in women of reproductive age, yet it is also frequently normalized by patients and, at times, by clinicians as an unremarkable gynecologic finding rather than recognized as a potential systemic hemostatic symptom. Objective indicators that distinguish pathologic from physiologic menstrual bleeding include the need to change menstrual protection more frequently than hourly, passage of clots larger than approximately one inch in diameter, bleeding lasting longer than seven days, and iron deficiency anemia attributable to menstrual loss.

Population studies of women presenting to gynecology clinics for heavy menstrual bleeding have consistently identified von Willebrand disease and other inherited bleeding disorders in a meaningful minority of patients who had not previously undergone hematologic evaluation, supporting current guidance that women with heavy menstrual bleeding, particularly when present since menarche or accompanied by other bleeding symptoms elsewhere in the structured history, should be screened for an underlying bleeding disorder rather than proceeding directly to gynecologic intervention alone.

Age-Specific Considerations in Bleeding History

The bleeding history must be interpreted against age-appropriate expectations, since the hemostatic challenges an individual has faced, and therefore the diagnostic weight of an unremarkable history, differ substantially across the lifespan. A young child who has not yet undergone a significant hemostatic challenge such as surgery, dental extraction, or, in girls, menarche, has had comparatively few opportunities to reveal an underlying inherited disorder, so a benign history in this age group carries less reassurance than the same history in an adult, and the family history and any history of bleeding with minor procedures such as circumcision or venipuncture take on correspondingly greater diagnostic weight.

Older adults, conversely, often carry a lifetime of unremarkable hemostatic challenges that substantially lowers the pretest probability of a previously unrecognized inherited disorder, making a new bleeding symptom in this population more likely to reflect an acquired process, including medication effect, an acquired platelet function disorder, or, less commonly, an acquired von Willebrand syndrome associated with an underlying lymphoproliferative or myeloproliferative disorder or with aortic stenosis through a shear-related mechanism analogous to that discussed for mechanical circulatory support in Chapter 3.

Differential Diagnostic Framework: Localizing the Bleeding Tendency

Primary Versus Secondary Hemostatic Bleeding Patterns

Once the structured history and family history have been obtained, the clinician's next task is to localize the bleeding tendency to the primary hemostatic system, comprising platelets and von Willebrand factor as developed throughout Part I, or to the secondary hemostatic system of coagulation factors and the fibrin-generating cascade, since these two categories carry distinct bleeding phenotypes, distinct laboratory pathways, and distinct urgency profiles. Primary hemostatic bleeding characteristically presents immediately after an inciting injury, involves mucocutaneous sites including the skin, gums, nose, and gastrointestinal or genitourinary mucosa, and produces petechiae and superficial ecchymoses, while secondary hemostatic bleeding characteristically presents in a delayed fashion hours after injury, favors deep soft tissue, joints, and body cavities, and rarely produces petechiae.

This distinction, though useful as an organizing framework, is not absolute, since severe deficiencies of either system can eventually produce overlapping features, and combined defects, including the acquired coagulopathy of liver disease discussed in Chapter 14 and disseminated intravascular coagulation, which simultaneously consumes platelets and coagulation factors, blur this clean separation in critically ill patients. Nonetheless, the pattern recognition this framework provides is clinically valuable at the point of initial evaluation, directing the clinician toward a platelet count and platelet function assessment when the pattern favors primary hemostatic bleeding, and toward coagulation factor testing, including prothrombin time and activated partial thromboplastin time, when the pattern instead favors a secondary hemostatic process.

Feature	Primary Hemostatic (Platelet/vWF) Pattern	Secondary Hemostatic (Coagulation Factor) Pattern
Onset after injury	Immediate	Delayed, often hours later
Characteristic sites	Skin, mucosa, gingiva, GI/GU tract	Deep soft tissue, joints, body cavities
Petechiae	Characteristic	Rare
Hemarthrosis	Rare	Characteristic, particularly in hemophilia
Bleeding after superficial cuts	Prolonged, often immediate	Usually normal
Typical screening abnormality	Platelet count, PFA/aggregometry	Prothrombin time, activated partial thromboplastin time

Isolated Thrombocytopenia Versus Multilineage Cytopenia

A second axis of differential organization distinguishes isolated thrombocytopenia, in which the platelet count alone is reduced while hemoglobin and white cell count remain normal, from multilineage cytopenia, in which two or three blood cell lines are simultaneously reduced. Isolated thrombocytopenia points toward a process specific to platelet production or destruction, including immune thrombocytopenia, drug-induced thrombocytopenia, and most inherited thrombocytopenia syndromes, while multilineage cytopenia points toward a process affecting the marrow more broadly or a peripheral consumptive process affecting multiple lineages, including marrow infiltration by malignancy, myelodysplastic syndrome, aplastic anemia, vitamin deficiency, and hypersplenism from portal hypertension, each addressed in the diagnostic pathways of subsequent chapters.

This distinction should be drawn directly from the complete blood count differential at the initial encounter, since it substantially narrows the subsequent evaluation before any additional testing is ordered: an isolated thrombocytopenia with an otherwise unremarkable blood count and smear supports proceeding along the immune thrombocytopenia-focused pathway detailed in Chapter 9, while any accompanying anemia or leukopenia, particularly when accompanied by abnormal cell morphology on the peripheral smear, should redirect the evaluation toward the broader diagnostic algorithm in Chapter 8 and toward earlier consideration of a bone marrow examination.

Distinguishing Congenital From Acquired Presentations

A final organizing axis separates congenital, or inherited, presentations from acquired presentations, a distinction that draws directly on the family history, the age at first recognition, and the chronicity of the platelet count trend discussed earlier in this chapter. A platelet count abnormality first identified in childhood, particularly one that has remained stable over years of subsequent testing, and especially one accompanied by a supportive family history or syndromic features, favors an inherited disorder among those catalogued in Chapters 1, 2, and 15, and should prompt consideration of genetic evaluation even when the abnormality is mild.

Figure 5.1: Tourniquet (Hess) Test Technique for Eliciting Petechiae

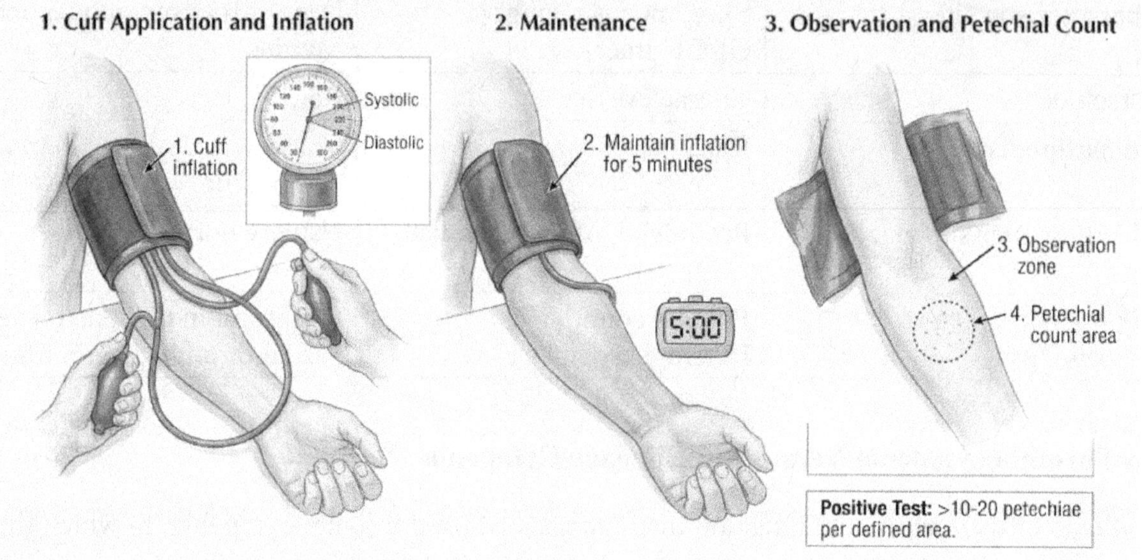

THE PLATELET CRISIS DECISION COMPASS — Recognizing a Bleeding History That Requires Same-Day Evaluation

The Presentation: A patient reports a bleeding history during a routine or urgent care visit, and the clinician must decide whether this can be evaluated through routine outpatient referral or requires same-day hematologic assessment.

Mimic Signature: Chronic, stable mucocutaneous bleeding consistent with a mild, longstanding inherited disorder appropriate for routine evaluation; an acute, evolving bleeding presentation suggesting a new severe thrombocytopenia or acute platelet function disorder; and a bleeding history that, on closer questioning, reflects normal physiologic variation rather than a true disorder.

The Decision: Obtain an immediate complete blood count with peripheral smear review in any patient reporting new-onset spontaneous bruising, petechiae, or mucosal bleeding, particularly if accompanied by systemic symptoms such as fever, fatigue, or bone pain; a severely low platelet count or an abnormal smear on this same-day testing should trigger urgent hematology involvement rather than routine outpatient referral.

Trap Logic: Deferring a same-day complete blood count in a patient with new, spontaneous, unexplained bruising or bleeding because the history sounds similar to a chronic, benign pattern risks missing an acute, rapidly evolving process such as immune thrombocytopenia, acute leukemia, or a thrombotic microangiopathy, each of which can progress rapidly if evaluation is delayed.

Crisis Anchor: New-onset spontaneous bruising or mucosal bleeding, as distinct from a chronic, stable bleeding pattern, warrants a same-day complete blood count and smear review, not routine outpatient scheduling.

Physical Examination in Suspected Platelet Disorders

Characterizing Cutaneous Findings

Physical examination findings, particularly the appearance and distribution of cutaneous bleeding, provide substantial diagnostic information when interpreted using the mechanistic framework developed in Chapter 4. Petechiae, defined as pinpoint, non-blanching hemorrhages typically one to two millimeters in diameter, reflect failure at the level of individual capillaries and are the most specific cutaneous finding for a primary hemostatic disorder, particularly thrombocytopenia; they characteristically appear in dependent areas subject to increased venous pressure, such as the lower extremities in an ambulatory patient, and can be provoked or accentuated by applying a blood pressure cuff between systolic and diastolic pressure for several minutes, the basis of the historical Hess or tourniquet test.

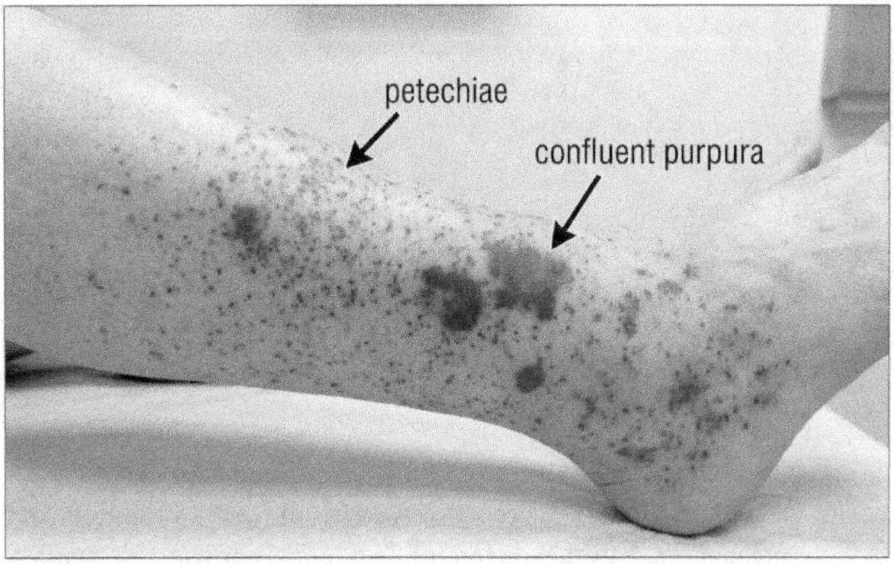

Figure 5.2: Petechial and Purpuric Distribution on the Lower Extremity

Purpura, larger areas of non-blanching hemorrhage generally exceeding several millimeters, and ecchymoses, still larger bruise-like collections, are less specific than petechiae and can arise from platelet disorders, coagulation factor deficiencies, or the vascular causes discussed in Chapter 4, so their presence alone carries less discriminating value than petechiae specifically; palpable purpura, in which the lesion can be felt as raised above the skin surface rather than flat, is instead a red flag for vasculitis, as introduced in Chapter 4, and should prompt consideration of that alternative diagnostic pathway rather than an intensified platelet-focused evaluation.

Mucosal and Ocular Examination

Direct examination of the oral mucosa for gingival bleeding, mucosal petechiae, and, most concerning, hemorrhagic bullae, sometimes termed wet purpura, provides both diagnostic and prognostic information; wet purpura in a patient with severe thrombocytopenia is a recognized clinical marker of substantially elevated bleeding risk, historically associated with an increased risk of subsequent major hemorrhage including intracranial hemorrhage in immune thrombocytopenia, and its presence should accelerate the urgency of both evaluation and treatment discussed in Chapter 9. Fundoscopic examination for retinal hemorrhage, though not always practical outside specialty settings, is similarly informative when available, since retinal hemorrhage indicates that the same microvascular vulnerability discussed in Chapter 4 is manifesting in an anatomic location where consequences can be severe and where intracranial hemorrhage risk may be correspondingly elevated.

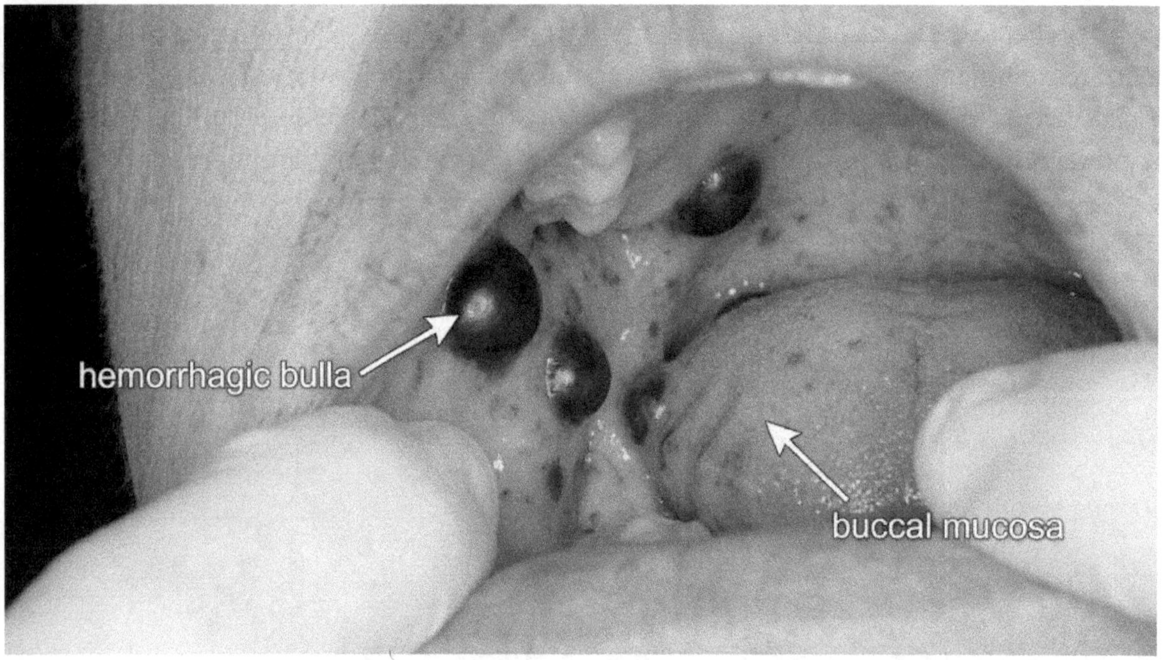

Lymphadenopathy, hepatosplenomegaly, and any evidence of a systemic illness identified on general physical examination carry substantial diagnostic weight in the evaluation of thrombocytopenia specifically, since their presence shifts the differential diagnosis toward secondary causes, including infection, malignant infiltration, or an underlying autoimmune or lymphoproliferative process, discussed further in the diagnostic algorithm developed in Chapter 8, rather than a primary, isolated platelet disorder such as immune thrombocytopenia, in which the physical examination beyond the bleeding manifestations themselves is otherwise characteristically unremarkable.

Examination Findings Suggesting an Inherited Syndrome

A focused examination for the syndromic features introduced throughout Part I of this book, including skeletal abnormalities such as absent or hypoplastic radii, sensorineural hearing loss, oculocutaneous albinism, eczema, and characteristic facial or skeletal dysmorphism, should be incorporated whenever an inherited platelet disorder is under consideration, since identification of an associated syndromic feature, as emphasized in Chapters 1 and 2, can substantially narrow subsequent genetic testing before it is even ordered. This syndromic examination is particularly important in the pediatric population, where an inherited disorder is proportionally more likely and where an early, accurate diagnosis has the greatest downstream benefit for family counseling and long-term surveillance planning.

Nail findings, including koilonychia suggesting iron deficiency, which can itself cause a mild secondary thrombocytosis or, through associated bleeding, contribute to a mixed clinical picture, and specific nail dystrophy patterns associated with certain inherited marrow failure syndromes, provide additional low-effort examination clues that are easily overlooked but occasionally prove diagnostically decisive, particularly in a patient whose presentation does not fit neatly into a single, more common diagnostic category.

Incidental Versus Symptomatic Thrombocytopenia

The Rising Frequency of Incidental Discovery

The widespread use of automated complete blood counts for reasons unrelated to hemostatic concern, including routine screening, preoperative evaluation, and monitoring of unrelated chronic conditions, has made incidental discovery of an abnormal platelet count an increasingly common clinical scenario, distinct from thrombocytopenia identified specifically because a patient presented with bleeding symptoms. This distinction matters because the pretest probability of specific diagnoses differs substantially between these two presentations: incidentally discovered, mild thrombocytopenia in an asymptomatic patient is more likely to reflect a benign or slowly progressive process, while thrombocytopenia identified during evaluation of active bleeding symptoms is more likely to reflect a more acute or severe underlying process, or simply a lower platelet count at the more severe end of the same disease spectrum.

This distinction should inform, though never entirely determine, the urgency and intensity of subsequent evaluation: an asymptomatic patient with a first, incidentally discovered platelet count of 130 x10^9/L generally warrants confirmatory repeat testing and a reasonably paced outpatient evaluation, while a patient presenting with active mucocutaneous bleeding and a platelet count in a similar or lower range warrants a more urgent, same-day evaluation pathway, reflecting the different pretest probabilities and different immediate risks these two presentations carry despite a potentially similar numeric platelet count.

The Danger of Anchoring on a Reassuring Presentation

Despite the general pattern described above, clinicians should resist the temptation to assume that an asymptomatic presentation guarantees a benign underlying process, since several of the more serious conditions discussed later in this book, including early clonal thrombocytosis discussed in Chapter 1, certain myelodysplastic syndromes, and some cases of chronic immune thrombocytopenia, can present with an incidentally discovered abnormal count in an entirely asymptomatic patient. The absence of symptoms lowers, but does not eliminate, the probability of a clinically significant underlying process, and the diagnostic evaluation detailed in Chapter 8 should proceed on the same systematic basis regardless of whether the presentation was incidental or symptomatic, with urgency, rather than diagnostic thoroughness, being the primary variable that differs between these two scenarios.

This principle parallels the reasoning developed in Chapter 1 around isolated, asymptomatic thrombocytosis, where the absence of symptoms similarly does not exclude a clinically important underlying clonal process, and it reflects a broader theme of this book: platelet count abnormalities are best evaluated according to a systematic, mechanism-based diagnostic framework rather than triaged primarily on the basis of how the abnormality happened to be discovered.

Confirming a Genuinely Abnormal Result Before Extensive Evaluation

Before committing a patient to an extensive diagnostic evaluation, the first and most important step is confirming that the abnormal platelet count is genuine rather than a preanalytic artifact, most commonly pseudothrombocytopenia from ethylenediaminetetraacetic acid-induced platelet clumping, addressed in full mechanistic and practical detail in Chapter 6. A single, unconfirmed low platelet count, particularly one discovered incidentally without a clear clinical correlate, should generally prompt review of the automated analyzer's flags and, when available, direct smear examination before an extensive workup is initiated, since a substantial proportion of apparently new thrombocytopenia identified on routine testing reflects this artifact rather than a genuine hematologic abnormality.

This confirmation step is not merely a matter of laboratory precision; it has direct consequences for patient experience and resource utilization, since an unconfirmed pseudothrombocytopenia that proceeds to extensive hematologic evaluation, including in some reported cases unnecessary bone marrow biopsy, represents an avoidable burden on both the patient and the health system that a simple repeat sample collected into an alternative anticoagulant, discussed in Chapter 6, can prevent in the substantial majority of cases.

THE PLATELET CRISIS DECISION COMPASS — A Markedly Low Platelet Count in an Asymptomatic Patient

The Presentation: A platelet count in the range of 10 to 30 x10^9/L is reported on a routine or incidental complete blood count in a patient who denies any bleeding symptoms and appears clinically well.

Mimic Signature: Pseudothrombocytopenia from ethylenediaminetetraacetic acid-induced clumping, which can produce an artifactually severe count in an entirely well patient; genuine severe thrombocytopenia from immune thrombocytopenia or another process that has not yet produced clinically apparent bleeding despite the low count; and, less commonly, an underlying marrow infiltrative process discovered before symptoms have developed.

The Decision: Request immediate smear review specifically to assess for platelet clumping before accepting the automated count as accurate; if clumping is absent and the count is confirmed genuinely low, proceed the same day to a full clinical evaluation and physical examination for bleeding stigmata, since a platelet count this low, even without current symptoms, carries meaningful imminent bleeding risk and should not be managed on a routine outpatient timeline.

Trap Logic: Treating an asymptomatic presentation as evidence that a markedly low reported count can safely wait for routine follow-up conflates the patient's current symptom status with the count's underlying accuracy and risk, when in fact a genuinely severe, confirmed thrombocytopenia carries substantial near-term bleeding risk regardless of whether symptoms have yet appeared.

Crisis Anchor: A platelet count below 30 x10^9/L is confirmed via smear review for clumping and evaluated urgently the same day, regardless of the patient's current symptom status.

Constructing an Efficient Initial Evaluation

A Stepwise Framework for the First Encounter

Bringing together the elements developed throughout this chapter, an efficient initial evaluation of a patient with a suspected platelet disorder proceeds through a defined sequence: confirm the abnormal finding is genuine (via smear review or repeat testing as appropriate), obtain a structured bleeding history including a validated bleeding assessment tool score where the presentation is ambiguous, perform a focused physical examination for the localizing findings described above, and use the resulting composite clinical picture to direct laboratory evaluation toward the specific diagnostic pathway most likely to be productive, whether that is the thrombocytopenia algorithm in Chapter 8, the platelet function testing pathway in Chapter 7, or a vascular or non-hematologic evaluation as suggested by the findings in Chapter 4.

This stepwise approach deliberately front-loads history and examination before extensive laboratory testing, reflecting the evidence, discussed earlier in this chapter regarding preoperative bleeding time screening, that a well-structured clinical evaluation frequently outperforms indiscriminate laboratory testing in both diagnostic yield and resource efficiency, and it establishes the clinical scaffolding onto which the specific laboratory and diagnostic algorithms of the following chapters are built.

When to Involve Hematology Immediately Versus When to Proceed Independently

Not every abnormal platelet finding requires immediate subspecialty involvement, and part of constructing an efficient evaluation is recognizing which findings a generalist clinician can appropriately evaluate independently versus which warrant same-day hematology consultation. Findings warranting immediate hematology involvement generally include active, clinically significant bleeding at any platelet count, a platelet count below approximately 20 to 30 x10^9/L regardless of symptoms as discussed in the Compass instance above, evidence of a possible thrombotic microangiopathy including schistocytes on smear, and any presentation suggesting a possible underlying hematologic malignancy such as accompanying anemia, leukopenia, or abnormal white cell morphology.

Findings that can generally proceed through an initial evaluation without immediate subspecialty involvement include mild, stable, incidentally discovered thrombocytopenia in an asymptomatic patient after pseudothrombocytopenia has been excluded, and a mild bleeding history with a low validated bleeding assessment tool score, both of which can reasonably proceed through the confirmatory laboratory testing described in Chapters 6 and 7 before subspecialty referral is considered, reserving hematology consultation for cases in which this initial evaluation itself proves abnormal or remains diagnostically unclear.

Documentation and Longitudinal Tracking

Because many platelet disorders, particularly the inherited conditions discussed throughout Part I of this book, are chronic and require longitudinal management, establishing clear, structured documentation at the initial encounter, including the bleeding assessment tool score, specific examination findings, and the platelet count trend if prior values are available, provides substantial value for future encounters, particularly when a patient is subsequently evaluated by a different clinician or presents urgently to an unfamiliar setting. A platelet count trend over time is often more diagnostically informative than any single value, since a stable, mildly low count over years points toward a chronic, likely benign process, while a progressively falling count points toward an active, evolving process requiring more urgent evaluation, a distinction that is only possible to make when prior values have been documented and are readily retrievable.

This longitudinal perspective closes the loop back to the chapter's opening emphasis on structured history-taking: just as a single bleeding symptom is best interpreted in the context of a full, structured bleeding history, a single platelet count is best interpreted in the context of its trend over time, and both principles reflect the same underlying clinical discipline of resisting premature conclusions drawn from an isolated data point in favor of a more complete, contextualized clinical picture.

Special Populations in the Initial Clinical Encounter

Pediatric Evaluation

The initial evaluation of a child with a suspected platelet disorder requires adjustments beyond the age-specific history considerations already discussed, since the differential diagnosis in this population weights differently toward inherited conditions and toward a small number of acute pediatric-specific presentations, most notably acute immune thrombocytopenia following a viral illness, which is discussed in detail in Chapter 9 and which typically follows a substantially more self-limited course in children than the chronic pattern more common in adults. A thorough birth history, including any bleeding at circumcision, any need for vitamin K administration, and any neonatal bruising or cephalohematoma out of proportion to the delivery course, adds diagnostic value in children that has no direct counterpart in the adult history.

Growth and developmental assessment should be incorporated into the examination of a child with suspected inherited thrombocytopenia, since several of the inherited marrow failure syndromes discussed in Chapter 15 are associated with short stature, developmental delay, or other systemic findings that, when present, substantially raise the likelihood of a syndromic rather than isolated inherited platelet disorder and should prompt early genetics involvement alongside hematology rather than a hematology-only referral pathway.

Pregnancy and the Peripartum Period

Thrombocytopenia identified during pregnancy requires a distinct evaluation framework, developed in full in Chapter 13, but several principles are relevant to the initial encounter regardless of gestational timing: gestational thrombocytopenia, a benign, mild, and self-limited decline in platelet count of no clinical consequence to mother or fetus, accounts for the substantial majority of thrombocytopenia first identified during pregnancy and must be distinguished from the hypertensive and thrombotic microangiopathic syndromes of pregnancy, which share overlapping laboratory features but carry materially different maternal and fetal risk and require materially different management urgency.

The distinguishing features that separate benign gestational thrombocytopenia from these more concerning pregnancy-specific syndromes, including the platelet count nadir typically observed, the trimester of onset, and the presence or absence of accompanying hypertension, proteinuria, hemolysis, or elevated liver enzymes, are addressed in the dedicated diagnostic algorithm in Chapter 13; the key point for the initial encounter is that a pregnant patient with a new platelet count abnormality should have blood pressure, urine protein, and a basic metabolic and hepatic panel obtained at the same visit as the platelet count, since these additional data points are often decisive in determining the correct diagnostic pathway and cannot efficiently be obtained after the fact.

Perioperative and Preprocedural Assessment

A patient scheduled for an elective surgical or invasive procedure who is found to have an abnormal platelet count, or who reports a bleeding history during preoperative evaluation, presents a distinct clinical challenge, since the evaluation must be completed with adequate time before the scheduled procedure while avoiding unnecessary delay for a patient whose bleeding risk, on structured evaluation, proves unremarkable. The stepwise framework developed earlier in this chapter applies directly to this setting, with the structured bleeding history and validated bleeding assessment tool serving as the primary triage instrument, reserving extensive preoperative laboratory testing, discussed further in Chapter 18, for patients whose structured history or known platelet count abnormality places them at genuinely elevated risk.

Coordination between the proceduralist, anesthesiology, and hematology, when hematology involvement is warranted, should occur with sufficient lead time to allow any additional testing, subspecialty optimization, or procedural modification to be completed without last-minute cancellation, a coordination failure that remains a common and largely avoidable source of both patient inconvenience and health system inefficiency, and one that a structured, early preoperative bleeding assessment, applied consistently as described in this chapter, substantially reduces.

Point-of-Care Tools and Communicating Uncertainty to the Patient

Point-of-Care and Rapid Assessment Adjuncts

A small number of point-of-care instruments, most notably the platelet function analyzer discussed mechanistically in Chapter 7, can supplement the structured history and examination described in this chapter when a rapid functional assessment is needed before a procedure, though these instruments are best understood as an adjunct that refines pretest probability rather than a substitute for the structured history itself, since their sensitivity and specificity for clinically significant bleeding risk remain imperfect and highly dependent on the pretest probability established through careful clinical evaluation. A normal point-of-care functional assay in a patient with a strongly positive structured bleeding history should not be taken as definitively excluding an underlying disorder, particularly a mild von Willebrand disease or a subtle inherited platelet function defect, both of which may require the more specific laboratory evaluation detailed in Chapter 7 regardless of a reassuring point-of-care result.

Conversely, an isolated abnormal point-of-care result in a patient with an unremarkable structured bleeding history and no personal or family history of bleeding more often reflects a preanalytic variable, including recent aspirin or nonsteroidal anti-inflammatory drug exposure, anemia, or sample handling artifact, than a genuine underlying platelet function disorder, reinforcing the principle developed throughout this chapter that laboratory results are interpreted within, rather than in place of, the clinical picture the history and examination establish.

Explaining an Ambiguous Result to the Patient

Many patients evaluated under the framework developed in this chapter will not receive a definitive diagnosis at the initial encounter, since confirmatory laboratory testing, genetic evaluation, or a period of longitudinal observation is frequently required before a specific diagnosis can be established with confidence, and clear communication of this uncertainty is itself an important clinical skill. Patients generally tolerate diagnostic uncertainty well when it is explained in terms of a clear plan, including what has already been ruled out, what remains under consideration, what testing is pending, and what specific new symptom should prompt them to seek care before the next scheduled follow-up, rather than being left with an unexplained abnormal result and no clear sense of what happens next.

This communication should also address the practical implications of the working differential for the patient's immediate activities, including guidance on activity restriction, medication avoidance where relevant, such as counseling against new aspirin or nonsteroidal anti-inflammatory drug use pending further evaluation, and, in women of reproductive age, guidance regarding menstrual bleeding management and any implications for future pregnancy planning, since these practical questions are frequently the patient's most immediate concern and deserve direct attention even before a final diagnosis is reached.

When Structured Tools Disagree With Clinical Gestalt

Occasionally a patient's overall clinical impression, formed through experienced clinical judgment, diverges from the result produced by a validated bleeding assessment tool or an initial laboratory screen, and the framework developed in this chapter does not suggest that structured tools should mechanically override clinical judgment in every instance. A patient with a low bleeding assessment tool score but a compelling, specific bleeding history involving a documented episode of major hemorrhage, or a family history of a well-characterized inherited disorder, warrants continued evaluation despite a reassuring score, since validated tools are population-level instruments that improve average diagnostic accuracy without perfectly capturing every individual clinical scenario.

The structured approach described throughout this chapter is best understood as a discipline that reduces variability and oversight, not as a rigid algorithm that supersedes clinical reasoning, and the most effective use of these tools combines their quantitative rigor with the qualitative clinical judgment that experienced evaluation of the whole patient, including elements that a checklist cannot fully capture, continues to provide.

Patients Already on Antiplatelet or Anticoagulant Therapy

A patient who presents for evaluation of a new bleeding symptom or abnormal platelet count while already established on antiplatelet or anticoagulant therapy for an unrelated indication requires an additional layer of assessment, since the clinician must determine whether the presenting symptom reflects an expected, dose-related consequence of the known therapy, an idiosyncratic exaggeration of that expected effect, or a superimposed, previously unrecognized primary hematologic disorder that has been unmasked or aggravated by the antithrombotic exposure. The structured history developed in this chapter remains fully applicable in this setting, with particular attention to whether the bleeding pattern and severity are proportionate to the known pharmacologic effect of the specific agent, discussed in full in Chapter 18, or instead exceed what that mechanism alone would be expected to produce.

A platelet count obtained in this setting should always be interpreted before assuming the antithrombotic agent alone explains the presentation, since antiplatelet and anticoagulant therapy do not typically reduce the platelet count itself, and a genuinely low count in a patient on these therapies should still prompt the same systematic evaluation for an independent thrombocytopenic process described throughout this chapter, rather than being attributed reflexively to the known medication without further scrutiny.

CLINICAL CASE: A 24-year-old woman presents to primary care for evaluation before starting combined oral contraception, and a routine complete blood count obtained as part of this visit incidentally reveals a platelet count of 145 x10^9/L, just below the lower limit of the local laboratory's reference range. She reports no bleeding symptoms on direct questioning, but when the clinician applies a structured bleeding assessment tool as taught in this chapter, she reports needing to change menstrual protection hourly during the heaviest days of her period since menarche, occasional gum bleeding with brushing, and a memorable episode of prolonged bleeding after a wisdom tooth extraction three years earlier that required the dentist to place additional sutures, findings she had never previously connected or considered worth mentioning because each seemed individually minor. Her family history reveals that her mother has a similar history of heavy menstrual bleeding, and her platelet count, though at the low end of normal, does not fully explain a bleeding history of this severity on its own. Applying the framework developed in this chapter, the mildly low platelet count is treated as one data point within a larger clinical picture rather than the primary focus of concern, and the constellation of a structured bleeding history score in the abnormal range, a suggestive family history, and a platelet count that is only mildly reduced together raise specific concern for von Willebrand disease rather than a primary quantitative platelet disorder, prompting the clinician to order von Willebrand factor antigen, activity, and factor VIII level as the appropriately directed first-line test discussed in Chapter 2, rather than proceeding directly to platelet-specific testing or dismissing the mildly low count as an isolated, inconsequential finding. This case illustrates the central lesson of this chapter: a structured bleeding history, applied systematically rather than relying on a patient's own unprompted symptom reporting, frequently reveals a clinically significant pattern that neither an isolated laboratory value nor an unstructured conversation would have uncovered. Her physical examination, performed at the same visit, reveals no petechiae, purpura, or wet purpura, consistent with the localization framework developed earlier in this chapter, since a mild von Willebrand disease of this severity does not typically produce these more dramatic cutaneous findings, which are more characteristic of severe thrombocytopenia; this negative examination does not argue against the working diagnosis and instead simply reflects the expected examination in a mild primary hemostatic disorder of this type. The clinician documents the bleeding assessment tool score, the family history, and the differential diagnosis in the chart, explains to the patient that her constellation of findings raises a specific, testable hypothesis rather than a certain diagnosis, and provides clear guidance to avoid aspirin and nonsteroidal anti-inflammatory drugs pending the results and to seek urgent care for any heavy bleeding before then, illustrating the communication principles addressed later in this chapter.

KEY POINT: A structured bleeding history frequently uncovers a clinically significant pattern in a patient who denied bleeding symptoms on open-ended questioning, underscoring why directed, tool-based questioning is preferred over unstructured history-taking whenever a platelet count abnormality or bleeding concern is under evaluation.

THE PLATELET CRISIS DECISION COMPASS — Clinical Recognition and Triage

Compass Recap: Same-Day Evaluation Threshold: New-onset spontaneous bruising or mucosal bleeding warrants a same-day complete blood count and smear review, not routine outpatient scheduling, regardless of how mild the history initially sounds.

Compass Recap: Asymptomatic Severe Thrombocytopenia: A confirmed platelet count below approximately 30 x10^9/L is evaluated urgently the same day regardless of current symptom status, since absence of symptoms does not equal absence of imminent risk.

Chapter Anchor: A structured bleeding history, a validated bleeding assessment tool score, and a focused, mechanism-informed physical examination together outperform an unstructured conversation and indiscriminate laboratory testing in directing an efficient, correctly targeted evaluation of a suspected platelet disorder.

Summary and Key Concepts

A structured bleeding history, incorporating spontaneous bleeding, disproportionate bleeding, multi-site bleeding, and prior hemostatic challenges (surgery, dental extraction, childbirth), outperforms unstructured questioning in distinguishing pathologic from physiologic bleeding tendency.

Validated bleeding assessment tools, most notably the ISTH Bleeding Assessment Tool, quantify bleeding history across defined anatomic categories and carry substantial negative predictive value when normal.

Heavy menstrual bleeding is a sensitive, frequently underrecognized indicator of an underlying primary hemostatic disorder and should prompt directed hematologic screening rather than gynecologic management alone.

Petechiae are the most specific cutaneous finding for a primary hemostatic disorder; palpable purpura instead suggests vasculitis; wet purpura (oral hemorrhagic bullae) is a marker of substantially elevated bleeding risk in severe thrombocytopenia.

Incidentally discovered thrombocytopenia carries a different pretest probability distribution than symptomatic thrombocytopenia but must still be confirmed (excluding pseudothrombocytopenia) and evaluated systematically, since absence of symptoms does not exclude a clinically significant process.

An efficient initial evaluation confirms the abnormal finding, obtains structured history and examination, and directs laboratory testing toward the most likely diagnostic pathway, reserving immediate hematology involvement for defined high-risk findings rather than every abnormal platelet result.

CHAPTER 6: LABORATORY EVALUATION: PLATELET COUNT, MORPHOLOGY, AND PSEUDOTHROMBOCYTOPENIA

Learning Objectives

1. Explain the impedance and optical methods used by automated hematology analyzers to generate the platelet count and the specific circumstances under which each method is prone to error.
2. Recognize the peripheral blood smear findings that confirm, refute, or explain an automated platelet count.
3. Identify pseudothrombocytopenia from ethylenediaminetetraacetic acid-induced platelet clumping and apply the correct confirmatory testing sequence.
4. Interpret platelet indices, including mean platelet volume and platelet distribution width, and describe their incremental diagnostic value.
5. Apply age-, sex-, and population-adjusted reference ranges when interpreting a platelet count.
6. Construct an efficient confirmatory and trending strategy for a newly identified platelet count abnormality.

Chapter Outline

This chapter develops the laboratory science underlying the single most common data point in platelet medicine: the platelet count itself. It addresses the automated methods used to generate this number, the peripheral smear examination that confirms or refutes it, the pseudothrombocytopenia artifact that remains the most common cause of a spuriously abnormal result, the platelet indices that add incremental diagnostic information, and the population-specific reference ranges required for correct interpretation. Two Platelet Crisis Decision Compass instances address the recognition of an analyzer flag warranting smear review and the correct resolution pathway once ethylenediaminetetraacetic acid-induced clumping is suspected.

The clinical framework developed in Chapter 5 is only as reliable as the laboratory value it is built upon, and a substantial proportion of diagnostic error in platelet medicine originates not from flawed clinical reasoning but from an uncritically accepted laboratory number that was, in fact, inaccurate. This chapter equips the reader to interrogate a platelet count with the same rigor applied to the clinical history, recognizing when the number can be trusted and when it demands confirmation before any clinical decision is built upon it.

Automated Platelet Counting: Technology and Limitations

Impedance-Based Counting

Most automated hematology analyzers determine the platelet count using electrical impedance technology, in which cells suspended in a conductive diluent are passed individually through a small aperture across which a current flows, and each cell's passage produces a brief voltage pulse whose amplitude is proportional to cell volume. Particles within a defined size threshold, conventionally between two and twenty femtoliters, are classified as platelets, and the instrument reports both the platelet count and the volume distribution histogram from which the platelet indices discussed later in this chapter are derived.

This size-based classification is the fundamental vulnerability of impedance counting, since any particle falling within the platelet size threshold, regardless of its true identity, is counted as a platelet, and any true platelet whose volume falls outside this threshold, whether unusually large or aggregated with other platelets, is misclassified. Microcytes, red cell fragments, cryoglobulin precipitates, and cellular debris can each spuriously elevate the impedance platelet count, while giant platelets, seen in several inherited macrothrombocytopenia syndromes discussed in Chapter 15, and platelet clumps or satellites can each spuriously lower it, producing the two directions of analytic error the clinician must recognize.

Optical and Fluorescence-Based Counting

Many contemporary analyzers supplement or replace impedance counting with an optical method, in which platelets are identified using light scatter properties, or with a fluorescence method, in which a fluorescent dye binds RNA or other intracellular constituents to positively identify platelets rather than relying on size alone. These optical and fluorescence platelet counts are generally more accurate than impedance counting in the presence of confounding factors such as microcytosis or red cell fragmentation, since they identify platelets based on additional characteristics beyond volume, and most modern analyzers automatically flag a discrepancy between the impedance and optical platelet counts, a flag that should itself prompt smear review.

Despite this improved accuracy, optical and fluorescence counting methods remain imperfect, and severe thrombocytopenia, marked platelet clumping, or an unusual population of circulating cells can still produce discordant or inaccurate results even with these more sophisticated methods, reinforcing the principle, developed throughout this chapter, that no automated platelet count, regardless of the underlying technology, should be treated as unquestionably accurate when it is unexpected, discordant with the clinical picture, or accompanied by an instrument flag.

Instrument Flags and When They Demand Action

Modern hematology analyzers generate a range of flags intended to alert the operator to a result that may not be analytically reliable, including flags for platelet clumping, giant platelets, an abnormal platelet histogram, and discordance between counting methods, and institutional laboratory policy generally mandates smear review whenever one of these flags accompanies a low platelet count. Clinicians ordering and interpreting a complete blood count should understand that these flags exist and should specifically request or confirm smear review when a low platelet count is reported without clear documentation that flagging criteria were addressed, since relying solely on the numeric result without attention to the accompanying flags is a recognized and avoidable source of diagnostic error.

This principle applies with particular force to a first, unexpected low platelet count in an asymptomatic patient, precisely the scenario introduced in the Chapter 5 Decision Compass instance addressing incidental severe thrombocytopenia, where the clinical stakes of an inaccurate result, whether falsely reassuring or falsely alarming, are highest and where the modest additional effort of confirming smear review is most clearly justified by the diagnostic and management consequences that follow.

Figure 6.1: Automated Analyzer Platelet Histogram: Normal Versus Clumped Sample

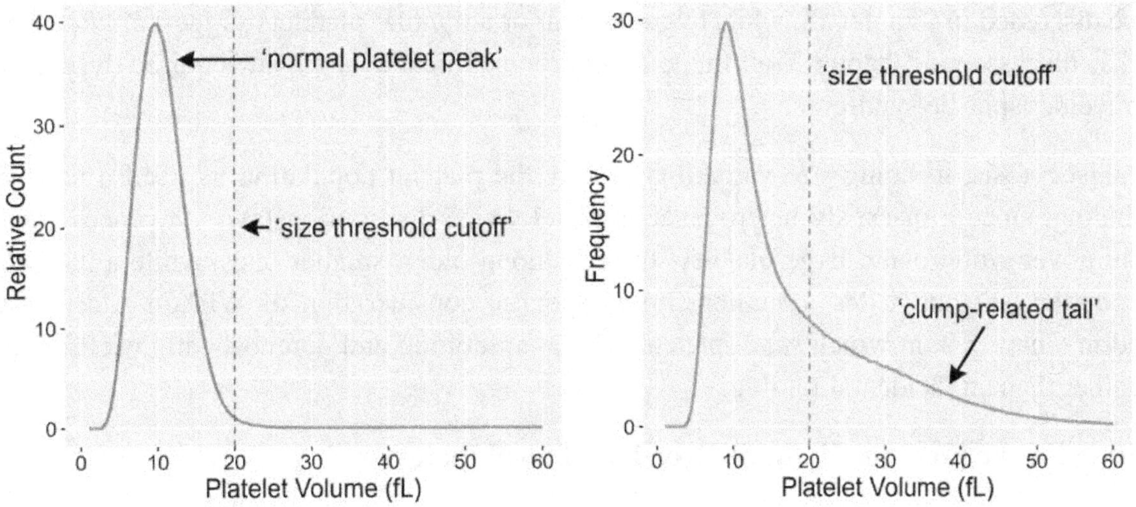

Peripheral Blood Smear Examination and Platelet Morphology

Systematic Approach to Smear Review

A systematic peripheral smear review for a suspected platelet disorder proceeds through a defined sequence: low-power scan of the feathered edge specifically for platelet clumps or satellites, estimation of the platelet count from multiple oil-immersion fields using the standard multiplier appropriate to the analyzer and stain, assessment of platelet size and granularity, and examination of the red and white cell lines for any accompanying abnormality that would redirect the evaluation toward the multilineage diagnostic pathway discussed in Chapter 8. This sequence should be followed in order, since clumping identified early in the review changes the interpretation of every subsequent step and should prompt the confirmatory pathway detailed later in this chapter before the remainder of the smear is over-interpreted.

Estimating the platelet count from the smear provides an independent check on the automated result and is performed by counting platelets across several oil-immersion fields and multiplying by a standard factor, typically fifteen to twenty thousand per platelet per field depending on the specific microscope and analyzer combination in use, to derive an estimated count per microliter; a smear estimate that broadly agrees with the automated count supports its accuracy, while a substantial discrepancy, particularly one in which the smear estimate is higher than the automated count, raises specific concern for an artifact such as clumping that the automated instrument has undercounted.

Normal and Abnormal Platelet Morphology

Normal platelets on a well-prepared smear appear as small, anucleate, discoid fragments with fine azurophilic granules distributed throughout a pale blue-grey cytoplasm, typically one to three micrometers in diameter, roughly one-fifth to one-third the diameter of an adjacent red cell. Morphologic assessment of platelet size and granularity provides diagnostically useful information beyond the numeric count: giant platelets approaching or exceeding the size of a red cell suggest either a compensatory response to increased platelet turnover, as in immune thrombocytopenia, or an inherited macrothrombocytopenia syndrome discussed in Chapter 15, while hypogranular or agranular platelets suggest either a storage pool disorder, as discussed in Chapter 2, or, in the appropriate clinical context, an acquired dysplastic process such as myelodysplastic syndrome.

Platelet anisocytosis, meaning size variability among the platelet population, is itself a nonspecific but useful finding, since a markedly heterogeneous platelet size distribution favors a process of increased platelet turnover with young, large platelets mixed among older, smaller ones, while a uniformly small platelet population, though less common, raises specific consideration of Wiskott-Aldrich syndrome, discussed in Chapter 2, in which small platelet size is a defining and diagnostically useful morphologic feature rather than an incidental finding.

Correlating Smear Findings With the Broader Clinical Picture

Smear examination should never be performed or interpreted in isolation from the platelet count and the clinical history developed in Chapter 5, since the diagnostic value of a specific morphologic finding depends substantially on the count and clinical context in which it appears: giant platelets accompanying a markedly reduced count in a young patient with a lifelong bleeding history suggest a specific inherited disorder worth pursuing genetically, while the same giant platelets accompanying a mildly reduced count in an older patient with a recent viral illness more likely reflect the compensatory response of an acute, self-limited immune thrombocytopenia.

This integrated interpretation extends to the accompanying red and white cell findings as well; schistocytes accompanying thrombocytopenia raise urgent concern for a thrombotic microangiopathy, discussed in full in Chapter 12, and this specific combination should be treated as a hematologic emergency regardless of how mild the platelet count reduction otherwise appears, illustrating how a single smear finding, properly integrated with the rest of the clinical and laboratory picture, can decisively redirect the urgency and direction of the entire evaluation.

THE PLATELET CRISIS DECISION COMPASS — An Analyzer Flag Accompanying a Low Platelet Count

The Presentation: An automated complete blood count reports a platelet count of 45 x10^9/L accompanied by an instrument flag for possible platelet clumping.

Mimic Signature: Genuine ethylenediaminetetraacetic acid-induced pseudothrombocytopenia; genuine thrombocytopenia with a coincidental instrument flag unrelated to the true count; and a partially clotted or improperly mixed sample producing an artifactually low count through a distinct preanalytic mechanism.

The Decision: Do not report or act upon the flagged count until smear review has specifically assessed for platelet clumps and satellitism; if clumping is confirmed, proceed to the citrate or alternative-anticoagulant confirmatory pathway detailed later in this chapter before accepting any platelet count as accurate.

Trap Logic: Accepting a flagged platelet count at face value because the flag seems like a routine laboratory technicality, rather than treating it as a specific instruction to confirm the result before clinical action, risks initiating an unnecessary and potentially invasive workup for an artifactual finding.

Crisis Anchor: Any platelet count accompanied by a clumping flag is confirmed by smear review before it is treated as clinically actionable.

Pseudothrombocytopenia: Mechanism, Recognition, and Resolution

The Mechanism of Ethylenediaminetetraacetic Acid-Induced Clumping

Ethylenediaminetetraacetic acid, the standard anticoagulant used in the lavender-top tube for complete blood count collection, occasionally exposes a cryptic epitope on the platelet glycoprotein IIb/IIIa complex in susceptible individuals through calcium chelation-dependent conformational change, and this exposed epitope is recognized by naturally occurring autoantibodies present in a small subset of the population, producing in vitro platelet agglutination that has no counterpart or clinical significance in the patient's actual circulating blood. This phenomenon is entirely an artifact of the anticoagulant used for sample collection and does not reflect any pathologic process occurring within the patient, a distinction that is essential to communicate clearly once the artifact has been confirmed.

The resulting platelet clumps are counted by impedance-based analyzers as single large particles falling outside the platelet size threshold, producing an artifactually low platelet count that can be dramatic, occasionally falling below 20 x10^9/L in a patient whose true platelet count is entirely normal, a magnitude of discordance that underscores why this artifact cannot be reliably distinguished from genuine severe thrombocytopenia on the basis of the numeric count alone and specifically requires the confirmatory evaluation described in this section.

Recognizing Pseudothrombocytopenia on Smear Review

Pseudothrombocytopenia is recognized on peripheral smear as clusters of platelets adherent to one another, often at the feathered edge of the smear where cells concentrate during preparation, sometimes accompanied by platelet satellitism, in which platelets adhere to the surface of circulating neutrophils, forming a rosette-like pattern around the leukocyte. Both findings confirm that the low automated count reflects a counting artifact rather than a genuine reduction in circulating platelet number, and their identification should prompt immediate correction of the reported result rather than initiation of a thrombocytopenia workup.

The time interval between sample collection and smear preparation influences the degree of clumping observed, since the agglutination reaction develops progressively after ethylenediaminetetraacetic acid exposure, meaning a smear prepared very soon after collection may show less pronounced clumping than one prepared after a delay, a practical consideration relevant to laboratories troubleshooting an ambiguous or borderline case where clumping is suspected but not immediately obvious on initial review.

Confirmatory Testing and Reporting the Corrected Result

Once pseudothrombocytopenia is suspected, the standard confirmatory approach is to redraw the sample into an alternative anticoagulant, most commonly sodium citrate, which does not chelate calcium in the same manner and typically prevents the agglutination reaction, allowing an accurate platelet count to be obtained; when a citrate tube is used, the reported platelet count should be adjusted by a standard correction factor to account for the dilutional effect of the citrate anticoagulant relative to the ethylenediaminetetraacetic acid tube. Alternative approaches include collection into a heparin anticoagulant or, in some laboratories, a specialized magnesium-based anticoagulant, each of which similarly circumvents the calcium-dependent mechanism underlying the artifact.

Once a corrected, accurate platelet count is obtained, this finding should be clearly documented in the medical record, ideally in a manner that will be visible to any future clinician ordering a complete blood count on this patient, since ethylenediaminetetraacetic acid-induced pseudothrombocytopenia is a reproducible, patient-specific phenomenon that will recur on every subsequent standard blood draw; clear documentation prevents the same unnecessary evaluation from being repeated at a future encounter, a practical benefit that directly parallels the longitudinal documentation principle developed in Chapter 5.

THE PLATELET CRISIS DECISION COMPASS — Resolving a Suspected Pseudothrombocytopenia Result

The Presentation: Smear review of a patient with an automated platelet count of 32 x10^9/L reveals prominent platelet clumping at the feathered edge with associated platelet satellitism around several neutrophils.

Mimic Signature: Isolated ethylenediaminetetraacetic acid-induced pseudothrombocytopenia in an otherwise well patient; a mixed picture in which genuine mild thrombocytopenia is present alongside superimposed clumping, potentially masking the true severity; and a delayed or mishandled sample producing clot-related artifact rather than a true ethylenediaminetetraacetic acid-antibody phenomenon.

The Decision: Redraw the sample into sodium citrate or an alternative anticoagulant, apply the appropriate correction factor, and report the corrected count as the accurate result; document the phenomenon prominently in the chart for future reference.

Trap Logic: Assuming that clumping fully explains the low count without obtaining a corrected value risks missing a mixed picture in which a genuinely low, clinically significant platelet count is present beneath the artifact, particularly in a patient with an independent reason for thrombocytopenia.

Crisis Anchor: A confirmed clumping artifact is resolved with a corrected count from an alternative anticoagulant, not simply disregarded as falsely low without verification of the true value.

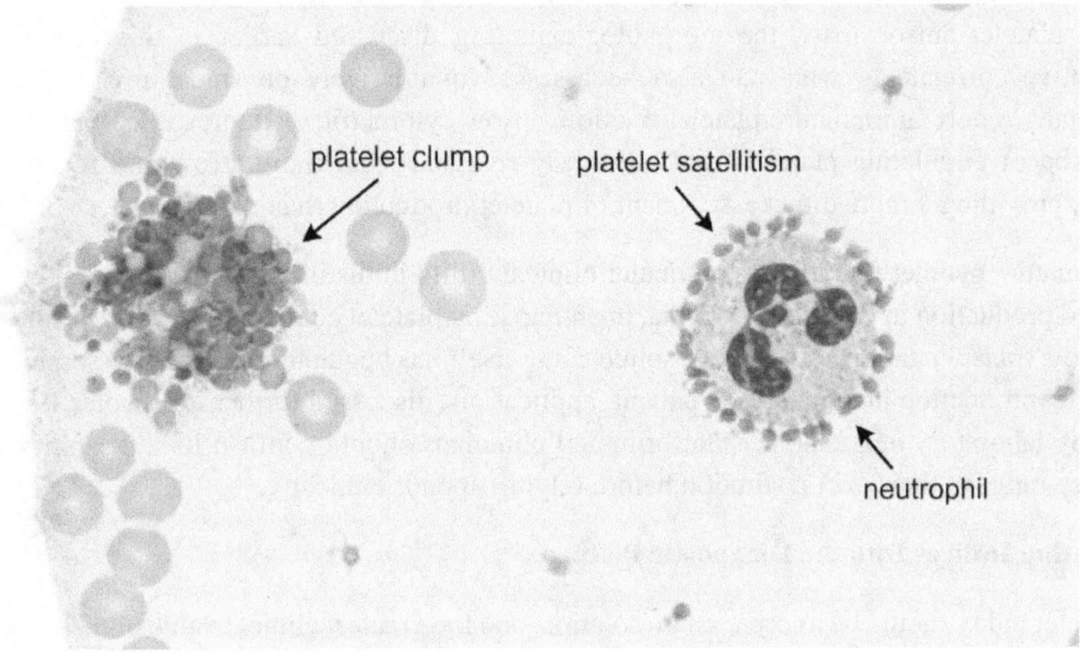

Platelet Indices and Their Clinical Utility

Mean Platelet Volume

Mean platelet volume, derived directly from the platelet volume histogram generated during automated counting, reflects the average size of the circulating platelet population and provides indirect information about platelet production and turnover: an elevated mean platelet volume in the setting of thrombocytopenia suggests a peripheral destructive process with compensatory release of young, large platelets from the marrow, as occurs in immune thrombocytopenia, while a low or inappropriately normal mean platelet volume in the setting of thrombocytopenia suggests impaired marrow production, as occurs in aplastic anemia or marrow infiltration, discussed further in Chapter 8.

This inference must be applied cautiously, since mean platelet volume is influenced by numerous preanalytic variables, including the anticoagulant used and the time elapsed between collection and analysis, as platelets progressively swell in ethylenediaminetetraacetic acid over time, and by technical variability between different analyzer platforms that limits direct comparison of values obtained on different instruments; mean platelet volume is therefore best interpreted as a supportive, trend-based data point within the broader clinical and laboratory picture rather than as a standalone diagnostic test.

Platelet Distribution Width and Other Derived Indices

Platelet distribution width quantifies the degree of variation in platelet size across the population, analogous to red cell distribution width in red cell indices, and an elevated platelet distribution width reflects platelet anisocytosis, the morphologic finding discussed earlier in this chapter, providing a quantitative correlate to what can also be assessed qualitatively on smear review. Some analyzers additionally report an immature platelet fraction, a flow cytometric or fluorescence-based estimate of the proportion of circulating platelets that are newly released from the marrow and retain residual RNA content, providing a more direct assessment of platelet production than mean platelet volume alone.

The immature platelet fraction has particular clinical utility in distinguishing peripheral destruction from impaired production in thrombocytopenia, in anticipating platelet count recovery following chemotherapy or marrow transplantation before the absolute count itself has begun to rise, and in assessing the adequacy of platelet production in a transfused patient, applications discussed further in Chapter 19; its availability varies by laboratory and analyzer platform, and clinicians should confirm its availability and validated reference range at their own institution before relying upon it clinically.

Integrating Indices Into the Diagnostic Picture

No platelet index should be interpreted in isolation, and the greatest clinical value of these indices emerges when they are considered together with the platelet count, the smear morphology, and the clinical history developed in Chapter 5: a low platelet count with an elevated mean platelet volume, elevated platelet distribution width, and elevated immature platelet fraction together paint a coherent picture of peripheral destruction with an appropriately responsive marrow, supporting a diagnosis such as immune thrombocytopenia, while the same low platelet count with a normal or low mean platelet volume and low immature platelet fraction instead suggests impaired production, redirecting the evaluation toward the marrow-focused pathway in Chapter 8.

This integrated interpretation exemplifies the broader diagnostic philosophy of this book: no single laboratory value, however sophisticated, substitutes for the systematic, mechanism-based integration of multiple data points, and the platelet indices are most valuable not as isolated numbers but as additional inputs into the same clinical reasoning framework developed throughout Chapter 5 and continued here.

Index	Typical Reference Range	Elevated Suggests	Low Suggests
Mean platelet volume	7.5-11.5 fL (platform-dependent)	Peripheral destruction, compensatory turnover	Impaired marrow production
Platelet distribution width	9-17% (platform-dependent)	Platelet anisocytosis, active turnover	Uniform, less heterogeneous population
Immature platelet fraction	1-8% (platform-dependent)	Active marrow production, early recovery	Impaired or suppressed production

Reference Ranges and Interpretation Across Populations

Establishing and Applying a Population-Appropriate Reference Range

Platelet count reference ranges are derived from population studies of presumed healthy individuals and conventionally span approximately 150 to 400 or 450 x10^9/L, though the precise lower and upper limits vary modestly between laboratories, analyzer platforms, and reference populations; clinicians should always interpret a platelet count against the specific reference range reported by the laboratory that generated the result rather than a memorized universal cutoff, since minor variation between platforms and populations can meaningfully affect classification of a borderline value.

The reference range itself, by statistical convention, is generally derived to capture the central ninety-five percent of a healthy reference population, meaning that approximately two and one-half percent of entirely healthy individuals will have a platelet count below the lower reference limit and a similar proportion above the upper limit purely as a matter of normal population variation, a statistical reality that supports the general principle, developed in Chapter 5, that a single mildly abnormal value in an asymptomatic patient warrants confirmation and contextualization rather than an immediate, alarmed response.

Ancestry and Population-Specific Variation

Population studies have identified modest but reproducible differences in baseline platelet count across ancestral populations, most notably a somewhat lower average platelet count reported in individuals of African ancestry compared with reference ranges derived predominantly from European ancestry populations, a difference attributed at least in part to genetic variation, including the atypical chemokine receptor variant more prevalent in this population and associated independently with lower baseline neutrophil and platelet counts without conferring any corresponding increase in bleeding risk. Clinicians should be aware of this population variation, since applying a single, non-representative reference range uniformly across all patients risks over-labeling a normal population variant as pathologic thrombocytopenia, a diagnostic error with potential downstream consequences including unnecessary evaluation, and in some settings, inappropriate delay or denial of otherwise indicated therapy.

This principle does not imply that a low platelet count in a patient from an ancestral group with a lower population average should be dismissed without appropriate evaluation, but rather that the pretest probability of a genuinely pathologic process at a given platelet count should be calibrated against a reference range and clinical context appropriate to that patient, a nuance increasingly incorporated into population-specific reference range studies and into individual laboratory reporting practices as this evidence base continues to mature.

Age, Sex, and Physiologic Variation

Platelet counts vary modestly but measurably across the lifespan and between sexes: neonates and young infants have platelet count reference ranges that differ from those of older children and adults, discussed further in the context of neonatal thrombocytopenia in Chapter 13, and healthy women on average carry a slightly higher platelet count than healthy men, a difference of uncertain full mechanistic explanation but consistently reproduced across population studies. Platelet count also varies modestly within an individual across the menstrual cycle and can fall modestly during the later stages of a normal pregnancy, the gestational thrombocytopenia phenomenon introduced in Chapter 5 and developed fully in Chapter 13.

These physiologic sources of variation reinforce a theme woven throughout this chapter: a platelet count is not a single, universally applicable number to be checked against one fixed threshold, but a laboratory value whose correct interpretation depends on the specific analytic method that generated it, the population-appropriate reference range against which it is compared, and the individual patient's own baseline and physiologic context, all of which the careful clinician integrates before assigning clinical significance to an isolated result.

Confirming and Trending an Abnormal Platelet Count

When and How to Repeat a Platelet Count

A newly identified, unexpected platelet count abnormality, particularly one discovered incidentally and without a clear clinical correlate, generally warrants repeat testing before it is accepted as representing a genuine, new clinical finding, both to exclude the preanalytic artifacts discussed throughout this chapter and to establish whether the abnormality is an isolated occurrence or the first observation of a persistent or progressive process. The interval before repeat testing should be guided by clinical urgency: a markedly abnormal count, particularly one accompanied by any bleeding symptom, warrants same-day or next-day repeat testing as discussed in the Chapter 5 Decision Compass instance addressing same-day evaluation, while a mildly abnormal, asymptomatic, incidental finding can generally be repeated within several weeks without meaningful risk of missing a time-sensitive diagnosis.

Repeat testing should, whenever feasible, be accompanied by direct smear review rather than relying solely on the repeat automated count, since a single confirmatory result that itself carries an unrecognized artifact provides false reassurance rather than genuine confirmation, and the modest additional effort of smear review at this confirmatory step substantially strengthens the reliability of the conclusion drawn from it.

Establishing and Interpreting a Platelet Count Trend

Once an abnormal platelet count has been confirmed as genuine, establishing a trend over time, whenever prior values are available through the medical record, provides diagnostic information that a single value, however accurately measured, cannot supply on its own, directly extending the longitudinal documentation principle introduced in Chapter 5. A platelet count that has remained stable within a narrow range over months or years supports a chronic, likely benign or at least indolent process and generally does not require urgent re-evaluation absent a new clinical change, while a platelet count that is progressively declining across sequential measurements, even if each individual value remains within a technically normal or only mildly abnormal range, suggests an active, evolving process that warrants more urgent attention than the absolute value alone would suggest.

This trend-based reasoning applies with particular importance to a patient approaching a specific numeric threshold relevant to management, such as the platelet count thresholds relevant to periprocedural risk discussed in Chapter 5 and further developed in Chapter 18, since a count trending steadily downward toward such a threshold warrants closer monitoring and earlier intervention planning than an isolated measurement at a similar level with no established trend.

Coordinating Laboratory Findings With the Clinical Evaluation

The laboratory principles developed in this chapter are not a self-contained diagnostic exercise but are designed to integrate directly with the clinical framework established in Chapter 5, and the two together form the complete initial evaluation of a suspected platelet disorder: the clinical history and examination establish the pretest probability and urgency of the presentation, while the laboratory evaluation confirms, refines, or occasionally overturns the clinical impression through accurate, correctly interpreted numeric and morphologic data. A confirmed, accurately trended, population-appropriately interpreted platelet count, combined with smear morphology and the relevant indices, positions the clinician to proceed confidently to the more advanced functional and diagnostic testing developed in Chapters 7 and 8.

This integration also has direct implications for how results are communicated to the patient, extending the principles of transparent communication about diagnostic uncertainty developed in Chapter 5; a patient told simply that their platelet count is low, without the context of whether this has been confirmed, whether it represents a new or chronic finding, and what it means for their immediate risk, is left with considerably more anxiety and considerably less actionable information than a patient given the fuller, integrated picture this chapter's laboratory framework makes possible.

Special Analytic Circumstances: Severe Thrombocytopenia, Macrothrombocytopenia, and Interfering Samples

Counting Accuracy at Very Low Platelet Counts

Automated platelet counting becomes progressively less precise as the true platelet count falls toward the lower limits of analyzer detection, since the statistical reliability of any particle count depends on the absolute number of particles enumerated, and a severely thrombocytopenic sample presents comparatively few platelets for the instrument to sample within a given analyzed volume. At platelet counts below approximately 10 to 20 x10^9/L, the coefficient of variation of the automated count widens substantially, meaning two sequential measurements on the identical sample can differ by a clinically meaningful margin purely from counting statistics rather than any true biological change, a limitation that has direct implications for the transfusion threshold decisions addressed in Chapter 19.

For this reason, many laboratories perform a manual platelet count, using a hemocytometer under phase-contrast microscopy, as the reference method whenever the automated count falls below a locally defined critical threshold, since manual counting, though more labor-intensive, avoids the size-threshold misclassification vulnerabilities of impedance counting and provides a more reliable value at the extremes of the clinically important range where transfusion and treatment decisions are most consequential. Clinicians managing a patient with severe, borderline-critical thrombocytopenia should be aware that the reported automated value carries wider uncertainty at this range and should request manual confirmation when a specific numeric threshold is about to drive an irreversible clinical decision.

Macrothrombocytopenia and Undercounting of Giant Platelets

The inherited macrothrombocytopenia syndromes introduced in Chapter 2 and developed fully in Chapter 15 produce platelets that may approach or exceed the size of a red cell, and because impedance analyzers classify particles by a fixed upper size threshold, a substantial proportion of these giant platelets can be misclassified as red cells rather than platelets, producing an automated platelet count that underrepresents the true circulating platelet mass, sometimes dramatically. This systematic undercounting means that a patient with a macrothrombocytopenia syndrome may appear, by automated count alone, to have more severe thrombocytopenia than is functionally the case, a discrepancy that smear review reliably identifies through direct visualization of the abnormally large platelet population.

This phenomenon has direct clinical significance beyond diagnostic classification, since a patient with a chronic, stable macrothrombocytopenia whose automated count appears alarmingly low may in fact have adequate hemostatic platelet mass and minimal bleeding risk once the true, smear-corrected platelet burden is accounted for, and recognizing this pattern can prevent unnecessary escalation of care, including inappropriate platelet transfusion, in a patient whose baseline laboratory pattern, once correctly understood, is not actually indicative of an acute or dangerous process.

Figure 6.3: Manual Hemocytometer Platelet Counting Technique

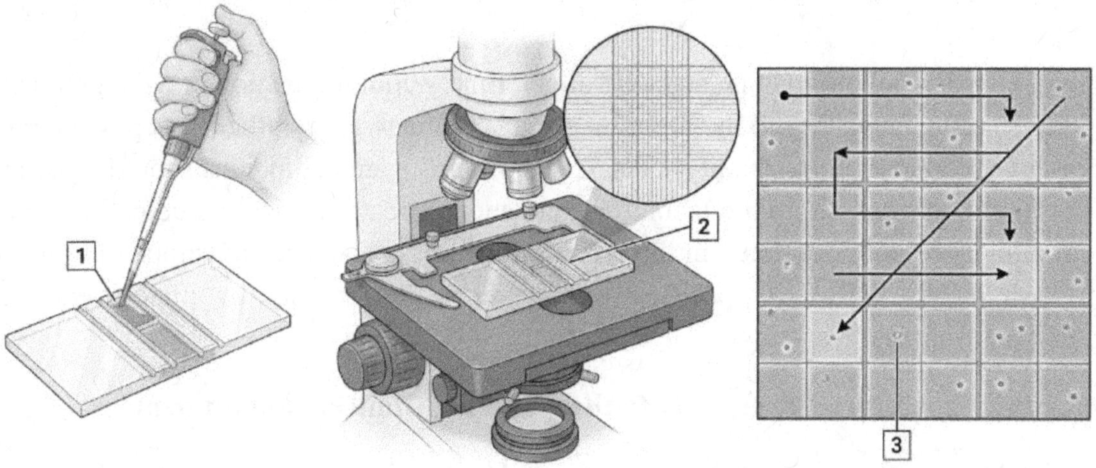

1 Sample loading 2 Counting grid 3 Phase-contrast platelet identification

Lipemic, Icteric, and Otherwise Interfering Samples

Severely lipemic samples, most often encountered in patients with marked hypertriglyceridemia or those sampled shortly after a fat-containing meal or intravenous lipid infusion, can interfere with optical and impedance platelet counting through light scatter and particle interference effects, occasionally producing spuriously elevated platelet counts as lipid particles fall within the platelet size and optical detection range. Similarly, severe icterus, marked leukocytosis with fragile or fragmenting white cells, and cryoglobulinemia can each interfere with accurate platelet enumeration through mechanisms analogous to those already discussed for red cell fragments and cellular debris earlier in this chapter.

Recognition of these less common interfering circumstances depends on awareness of the patient's broader clinical context, including recent oral intake, known hyperlipidemia, hepatic dysfunction, and any known paraprotein-associated condition, combined with laboratory-reported flags and, when the clinical picture and reported count are discordant, direct communication with the laboratory to discuss the specific interference pattern observed and the most appropriate corrective or confirmatory testing strategy for that specific analytic circumstance.

Quality Assurance and Laboratory-Clinician Communication

Delta Checks and Critical Value Reporting

Most clinical laboratories incorporate a delta check into their quality assurance process, an automated comparison between a patient's current result and their most recent prior result that flags an unexpectedly large change for additional review before the result is released, a safeguard directly relevant to the trend-based interpretation developed earlier in this chapter, since a delta check failure for platelet count often prompts the same smear review and confirmatory steps this chapter has emphasized before the laboratory even releases the result to the ordering clinician. Understanding that this safeguard exists helps the clinician interpret a delayed or amended platelet count result appropriately, recognizing that a delay in reporting a markedly changed value often reflects appropriate laboratory diligence rather than a system failure.

Critical value reporting policies, which mandate direct, timely communication of a dangerously abnormal platelet count from the laboratory to the ordering clinician or care team rather than passive result posting alone, represent a second essential quality and safety mechanism, and clinicians should ensure that current contact information is available to the laboratory and should treat a critical value call as warranting the same urgent clinical response outlined in the Decision Compass instances developed in this chapter and in Chapter 5, since these calls exist specifically to prevent a dangerously low platelet count from going unnoticed in a busy clinical workflow.

Communicating Laboratory Uncertainty to the Ordering Clinician and Patient

When a platelet count result carries meaningful analytic uncertainty, whether from severe thrombocytopenia at the limits of counting precision, suspected macrothrombocytopenia, or an unresolved interference pattern, effective communication between the laboratory and the ordering clinician, and in turn between the clinician and the patient, is essential to avoid either false reassurance or unwarranted alarm. A laboratory report that simply states a numeric platelet count without conveying an accompanying flag or interpretive comment leaves the ordering clinician without the information needed to judge how much confidence to place in that number, underscoring the value of laboratory information systems and reporting practices that surface flags and interpretive comments prominently rather than as easily overlooked footnotes.

This communication principle extends the transparency-in-uncertainty framework introduced in Chapter 5: just as a patient benefits from a clear explanation of diagnostic uncertainty in their clinical evaluation, a clinician benefits from a clear explanation of analytic uncertainty in a laboratory result, and building both forms of communication into routine practice reduces the diagnostic errors, unnecessary interventions, and patient anxiety that can otherwise follow from a laboratory value treated as more definitive than the underlying methodology actually supports.

Building an Institutional Reflex for Platelet Count Verification

The principles developed throughout this chapter are most effective when embedded as an institutional reflex rather than relying on individual clinician vigilance at each encounter: standing laboratory protocols mandating smear review for flagged or markedly abnormal platelet counts, electronic health record prompts that surface a patient's known pseudothrombocytopenia or macrothrombocytopenia history when a new low count is reported, and structured handoff communication that includes recent platelet count trends each reduce the likelihood that an inaccurate or unconfirmed count drives an inappropriate clinical decision.

Institutions that have implemented these systematic safeguards report measurable reductions in unnecessary hematology consultation, avoidable bone marrow biopsy, and inappropriate platelet transfusion attributable to unconfirmed analytic artifact, a body of quality improvement evidence that reinforces the central message of this chapter: the platelet count is a powerful and generally reliable laboratory value, but its full clinical value is only realized when the analytic principles developed here are applied systematically rather than left to inconsistent individual practice.

Historical Methods and the Evolution of Platelet Counting Technology

From Manual Counting to Automated Impedance Technology

Before the widespread adoption of automated hematology analyzers beginning in the latter decades of the twentieth century, platelet enumeration relied exclusively on manual hemocytometer counting under phase-contrast microscopy, a technically demanding and time-consuming method subject to substantial interobserver variability, particularly at the modest platelet concentrations that made accurate visual identification difficult against a background of red cells and cellular debris. The introduction of impedance-based automated counting represented a major advance in both speed and reproducibility, allowing a platelet count to be generated in seconds as part of a routine complete blood count rather than requiring a dedicated, specialized manual procedure, and this technological shift is directly responsible for the platelet count becoming the ubiquitous, routinely available screening value it is in contemporary practice.

This historical transition also explains why manual counting, though now reserved for the specific confirmatory circumstances discussed earlier in this chapter, remains the reference method against which automated technologies continue to be validated, since the fundamental principle of direct visual platelet identification under phase-contrast microscopy has not been superseded in accuracy, only in throughput, by the automated methods that have replaced it for routine use.

Ongoing Technological Refinement

Contemporary hematology analyzer development continues to refine platelet enumeration accuracy, with newer platforms increasingly combining multiple detection principles, including impedance, optical scatter, and fluorescence, within a single analyzer and using algorithmic reconciliation between these methods to flag discordant results automatically rather than relying solely on operator recognition of a suspicious count. Some newer platforms additionally incorporate machine learning-based image analysis of digital smear images, allowing automated morphologic screening for clumping, giant platelets, and other confounding findings to be performed at a scale not previously practical with manual smear review alone, though these digital morphology systems remain adjuncts to, rather than replacements for, expert manual review in ambiguous or clinically significant cases.

Clinicians should expect continued evolution in this technology over the course of their careers and should maintain the underlying diagnostic principles developed throughout this chapter, rather than platform-specific technical details alone, as the durable foundation of their approach to an abnormal platelet count, since the specific instruments in use will continue to change while the fundamental need to confirm, contextualize, and trend a platelet count before acting upon it will not.

Implications for Resource-Limited Settings

In settings where automated hematology analyzers are unavailable, unreliable, or subject to frequent maintenance interruption, manual platelet counting and smear-based estimation, discussed earlier in this chapter, remain clinically essential and fully adequate skills, and clinicians training or practicing in these settings should maintain proficiency in manual smear-based platelet estimation as a primary, rather than backup, diagnostic method. The smear estimation technique described earlier in this chapter, appropriately performed, provides clinically actionable accuracy sufficient to guide the same triage and management decisions developed throughout this chapter and Chapter 5, even in the complete absence of automated analyzer support.

This point carries particular relevance for global health contexts and for disaster or resource-constrained response settings, where the diagnostic principles developed in this chapter, rooted in direct microscopic examination and structured clinical correlation rather than dependence on sophisticated automated technology, remain fully applicable and, in some respects, represent the more fundamental and universally transferable skill set that automated technology has supplemented rather than replaced.

CLINICAL CASE: A 58-year-old man undergoing a routine annual physical examination is found to have a platelet count of 58 x10^9/L on automated complete blood count, a marked decline from a count of 210 x10^9/L recorded eighteen months earlier during an unrelated hospitalization, though the patient reports feeling entirely well and denies any bleeding symptoms. Applying the framework developed in this chapter, the ordering clinician requests smear review before any further action, and the smear confirms a genuinely low platelet count without evidence of clumping or satellitism, with platelets appearing normal in size and granularity and no schistocytes, blasts, or other concerning morphologic findings on the accompanying red and white cell examination. The mean platelet volume is reported as low-normal and the immature platelet fraction, available at this laboratory, is reported as low, a combination suggesting impaired marrow production rather than peripheral destruction, in contrast to the pattern that would be expected in immune thrombocytopenia. This laboratory picture, combined with the substantial interval decline from a previously normal, documented count, redirects the evaluation away from the acute, immune-mediated pathway that might otherwise be the first consideration in an isolated low platelet count and toward the broader marrow-focused diagnostic algorithm developed in Chapter 8, prompting the clinician to obtain a complete blood count with full differential and to arrange hematology evaluation for consideration of bone marrow examination given the production-pattern indices and the magnitude of interval decline. This case illustrates how the platelet indices and immature platelet fraction, properly integrated with the trend and smear findings developed throughout this chapter, can meaningfully redirect a diagnostic pathway before any additional testing beyond the basic complete blood count has even been obtained.

KEY POINT: A platelet count should never be accepted as clinically actionable in isolation; smear confirmation, awareness of instrument flags, population-appropriate reference ranges, and, whenever available, a documented trend together determine whether a reported number reflects the patient's true circulating platelet mass.

THE PLATELET CRISIS DECISION COMPASS — Laboratory Confirmation and Interpretation

---

Compass Recap: Flagged Results: Any platelet count accompanied by a clumping flag is confirmed by smear review before it is treated as clinically actionable.

Compass Recap: Confirmed Clumping: A confirmed clumping artifact is resolved with a corrected count from an alternative anticoagulant, not simply disregarded as falsely low without verification of the true value.

Chapter Anchor: The platelet count is a laboratory result requiring active interrogation, not passive acceptance: smear morphology, platelet indices, population-appropriate reference ranges, and a documented trend together determine whether a reported value can be trusted as the foundation for clinical decision-making.

Summary and Key Concepts

Automated platelet counts are generated by impedance, optical, or fluorescence-based methods, each with distinct vulnerabilities to spurious elevation (debris, fragments) or spurious reduction (clumping, giant platelets).

Peripheral smear review, following a systematic sequence beginning with a low-power scan for clumping, confirms or refutes the automated count and adds morphologic information (size, granularity, anisocytosis) unavailable from the number alone.

Pseudothrombocytopenia from ethylenediaminetetraacetic acid-induced platelet clumping is recognized by clumps and satellitism on smear and resolved by redrawing into an alternative anticoagulant, most commonly sodium citrate, with appropriate correction and clear chart documentation for future encounters.

Mean platelet volume, platelet distribution width, and immature platelet fraction provide incremental information about platelet production versus destruction but must be interpreted as supportive, platform-dependent trend data rather than standalone diagnostic tests.

Platelet count reference ranges vary by age, sex, pregnancy status, and ancestral population; applying a non-representative reference range risks mislabeling normal population variation as pathologic thrombocytopenia.

A confirmed, accurately trended platelet count integrated with smear morphology and clinical findings from Chapter 5 forms the foundation for the more advanced functional and diagnostic evaluation developed in Chapters 7 and 8.

CHAPTER 7: PLATELET FUNCTION TESTING: AGGREGOMETRY, FLOW CYTOMETRY, AND POINT-OF-CARE ASSAYS

Learning Objectives

1. Describe the principle of light transmission aggregometry and the standard agonist panel used to characterize platelet function.
2. Recognize the characteristic aggregometry tracing patterns associated with major inherited platelet function disorders.
3. Identify the preanalytic variables that most commonly confound platelet function testing and the steps required to control for them.
4. Explain the role of flow cytometry in assessing platelet receptor expression and granule release.
5. Compare the clinical utility and limitations of point-of-care platelet function assays against laboratory-based aggregometry.
6. Construct an efficient, stepwise platelet function testing strategy for a patient with a suspected inherited or acquired platelet function disorder.

Chapter Outline

This chapter develops the specialized testing methods used to characterize platelet function beyond the count and morphology addressed in Chapter 6, building directly on the receptor biology, signaling cascades, and aggregation mechanisms developed in Chapters 2 and 3. It addresses light transmission aggregometry and its agonist panel, the preanalytic variables that most often confound this testing, flow cytometric and point-of-care alternatives, the specific application of function testing to antiplatelet therapy monitoring, and the genetic testing that increasingly complements or supersedes functional assays for a definitive diagnosis. Two Platelet Crisis Decision Compass instances address the recognition of an aggregometry pattern requiring urgent clinical correlation and the resolution of a discordant point-of-care result.

Platelet function testing occupies a technically demanding niche within hematology laboratory medicine, requiring careful attention to specimen handling, timing, and interpretation that, if neglected, produces results of limited or misleading clinical value. This chapter equips the reader to order, interpret, and troubleshoot platelet function testing with the same rigor developed for platelet count interpretation in Chapter 6, recognizing both the diagnostic power and the substantial pitfalls of this testing category.

Light Transmission Aggregometry: Principles and Technique

The Optical Principle of Aggregometry

Light transmission aggregometry, the reference standard for platelet function testing, measures the change in light transmittance through a stirred sample of platelet-rich plasma as platelets aggregate in response to an added agonist; unactivated platelets remain in suspension and scatter light, producing low baseline transmittance, while aggregating platelets clump together and fall out of the light path, producing a rising transmittance curve that the instrument records as a tracing over several minutes. The shape, amplitude, and, in many protocols, the presence or absence of a second wave following an initial primary aggregation wave together characterize the platelet response to each specific agonist tested.

This method directly interrogates the downstream functional consequence of the receptor and signaling pathways developed mechanistically in Chapter 3, translating molecular-level activation events into a measurable, clinically interpretable aggregation curve, and it remains the reference standard against which newer point-of-care and flow cytometric methods, discussed later in this chapter, continue to be validated despite its technical demands and comparatively long turnaround time.

Specimen Preparation Requirements

Aggregometry requires platelet-rich plasma prepared by careful, low-speed centrifugation of whole blood to sediment red and white cells while leaving platelets in suspension, a preparation step demanding precise timing and centrifugation parameters, since excessive force activates platelets prematurely and invalidates subsequent testing, while inadequate centrifugation leaves residual red or white cells that interfere with the optical measurement. The platelet count within the prepared platelet-rich plasma must additionally fall within a validated range, typically adjusted with autologous platelet-poor plasma when the count is too high, since aggregometry tracings are count-dependent and results obtained outside the validated range cannot be reliably interpreted against established reference patterns.

This specimen preparation burden is a primary reason aggregometry remains centralized in specialized coagulation laboratories rather than performed as a routine, widely available test, and it underscores why careful coordination between the ordering clinician and the performing laboratory, including confirmation of an adequate baseline platelet count before the sample is drawn, is essential to obtaining an interpretable result rather than an uninterpretable, wasted specimen.

The Aggregation Tracing and Its Components

A normal aggregometry tracing in response to a strong agonist such as thrombin or high-dose collagen typically shows a single, sustained wave of aggregation reaching a high maximal amplitude without disaggregation, reflecting the full, irreversible activation and aggregation response developed in Chapter 3, while weaker agonists such as low-dose adenosine diphosphate or epinephrine characteristically produce a biphasic response in normal individuals, consisting of an initial, reversible primary wave followed by a sustained secondary wave that depends on release of endogenous adenosine diphosphate and thromboxane A2 from platelet granules and subsequent recruitment of additional platelets into the aggregate.

The presence, absence, or attenuation of this secondary wave, along with the maximal amplitude achieved and the lag time before aggregation begins, together constitute the interpretive elements that distinguish a normal tracing from the specific abnormal patterns associated with the inherited and acquired platelet function disorders discussed throughout this chapter and in Chapter 16, making careful, standardized tracing interpretation, ideally by a laboratory professional experienced specifically in aggregometry, essential to accurate diagnosis.

Agonist Panels and Pattern Interpretation

The Standard Agonist Panel

A standard aggregometry panel tests platelet response to a defined set of agonists selected to interrogate distinct receptor and signaling pathways, typically including adenosine diphosphate at two concentrations, epinephrine, collagen, arachidonic acid, and ristocetin, with each agonist engaging the specific receptor systems developed in Chapter 2: adenosine diphosphate engages the P2Y12 and P2Y1 receptors, collagen engages glycoprotein VI and integrin alpha2beta1, arachidonic acid interrogates the cyclooxygenase-thromboxane pathway, and ristocetin uniquely interrogates the glycoprotein Ib-von Willebrand factor axis rather than intrinsic platelet activation, distinguishing it mechanistically from every other agonist in the panel.

Because each agonist interrogates a distinct pathway, the pattern of response across the full panel, rather than any single agonist result in isolation, provides the diagnostic signature of a specific platelet function disorder, and this pattern-based interpretation is the central analytic skill this chapter develops; a laboratory report listing individual agonist results without integrated pattern interpretation places the burden of this synthesis on the ordering clinician, making familiarity with the characteristic patterns discussed below clinically essential rather than merely academic.

Characteristic Patterns in Inherited Disorders

Glanzmann thrombasthenia, arising from glycoprotein IIb/IIIa deficiency or dysfunction as developed in Chapter 2, produces absent aggregation to all agonists except ristocetin, which remains normal since the glycoprotein Ib-von Willebrand factor axis it interrogates is intact, a distinctive and highly specific pattern that essentially confirms the diagnosis once pseudothrombocytopenia and other artifacts have been excluded. Bernard-Soulier syndrome, arising from glycoprotein Ib-IX-V deficiency, produces the mirror-image pattern: absent or markedly reduced ristocetin-induced aggregation with generally preserved aggregation to other agonists, since the defect specifically impairs von Willebrand factor-dependent adhesion rather than the downstream aggregation machinery.

Storage pool disorders, discussed mechanistically in Chapter 2, characteristically produce an absent or markedly attenuated secondary aggregation wave in response to weak agonists such as low-dose adenosine diphosphate and epinephrine, reflecting the impaired release of granule contents needed to sustain and amplify the aggregation response, while the primary wave and the response to strong agonists such as collagen and thrombin, which are less dependent on granule release, may remain relatively preserved, producing a subtler pattern that requires careful tracing interpretation to distinguish from a normal but variable response.

Patterns Associated With Acquired Platelet Dysfunction

Aspirin and other cyclooxygenase inhibitors produce a characteristic aggregometry pattern of markedly reduced or absent aggregation specifically in response to arachidonic acid, with relative preservation of the response to other agonists, directly reflecting the thromboxane synthesis blockade discussed pharmacologically in Chapter 18, while P2Y12 receptor antagonists such as clopidogrel produce a corresponding reduction specifically in the adenosine diphosphate-induced response. Uremia, discussed in the context of chronic kidney disease throughout this book, produces a more generalized pattern of reduced aggregation across multiple agonists, reflecting the multifactorial mechanism of uremic platelet dysfunction, including accumulated uremic toxins and altered nitric oxide and prostacyclin signaling, that does not localize as cleanly to a single receptor pathway as the inherited disorders or single-agent drug effects discussed above.

Recognizing these distinct patterns allows the clinician to distinguish an inherited disorder from an acquired, potentially reversible cause of platelet dysfunction, a distinction with direct management implications, since an acquired pattern attributable to a specific medication or a treatable metabolic derangement such as uremia may resolve with discontinuation of the offending agent or correction of the underlying condition, while an inherited pattern requires the longitudinal management approach developed in Chapter 16.

THE PLATELET CRISIS DECISION COMPASS — An Aggregometry Pattern Suggesting Glanzmann Thrombasthenia

---

The Presentation: A young patient with a lifelong severe mucocutaneous bleeding history undergoes aggregometry, which shows absent aggregation to adenosine diphosphate, collagen, epinephrine, and arachidonic acid, with a normal ristocetin-induced response.

Mimic Signature: Genuine Glanzmann thrombasthenia from glycoprotein IIb/IIIa deficiency; a technical or preanalytic error, such as an inadequately platelet-rich preparation, producing a spuriously flat tracing across all agonists; and a severe acquired platelet function defect, such as marked uremia, mimicking a similarly broad aggregation defect.

The Decision: Confirm the platelet-rich plasma preparation met technical validity criteria before accepting the pattern as diagnostic; if technically valid, proceed to flow cytometric quantification of surface glycoprotein IIb/IIIa expression and, where available, genetic testing to confirm the diagnosis and characterize the specific molecular defect.

Trap Logic: Accepting a flat, pan-agonist aggregometry tracing as diagnostic of Glanzmann thrombasthenia without confirming technical validity of the preparation risks a false-positive diagnosis when the true explanation is a technically inadequate specimen rather than a genuine inherited defect.

Crisis Anchor: A near-absent response to all agonists except ristocetin, in a technically valid preparation, is the aggregometry signature of Glanzmann thrombasthenia and warrants confirmatory glycoprotein IIb/IIIa flow cytometry.

Figure 7.1: Light Transmission Aggregometry Tracings: Normal, Glanzmann Thrombasthenia, and Bernard-Soulier Syndrome

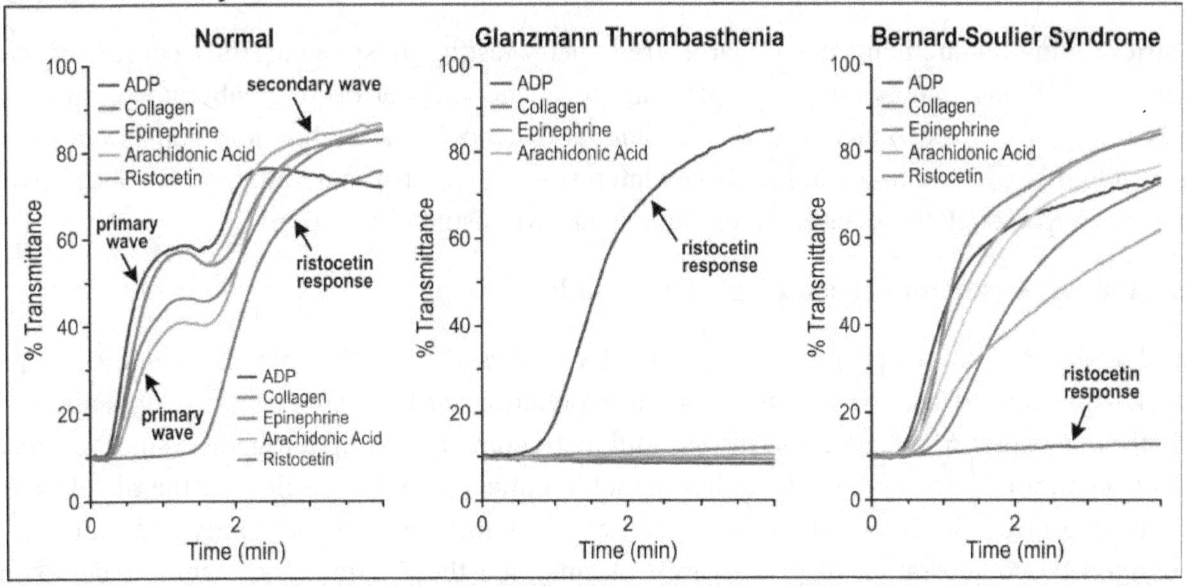

Figure 7.1: Light Transmission Aggregometry Tracings: Normal, Glanzmann Thrombasthenia, and Bernard-Soulier Syndrome

Preanalytic Variables Affecting Aggregometry

Medication and Dietary Interference

Aggregometry results are highly sensitive to recent medication and dietary exposure, and a standardized washout period, typically a minimum of ten to fourteen days for aspirin and other irreversible cyclooxygenase inhibitors and a shorter but still clinically important interval for many other agents, is required before testing to avoid attributing a medication-induced functional defect to an underlying inherited disorder. Patients should additionally be instructed to avoid other substances with recognized antiplatelet activity, including certain herbal supplements, prior to testing, and a careful, directed medication and supplement history, extending the principles developed in Chapter 5, should be obtained and documented at the time aggregometry is ordered.

Failure to observe an adequate washout period is among the most common preventable causes of a falsely abnormal aggregometry result, and a result obtained without documented confirmation of an adequate washout should be interpreted cautiously and, when clinically feasible, repeated after an appropriately confirmed washout period rather than accepted as diagnostic of an inherited disorder on the basis of a single, potentially confounded test.

Timing, Transport, and Sample Age

Aggregometry must be performed within a narrow window after specimen collection, typically within three to four hours, since platelets progressively lose functional responsiveness in vitro over time even under optimal storage conditions, and testing performed outside this window produces a falsely attenuated response that mimics a genuine functional disorder. Samples must be maintained at room temperature rather than refrigerated during this interval, since cold exposure itself activates and subsequently impairs platelet function, a preanalytic consideration distinct from, but analogous in clinical consequence to, the ethylenediaminetetraacetic acid clumping artifact discussed in Chapter 6.

These strict timing requirements mean that aggregometry testing must be carefully coordinated between the ordering clinician, phlebotomy, sample transport, and the performing laboratory, and testing is generally impractical for patients located a substantial distance from a laboratory capable of performing the assay, a logistical limitation that has driven interest in the point-of-care alternatives discussed later in this chapter, even though these alternatives carry their own distinct limitations.

Baseline Platelet Count and Hematologic Confounders

As introduced earlier in this chapter, an inadequate or excessive baseline platelet count in the prepared platelet-rich plasma invalidates aggregometry interpretation, and severe thrombocytopenia, discussed extensively in Chapter 6, can preclude meaningful aggregometry testing altogether, since an inadequate platelet concentration cannot generate an interpretable optical signal regardless of the platelets' intrinsic functional capacity. Severe anemia and marked leukocytosis can similarly interfere with the centrifugation-based separation of platelet-rich plasma, and these hematologic confounders should be assessed via a concurrent complete blood count before aggregometry is ordered, particularly in a patient with a known or suspected multilineage hematologic abnormality.

When aggregometry cannot be reliably performed due to severe thrombocytopenia, the flow cytometric methods discussed in the next section of this chapter offer a partial alternative, since flow cytometry requires substantially smaller platelet numbers and can, in some circumstances, provide functional information even when standard aggregometry is not technically feasible, illustrating the complementary rather than purely redundant relationship between these two testing modalities.

Flow Cytometric Assessment of Platelet Function

Principles of Flow Cytometric Platelet Analysis

Flow cytometry assesses platelet function by labeling platelets with fluorescently conjugated antibodies directed against specific surface receptors or activation-dependent epitopes and quantifying fluorescence intensity across thousands of individually analyzed platelets, providing single-cell resolution unavailable from the population-averaged signal generated by aggregometry. This single-cell approach allows flow cytometry to detect a subpopulation of abnormal platelets even when the majority population is functionally normal, a sensitivity advantage particularly relevant to detecting a partial or heterogeneous receptor deficiency that might be diluted below the detection threshold of a population-averaged aggregometry tracing.

Flow cytometric panels for platelet function assessment typically quantify surface expression of glycoprotein IIb/IIIa and glycoprotein Ib-IX-V, directly confirming or excluding Glanzmann thrombasthenia and Bernard-Soulier syndrome respectively with greater specificity than aggregometry alone, and can additionally assess activation-dependent markers such as P-selectin surface expression following in vitro agonist stimulation, providing a functional readout of granule release, developed mechanistically in Chapter 2, that complements the aggregation-based readout of standard aggregometry.

Clinical Applications Beyond Receptor Quantification

Beyond confirming specific inherited receptor deficiencies, flow cytometry has expanded clinical application in assessing platelet activation status in vivo, using markers such as surface P-selectin or activated glycoprotein IIb/IIIa conformation measured without in vitro agonist stimulation, providing information about ongoing platelet activation relevant to the procoagulant platelet phenomena discussed in Chapter 3 and to monitoring for platelet activation in specific clinical settings such as extracorporeal circulation or mechanical circulatory support. Flow cytometry additionally allows assessment of platelet-derived microparticles and platelet-leukocyte aggregates, markers of platelet activation with emerging, though not yet fully standardized, clinical applications in thrombotic and inflammatory conditions.

These expanded applications position flow cytometry as an increasingly versatile complement to traditional aggregometry, though its interpretation requires specialized expertise in flow cytometric methodology and careful attention to preanalytic handling similar in principle, though not identical in detail, to the preanalytic requirements developed earlier in this chapter for aggregometry, and clinicians ordering flow cytometric platelet studies should confirm with their laboratory the specific preanalytic requirements for the particular panel being requested.

Comparative Advantages and Limitations Relative to Aggregometry

Flow cytometry offers several practical advantages over aggregometry, including a smaller required blood volume and platelet count, greater specificity for confirming a specific receptor deficiency once suspected from an aggregometry pattern or clinical presentation, and somewhat more forgiving preanalytic handling requirements in some laboratories, but it does not fully substitute for aggregometry as a broad, unbiased screening test, since flow cytometry requires the laboratory to select specific antibody panels targeted at a hypothesized defect rather than surveying the full functional response across the broad agonist panel aggregometry provides.

For this reason, flow cytometry is most effectively used as a confirmatory, hypothesis-directed test following an abnormal or suggestive aggregometry pattern, or as an alternative when aggregometry is not technically feasible due to severe thrombocytopenia, rather than as a first-line, unbiased screening test in a patient with an undifferentiated bleeding history, a sequencing principle that the efficient testing strategy developed later in this chapter formalizes.

Point-of-Care Platelet Function Assays

The Platelet Function Analyzer and Similar Cartridge-Based Systems

Point-of-care platelet function assays, most widely represented by cartridge-based platelet function analyzer systems, measure the time required for platelets in citrated whole blood to occlude a small aperture coated with collagen and either epinephrine or adenosine diphosphate under high shear flow conditions, reported as a closure time, providing a rapid, whole-blood functional assessment that avoids the platelet-rich plasma preparation step required for aggregometry. This shear-dependent mechanism directly engages the glycoprotein Ib-von Willebrand factor adhesion axis developed in Chapters 2 and 3, making these assays particularly sensitive to von Willebrand disease and to Bernard-Soulier syndrome, though considerably less sensitive to some of the milder inherited platelet function disorders that aggregometry can detect.

A prolonged closure time on this point-of-care testing, particularly when confirmed on repeat testing and interpreted alongside the structured bleeding history developed in Chapter 5, appropriately prompts referral for confirmatory aggregometry or von Willebrand factor testing, while a normal closure time provides some reassurance but does not fully exclude a milder platelet function disorder or a mild von Willebrand disease, limiting its use as a standalone rule-out test in a patient with a strongly suggestive bleeding history.

Preanalytic Sensitivity of Point-of-Care Assays

Point-of-care platelet function assays share several of the preanalytic sensitivities discussed earlier in this chapter for aggregometry, including sensitivity to recent aspirin or other antiplatelet medication exposure, and additionally carry specific sensitivity to the patient's hematocrit and platelet count, since both anemia and thrombocytopenia can independently prolong the closure time through mechanisms unrelated to intrinsic platelet function, again illustrating that no platelet function assay, however rapid or convenient, can be interpreted without accounting for the broader hematologic context established through the complete blood count and history.

Von Willebrand factor level itself independently influences closure time, since the shear-dependent adhesion process these assays measure depends directly on von Willebrand factor concentration and multimer composition, meaning a low von Willebrand factor level from any cause, not only classic von Willebrand disease, can prolong the closure time, a consideration relevant when interpreting results in patients with conditions associated with acquired von Willebrand syndrome, including the aortic stenosis and mechanical circulatory support scenarios discussed in Chapter 3.

Viscoelastic Testing and Its Limited Platelet-Specific Utility

Viscoelastic testing methods, including thromboelastography and rotational thromboelastometry, widely used in perioperative and critical care settings to assess global clot formation and stability, provide some information relevant to platelet contribution to clot strength but were not designed as, and do not function as, platelet-specific function assays in the manner of aggregometry, flow cytometry, or the cartridge-based systems discussed above. Specialized platelet-mapping modifications of viscoelastic testing exist and can provide some additional platelet-specific information, particularly in monitoring antiplatelet therapy in select perioperative and critical care contexts discussed in Chapter 18, but these modified assays remain complementary to, rather than substitutes for, the dedicated platelet function testing methods that form the primary focus of this chapter.

Clinicians should be careful not to conflate a normal or abnormal viscoelastic study with a normal or abnormal platelet-specific functional assessment, since the global, composite nature of standard viscoelastic testing limits its specificity for isolating a platelet-attributable defect from the many other variables, including coagulation factor levels and fibrinogen concentration, that simultaneously influence the viscoelastic tracing.

THE PLATELET CRISIS DECISION COMPASS — A Discordant Point-of-Care Closure Time in a Patient on Antiplatelet Therapy

The Presentation: A patient on chronic low-dose aspirin therapy undergoes point-of-care platelet function testing before a planned procedure, and the closure time returns within the normal reference range despite the known antiplatelet exposure.

Mimic Signature: Genuine aspirin non-response, in which the medication has not produced the expected functional effect; a preanalytic issue such as inadequate medication adherence prior to testing; and inherent limitations of the specific point-of-care assay's sensitivity to the cyclooxygenase-mediated mechanism of aspirin, which may not reliably prolong closure time in all individuals despite adequate biochemical drug effect.

The Decision: Do not interpret a normal point-of-care closure time as definitive evidence that aspirin's antiplatelet effect is absent or that periprocedural bleeding risk from the medication is negligible; correlate with adherence history and, where the clinical stakes warrant, confirm with arachidonic acid-specific aggregometry, which more directly and reliably interrogates the cyclooxygenase pathway aspirin targets.

Trap Logic: Treating a normal point-of-care closure time as proof that a patient's aspirin therapy carries no periprocedural bleeding risk overstates the sensitivity of this specific assay for the cyclooxygenase-mediated mechanism and risks underestimating true bleeding risk before an invasive procedure.

Crisis Anchor: A normal point-of-care closure time on aspirin does not reliably exclude clinically relevant antiplatelet effect; arachidonic acid-specific aggregometry is the more direct confirmatory test when the clinical stakes require certainty.

Genetic and Molecular Testing for Platelet Function Disorders

The Expanding Role of Targeted Genetic Panels

Next-generation sequencing-based platelet gene panels, testing dozens of genes associated with inherited platelet function and production disorders simultaneously, have become increasingly accessible and increasingly integrated into the diagnostic pathway for a patient with a suggestive bleeding history and abnormal or equivocal functional testing, offering the potential to identify a specific molecular diagnosis even when aggregometry and flow cytometry produce an ambiguous or incompletely characteristic pattern. These panels are particularly valuable for the milder, more heterogeneous inherited platelet function disorders discussed in Chapter 16, many of which lack the sharply distinctive aggregometry signature that Glanzmann thrombasthenia and Bernard-Soulier syndrome characteristically produce.

Genetic testing also provides diagnostic and counseling value that functional testing alone cannot, including precise confirmation of inheritance pattern for family counseling, identification of variants associated with an increased malignancy risk in certain inherited platelet disorders discussed in Chapter 15, and, in some cases, identification of a specific pathogenic variant that carries prognostic or management implications beyond what the functional phenotype alone would suggest.

Variant Interpretation and Its Clinical Challenges

Genetic testing for platelet disorders shares the variant interpretation challenges common to genetic testing generally, including the frequent identification of variants of uncertain significance whose clinical relevance cannot be confidently determined at the time of testing, and results should be interpreted in close correlation with the functional testing and clinical phenotype developed throughout this chapter and Chapter 5, rather than treated as a standalone, definitive diagnostic answer independent of the broader clinical picture. A genetic variant of uncertain significance identified in a gene associated with platelet function, in a patient whose functional testing and clinical phenotype are strongly consistent with a specific disorder, provides supportive rather than independently diagnostic evidence, and formal reclassification of such variants often occurs over subsequent years as population and functional evidence accumulates.

Genetic counseling, ideally involving a counselor with specific expertise in inherited bleeding and platelet disorders, should accompany genetic testing whenever feasible, both to appropriately frame the pretest expectations and posttest implications for the patient and family and to ensure that a variant of uncertain significance is communicated with appropriate nuance rather than either false reassurance or false alarm.

Integrating Genetic Results With Functional and Clinical Data

The most robust diagnostic conclusions in inherited platelet function disorders emerge from the convergence of a suggestive clinical and family history, a characteristic or at least supportive functional testing pattern, and a genetic finding consistent with the suspected diagnosis, rather than reliance on any single data source in isolation, directly extending the multi-source integration principle developed throughout this book beginning with the structured clinical evaluation in Chapter 5. When genetic and functional findings are discordant, the discrepancy itself often provides diagnostically useful information, prompting reconsideration of the initial diagnostic hypothesis, additional functional testing, or extended genetic evaluation including family segregation studies where feasible.

This integrative approach positions genetic testing as a powerful complement to, rather than a replacement for, the functional testing methods developed throughout this chapter, and the efficient testing strategy presented in the final section of this chapter incorporates genetic testing at the appropriate sequential position within a broader, clinically directed diagnostic pathway rather than as an indiscriminate first-line test applied to every patient with a bleeding concern.

Interpreting Discordant or Borderline Results

Sources of Test-to-Test Discordance

Discordance between different platelet function testing modalities, such as a normal point-of-care closure time in a patient with an abnormal aggregometry pattern, or a borderline aggregometry result that does not clearly meet criteria for a specific diagnostic pattern, is a common and clinically important scenario that requires systematic rather than dismissive interpretation. Such discordance most often reflects the differing sensitivities and specificities of each testing modality discussed throughout this chapter rather than a laboratory error, and understanding the specific mechanism each test interrogates, developed section by section above, is essential to correctly interpreting an apparent discrepancy rather than simply selecting whichever result happens to align with the clinician's initial suspicion.

A structured approach to discordance begins with confirming that preanalytic requirements, including medication washout, sample timing, and adequate baseline platelet count, were met for each test in question, since a substantial proportion of apparent discordance resolves once a preanalytic confounder affecting one but not the other test is identified and addressed through repeat testing under controlled conditions.

The Role of Repeat Testing and Longitudinal Assessment

When discordance persists despite confirmed preanalytic adequacy, repeat testing, ideally performed on a separate occasion and, where feasible, at a laboratory with specific expertise in platelet function testing, provides additional diagnostic information and can clarify whether an initial abnormal or borderline result represents a reproducible finding or an isolated, potentially spurious result. This longitudinal approach to platelet function testing parallels the trend-based reasoning developed for platelet count interpretation in Chapter 6, reinforcing a consistent diagnostic philosophy across this book: a single laboratory result, whatever the specific test, is most reliably interpreted in the context of reproducibility and trend rather than as an isolated, definitive data point.

Reference laboratory consultation, including direct communication with the interpreting hematopathologist or laboratory director, is a valuable and underutilized resource when discordant or borderline platelet function results resist straightforward interpretation, since laboratory professionals with specific expertise in platelet function testing can often provide interpretive nuance, including technical caveats specific to the assay or platform used, that is not fully captured in a standard written laboratory report.

When to Accept Diagnostic Uncertainty and Proceed Empirically

In a subset of patients, careful, repeated, and appropriately interpreted platelet function testing will nonetheless fail to yield a definitive diagnosis, and the framework developed throughout this book supports proceeding with an empiric, symptom-directed management approach in this circumstance rather than pursuing an indefinite escalation of testing, particularly when the patient's bleeding phenotype is mild and the primary clinical goal is practical bleeding risk management rather than an exhaustive mechanistic diagnosis. This pragmatic acceptance of diagnostic uncertainty, communicated transparently to the patient using the communication principles developed in Chapter 5, respects both the genuine limitations of current platelet function testing technology and the primary clinical goal of safe, effective patient management.

This is not an argument for diagnostic complacency, and a patient with a severe or progressive bleeding phenotype that remains unexplained after the structured evaluation developed in this chapter warrants continued reassessment, including periodic reconsideration as testing technology and genetic knowledge continue to advance, but it does reflect an honest acknowledgment that the diagnostic yield of even a thorough, correctly performed platelet function evaluation is not unlimited, a nuance this book aims to convey rather than obscure behind an artificially confident diagnostic algorithm.

Constructing an Efficient Platelet Function Testing Strategy

A Stepwise, Clinically Directed Testing Sequence

Bringing together the elements developed throughout this chapter, an efficient platelet function evaluation begins with the structured bleeding history and platelet count evaluation established in Chapters 5 and 6, proceeds to von Willebrand factor testing given its high prevalence relative to other inherited platelet disorders, and, when von Willebrand disease has been reasonably excluded or a distinct platelet-specific pattern is suspected, proceeds to light transmission aggregometry as the primary functional screening test, reserving flow cytometry, point-of-care testing, and genetic panels for the specific, targeted roles developed in this chapter rather than ordering all available tests simultaneously and indiscriminately.

This sequential approach reflects both diagnostic efficiency and resource stewardship, since indiscriminate simultaneous testing across every available modality substantially increases cost and the likelihood of encountering an uninterpretable discordant result without a clear preanalytic explanation, while a stepwise, hypothesis-directed approach, informed at each step by the result of the preceding test, more efficiently converges on an accurate diagnosis while minimizing unnecessary testing burden on the patient and the health system.

Coordinating With the Performing Laboratory

Given the substantial preanalytic sensitivity of aggregometry and, to a lesser extent, the other testing modalities developed in this chapter, direct coordination with the performing laboratory before testing is initiated, confirming medication washout requirements, sample timing logistics, and any specific preparation instructions for the patient, substantially improves the likelihood of obtaining an interpretable, clinically actionable result on the first attempt rather than requiring repeat testing due to an avoidable preanalytic confounder.

This coordination is particularly important for patients traveling a substantial distance to a specialized coagulation laboratory, for whom a repeat visit due to an avoidable preanalytic error carries meaningful burden, and many specialized hemostasis and thrombosis centers provide structured preparation instructions and dedicated scheduling coordination specifically to minimize this avoidable source of diagnostic delay and patient inconvenience.

Communicating the Testing Plan and Expected Timeline to the Patient

Because platelet function testing frequently requires a medication washout period, coordinated specimen collection, and, in the case of genetic testing, a turnaround time of several weeks, setting clear expectations with the patient about the overall evaluation timeline at the outset, extending the transparent communication principles developed in Chapter 5, meaningfully improves the patient experience and reduces the anxiety that an unexplained delay between visits can otherwise produce. Patients should understand not only what each test will assess but also why the tests are being sequenced in a particular order, reinforcing that a stepwise evaluation reflects deliberate diagnostic efficiency rather than an indication that their case has been deprioritized or overlooked.

This complete testing strategy, integrating the structured clinical evaluation of Chapter 5, the platelet count and morphologic evaluation of Chapter 6, and the functional and genetic testing developed in this chapter, equips the reader to evaluate a patient with a suspected platelet function disorder from initial presentation through to a confirmed, or appropriately provisional, final diagnosis, establishing the complete diagnostic toolkit that the disease-specific chapters beginning with Chapter 8 will apply to the full range of clinical presentations this book addresses.

Quality Assurance, Standardization, and Emerging Technologies

Interlaboratory Variability and Standardization Efforts

Light transmission aggregometry has historically suffered from substantial interlaboratory variability, reflecting differences in agonist concentration, instrument platform, platelet-rich plasma preparation technique, and criteria used to define a normal versus abnormal response, and this variability has meaningfully limited the ability to directly compare results obtained at different institutions or to pool aggregometry data across multicenter research studies. International working groups within the field of hemostasis and thrombosis have published standardization guidelines addressing agonist concentrations, preanalytic handling, and reporting terminology, and laboratories increasingly participate in external proficiency testing programs specifically designed to benchmark aggregometry performance against reference standards.

Clinicians referring patients for aggregometry should be aware that meaningful variability in reference ranges and interpretive criteria can exist between different performing laboratories, and results obtained at one institution should generally be interpreted using that institution's own validated reference ranges rather than a generic textbook threshold, a nuance directly relevant when a patient transfers care or seeks a second opinion at a different center after initial testing elsewhere.

Whole Blood Aggregometry as an Alternative Platform

Whole blood impedance aggregometry, a technically distinct method from light transmission aggregometry, measures the change in electrical impedance across a pair of electrodes as platelets aggregate and adhere to the electrode surface directly within whole blood, avoiding the platelet-rich plasma preparation step and its associated centrifugation-related preanalytic vulnerabilities discussed earlier in this chapter. This platform offers practical advantages, including compatibility with thrombocytopenic samples that would be difficult to prepare as adequately concentrated platelet-rich plasma, and has found particular application in some European centers and in specific research and clinical contexts including cardiac surgery-associated platelet dysfunction assessment.

Despite these practical advantages, whole blood aggregometry has not fully supplanted light transmission aggregometry as the reference standard in most centers, reflecting a smaller accumulated evidence base correlating specific whole blood aggregometry patterns with the inherited disorders whose diagnostic signatures are best characterized using light transmission methodology, and clinicians encountering a whole blood aggregometry result should confirm with the performing laboratory how its reported patterns and reference ranges relate to the light transmission aggregometry patterns emphasized throughout this chapter.

Emerging Microfluidic and Digital Platforms

Microfluidic platelet function assays, which flow whole blood through channels lined with physiologically relevant adhesive substrates under controlled, adjustable shear conditions while capturing platelet adhesion and aggregation through fluorescence or bright-field microscopy, represent an active area of technology development aiming to combine the physiologic relevance of shear-dependent testing with more detailed, spatially resolved functional information than either standard aggregometry or point-of-care closure time assays currently provide. These platforms remain predominantly research tools at present, with limited validated clinical reference ranges and limited widespread clinical availability, but ongoing development suggests they may play an expanded diagnostic role over the working lifetime of readers of this book.

Clinicians should approach emerging platelet function testing technologies with the same interpretive discipline developed throughout this chapter for established methods: understanding the specific mechanism a novel assay interrogates, its validated preanalytic requirements, and its demonstrated correlation with clinically meaningful outcomes before incorporating it into diagnostic decision-making, resisting the temptation to adopt a novel technology principally because of its convenience or novelty rather than its demonstrated diagnostic validity.

Assay	Sample Requirement	Primary Clinical Use	Key Limitation
Light transmission aggregometry	Platelet-rich plasma, adequate count	Broad functional screening, pattern diagnosis	Technically demanding, narrow testing window
Flow cytometry	Small whole blood volume	Receptor quantification, granule release	Requires targeted, hypothesis-directed panel
Point-of-care closure time	Citrated whole blood	Rapid screening, von Willebrand-sensitive	Limited sensitivity for milder disorders
Genetic panel	Whole blood or saliva	Molecular confirmation, family counseling	Variants of uncertain significance common

Special Considerations in Pediatric and Perioperative Testing

Practical Barriers to Aggregometry in Young Children

Light transmission aggregometry in young children is limited by the substantial blood volume required to prepare adequate platelet-rich plasma, a practical barrier that can preclude comprehensive aggregometry testing in infants and young children without resorting to a volume that would itself pose meaningful phlebotomy-related risk, and pediatric hematology centers have developed modified low-volume protocols and prioritized flow cytometric and point-of-care methods, which require substantially smaller sample volumes, as more practical first-line options in this population when feasible. Coordination with a pediatric hematology laboratory experienced in these modified low-volume approaches meaningfully improves the likelihood of obtaining interpretable results without requiring a blood draw disproportionate to the child's size and total blood volume.

Age-specific reference ranges are additionally essential when interpreting any platelet function assay in children, since platelet reactivity and the concentration of several relevant plasma proteins, including von Willebrand factor, change across early childhood development, and applying adult-derived reference ranges to a pediatric result risks both false-positive and false-negative interpretation; pediatric-specific reference ranges, validated at the performing laboratory, should be confirmed before a pediatric platelet function result is interpreted as normal or abnormal.

Timing Testing Relative to a Planned Procedure

When platelet function testing is pursued specifically to inform perioperative risk assessment, discussed further in Chapter 18, the testing timeline must accommodate both the medication washout requirements developed earlier in this chapter and any turnaround time required for genetic or specialized flow cytometric testing, meaning testing initiated only days before a scheduled procedure frequently cannot be completed and interpreted in time to meaningfully inform the surgical plan. Early identification of a patient who may warrant platelet function testing, ideally during initial preoperative evaluation well in advance of the scheduled procedure date, allows the stepwise testing sequence developed in this chapter to be completed without last-minute compromise or procedural delay.

When testing cannot be completed with adequate lead time before an urgent or semi-urgent procedure, the clinician must weigh the value of incomplete or expedited testing against proceeding empirically with perioperative precautions appropriate to the suspected, though not yet confirmed, underlying disorder, a judgment that should involve direct hematology consultation rather than either reflexive procedural delay or reflexive proceeding without adequate risk assessment.

Documenting Test Results for Future Perioperative Reference

Once a platelet function evaluation has been completed, whether the result is normal, abnormal, or inconclusive, clear documentation accessible to future perioperative teams, extending the longitudinal documentation principle developed in Chapters 5 and 6, prevents the same evaluation from needing to be repeated before each subsequent procedure across the patient's lifetime, a particularly valuable consideration for a patient with a confirmed inherited platelet function disorder who will likely require multiple procedures over their lifespan. This documentation should specify not only the final diagnostic conclusion but also the specific tests performed, the laboratory and reference ranges used, and any preanalytic caveats relevant to interpreting the result, providing future clinicians the full context needed to decide whether repeat testing is warranted or whether the existing evaluation remains sufficient.

This documentation practice closes the chapter's arc by returning to the same principle that opened the clinical evaluation in Chapter 5: a well-documented, structured evaluation performed once, correctly, and made accessible across the patient's future care, provides more lasting clinical value than a series of incomplete or undocumented evaluations repeated inefficiently at each new encounter.

CLINICAL CASE: A 19-year-old college student with a lifelong history of easy bruising and two prior episodes of prolonged bleeding after dental procedures presents for evaluation. Her structured bleeding assessment tool score, obtained using the framework from Chapter 5, is markedly elevated, and her platelet count and morphology on smear review, following the approach from Chapter 6, are entirely normal. Von Willebrand factor antigen, activity, and factor VIII level, obtained as the first-line test given the high prevalence of von Willebrand disease among patients with this presentation, return within normal limits after confirmed adequate washout from any interfering medication or recent illness known to transiently affect von Willebrand factor levels. Light transmission aggregometry is subsequently performed after a confirmed fourteen-day aspirin and nonsteroidal anti-inflammatory drug washout, revealing normal primary aggregation to all agonists but an absent secondary wave specifically in response to low-dose adenosine diphosphate and epinephrine, with a relatively preserved response to collagen and thrombin, a pattern consistent with a storage pool disorder as discussed earlier in this chapter and mechanistically in Chapter 2. Flow cytometric assessment of platelet dense granule content, performed as a confirmatory test, demonstrates reduced granule number consistent with delta storage pool deficiency, and a targeted genetic panel subsequently identifies a variant in a gene associated with dense granule biogenesis, providing molecular confirmation that also informs family counseling, since her younger sister has a similar but milder bleeding history. This case illustrates the complete stepwise diagnostic sequence developed in this chapter: structured history and bleeding assessment tool, exclusion of von Willebrand disease as the most prevalent inherited bleeding disorder, aggregometry pattern recognition pointing toward a specific diagnostic category, and targeted confirmatory flow cytometry and genetic testing converging on a specific, actionable diagnosis.

THE PLATELET CRISIS DECISION COMPASS — Functional Testing Interpretation

Compass Recap: Pan-Agonist Aggregation Failure: A near-absent response to all agonists except ristocetin, in a technically valid preparation, is the aggregometry signature of Glanzmann thrombasthenia and warrants confirmatory glycoprotein IIb/IIIa flow cytometry.

Compass Recap: Point-of-Care and Aspirin Monitoring: A normal point-of-care closure time on aspirin does not reliably exclude clinically relevant antiplatelet effect; arachidonic acid-specific aggregometry is the more direct confirmatory test when the clinical stakes require certainty.

Chapter Anchor: Platelet function testing is interpreted as an integrated pattern across a defined agonist panel, confirmed by preanalytic validity, and sequenced logically from bleeding history through von Willebrand testing, aggregometry, flow cytometry, and, where indicated, genetic testing — never as a single isolated result read in clinical isolation.

Summary and Key Concepts

Light transmission aggregometry measures platelet aggregation via optical transmittance change in response to a standard agonist panel (adenosine diphosphate, epinephrine, collagen, arachidonic acid, ristocetin), each interrogating a distinct receptor pathway.

Characteristic aggregometry patterns distinguish Glanzmann thrombasthenia (absent response to all agonists except ristocetin), Bernard-Soulier syndrome (absent ristocetin response, preserved others), and storage pool disorders (absent secondary wave to weak agonists).

Aggregometry is highly preanalytically sensitive: medication washout (10-14 days for aspirin), sample timing (within 3-4 hours, room temperature), and adequate baseline platelet count are all required for a valid, interpretable result.

Flow cytometry offers single-cell resolution for confirming specific receptor deficiencies and assessing granule release and platelet activation status, complementing rather than replacing aggregometry as a broad screening test.

Point-of-care platelet function assays (cartridge-based closure time systems) provide rapid, whole-blood functional screening particularly sensitive to von Willebrand disease and Bernard-Soulier syndrome, but carry limited sensitivity for milder disorders and should not be used to definitively exclude clinically relevant antiplatelet drug effect.

An efficient testing strategy proceeds stepwise: structured history and bleeding assessment tool, platelet count/morphology, von Willebrand factor testing, aggregometry, and, when indicated, flow cytometry and genetic panels — sequenced rather than ordered indiscriminately and simultaneously.

CHAPTER 8: DIAGNOSTIC APPROACH TO THROMBOCYTOPENIA IN ADULTS

Learning Objectives

1. Apply a mechanistic framework distinguishing decreased production, increased destruction, and distributional causes of thrombocytopenia.
2. Integrate the complete blood count, peripheral smear, and platelet indices developed in Chapter 6 into a systematic thrombocytopenia differential diagnosis.
3. Identify the clinical and laboratory findings that indicate the need for bone marrow examination in the evaluation of thrombocytopenia.
4. Construct a stepwise diagnostic algorithm for new-onset thrombocytopenia in the adult outpatient and hospitalized settings.
5. Distinguish the diagnostic priorities and common etiologies of thrombocytopenia specific to hospitalized versus ambulatory patients.
6. Determine when chronic or recurrent thrombocytopenia warrants hematology referral versus continued primary care monitoring.

Chapter Outline

This chapter opens Part III of the book and integrates the clinical framework of Chapter 5 and the laboratory framework of Chapter 6 into a comprehensive, mechanism-based diagnostic approach to thrombocytopenia in adults. It develops the three-category mechanistic framework of decreased production, increased destruction, and distributional abnormality; the specific findings that localize a patient's presentation within this framework; the role and timing of bone marrow examination; and distinct algorithmic considerations for the outpatient, hospitalized, and chronic longitudinal settings. Two Platelet Crisis Decision Compass instances address the recognition of a thrombocytopenia presentation requiring urgent bone marrow evaluation and the correct sequencing of testing in newly hospitalized thrombocytopenia.

The chapters that follow this one, addressing immune thrombocytopenia, drug-induced thrombocytopenia, heparin-induced thrombocytopenia, thrombotic microangiopathy, and the other specific causes of thrombocytopenia catalogued throughout Part III, each represent a single branch of the broader diagnostic tree this chapter constructs. Mastery of this chapter's organizing framework is what allows the specific disease chapters that follow to be applied efficiently and correctly to an individual patient rather than considered as an undifferentiated list of possibilities.

A Mechanistic Framework for Thrombocytopenia

The Three Fundamental Mechanistic Categories

Every cause of thrombocytopenia can be organized into one of three fundamental mechanistic categories, directly extending the platelet production and clearance physiology developed in Chapter 1: decreased platelet production, in which the marrow fails to generate an adequate number of platelets; increased platelet destruction or consumption, in which platelets are produced normally but removed from circulation prematurely through immune-mediated clearance, consumption in a thrombotic process, or another peripheral mechanism; and distributional abnormality, in which the total body platelet mass is normal or near-normal but an abnormally large proportion is sequestered outside the circulating peripheral blood, most commonly within an enlarged spleen.

This three-category framework, while not exhaustive of every diagnostic nuance, provides the organizing scaffold for the entire diagnostic approach developed in this chapter, and correctly localizing a patient's presentation within this framework, using the clinical and laboratory tools developed in this section and the next, substantially narrows the subsequent differential diagnosis before any single specific disease entity is even considered.

Combined and Overlapping Mechanisms

Many clinically important causes of thrombocytopenia involve more than one of these mechanisms simultaneously, and recognizing this overlap prevents the diagnostic error of forcing a patient's presentation into a single, artificially clean mechanistic category. Sepsis and critical illness, discussed in full in Chapter 14, frequently combine impaired marrow production from bone marrow suppression, increased peripheral consumption from disseminated intravascular coagulation or direct platelet activation, and occasionally a component of splenic sequestration, while advanced liver disease combines impaired thrombopoietin production, discussed mechanistically in Chapter 1, with splenic sequestration from portal hypertension.

This overlap does not diminish the clinical value of the mechanistic framework but instead reinforces the importance of applying it as an analytical starting point, identifying the dominant mechanism or mechanisms contributing to a given patient's presentation, rather than as a rigid classification system requiring every patient to fit neatly into exactly one category before proceeding with evaluation and management.

Using the Framework to Direct Testing

The primary clinical value of this mechanistic framework lies in its ability to direct testing efficiently toward the category or categories most consistent with a given patient's presentation, since the diagnostic tests most useful for confirming decreased production, developed later in this chapter around bone marrow examination, differ substantially from those most useful for confirming increased destruction, developed around the immune and non-immune destructive processes catalogued in the chapters that follow. A patient whose presentation clearly localizes to increased destruction on initial evaluation generally does not require immediate bone marrow examination, while a patient whose presentation suggests impaired production, particularly when accompanied by other cytopenias, more urgently warrants that specific evaluation.

This directed approach reflects the same diagnostic efficiency philosophy developed throughout Chapters 5 through 7: a structured, mechanism-based framework applied systematically outperforms an undirected battery of testing applied indiscriminately to every patient regardless of their specific clinical presentation, both in diagnostic yield and in responsible use of health system resources.

Localizing the Mechanism: Decreased Production Versus Increased Destruction

Findings Suggesting Decreased Production

Several clinical and laboratory findings, developed in detail using the platelet indices from Chapter 6, favor decreased production as the dominant mechanism: a low or inappropriately normal mean platelet volume and immature platelet fraction, accompanying anemia or leukopenia suggesting a broader marrow process rather than an isolated platelet abnormality, and a clinical history suggesting marrow-suppressive exposure, including recent chemotherapy, radiation, or a medication with recognized marrow-suppressive potential distinct from the immune-mediated drug reactions discussed in Chapter 10. A gradual, progressive decline in platelet count over weeks to months, rather than an abrupt drop, additionally favors a production-limited process, consistent with the gradual exhaustion of marrow reserve rather than the more acute peripheral consumption pattern characteristic of destructive processes.

Marrow infiltrative processes, including acute leukemia, myelodysplastic syndrome, lymphoma, and metastatic solid tumor involvement of the marrow, characteristically produce this production-limited pattern and frequently, though not universally, present with accompanying cytopenias and abnormal cell morphology on peripheral smear, findings that should prompt early consideration of bone marrow examination as developed later in this chapter rather than an extended trial of empiric management directed at a presumed peripheral destructive process.

Findings Suggesting Increased Destruction

Conversely, an elevated mean platelet volume and immature platelet fraction, an isolated thrombocytopenia without accompanying cytopenia, and a normal peripheral smear aside from the reduced platelet count together favor increased destruction, reflecting a marrow appropriately attempting to compensate for peripheral platelet loss by releasing young, large platelets, the same physiologic pattern developed in the context of immune thrombocytopenia mechanistically in the chapters that follow. An abrupt, acute decline in platelet count, particularly one temporally associated with a recent viral illness, new medication, or other identifiable trigger, similarly favors a destructive process over the more gradual decline typical of impaired production.

Schistocytes on peripheral smear specifically point toward a thrombotic microangiopathic destructive process, discussed as a hematologic emergency in Chapter 12, and this single morphologic finding should immediately elevate diagnostic urgency regardless of the platelet count's absolute severity, illustrating how the destructive category itself subdivides into immune-mediated, thrombotic, and other mechanisms whose distinction carries direct and urgent management consequences.

The Diagnostic Value of Tempo and Trajectory

Beyond the specific findings discussed above, the overall tempo of a patient's thrombocytopenia, meaning the rate and pattern of platelet count change over time when prior values are available, provides substantial independent diagnostic information that complements the specific mechanistic findings developed in this section, directly extending the trend-based reasoning established in Chapter 6. A patient with a documented, stable, mildly reduced platelet count over years is unlikely to have an acute, urgent process regardless of the specific mechanistic category their presentation might otherwise suggest, while a patient with a rapidly falling count over days, even to a similar absolute level, warrants urgent evaluation regardless of which mechanistic category the initial findings appear to favor.

This principle underscores that the mechanistic framework developed in this chapter functions best when integrated with, rather than substituted for, the longitudinal and trend-based clinical reasoning developed throughout this book, and the algorithm developed later in this chapter formally incorporates both the mechanistic localization and the temporal trajectory as parallel, complementary inputs into the overall diagnostic and triage decision.

Distributional Thrombocytopenia: Splenic Sequestration

The Physiology of Splenic Platelet Sequestration

The normal spleen sequesters approximately one-third of the total body platelet mass in a dynamic equilibrium with the circulating pool, a physiologic reservoir function introduced in Chapter 1, and splenomegaly from any cause can expand this sequestered fraction substantially, in severe splenomegaly sequestering up to eighty or ninety percent of total body platelet mass and producing thrombocytopenia through redistribution rather than any true reduction in total platelet production or accelerated destruction. This distributional mechanism is functionally and prognostically distinct from the production and destruction mechanisms discussed above, since the marrow in distributional thrombocytopenia is typically functioning normally and total body platelet mass, though redistributed, is often not meaningfully reduced.

Recognizing distributional thrombocytopenia is clinically important because it generally produces a milder bleeding phenotype than a comparable platelet count from a true production or destruction disorder, reflecting the larger functional platelet reserve, and because its management, addressed further in Chapters 14 and 17 in the context of the underlying conditions that produce splenomegaly, differs substantially from the immune-directed or marrow-directed therapies appropriate to the other mechanistic categories.

Clinical and Radiographic Assessment of Splenomegaly

Physical examination for splenomegaly, though useful, has recognized limited sensitivity, particularly for mild to moderate splenic enlargement, and abdominal ultrasound provides a more sensitive and reproducible assessment of spleen size when splenic sequestration is suspected as a contributing mechanism, with a spleen length exceeding approximately thirteen centimeters generally considered enlarged in an adult, though this threshold varies modestly with body habitus and should be interpreted alongside the ultrasound report's own reference standards. Cross-sectional imaging with computed tomography or magnetic resonance imaging provides additional information about splenic architecture and any focal abnormality when the ultrasound finding is equivocal or when the underlying cause of splenomegaly itself requires further characterization.

The degree of thrombocytopenia attributable to splenomegaly correlates imperfectly with spleen size alone, since the underlying condition driving splenic enlargement, whether portal hypertension, myeloproliferative disease, lymphoproliferative infiltration, or an infectious or infiltrative process, often contributes additional production or destructive mechanisms simultaneously, again illustrating the mechanistic overlap principle developed earlier in this chapter and reinforcing the need to evaluate the underlying cause of splenomegaly rather than attributing thrombocytopenia to splenic sequestration by imaging finding alone.

Distinguishing Distributional From Other Mechanisms in Practice

A pragmatic approach to suspected distributional thrombocytopenia integrates spleen size on imaging, the platelet indices developed in Chapter 6, and the broader clinical context, since a patient with confirmed splenomegaly, a platelet count in the mild to moderate range, and no other cytopenia or concerning smear finding can often be reasonably attributed to splenic sequestration without further invasive evaluation, while a patient with splenomegaly and a more severe thrombocytopenia, or with accompanying cytopenias suggesting an additional production-limiting process, warrants further evaluation of the underlying cause of splenomegaly itself, including consideration of the myeloproliferative and lymphoproliferative processes discussed in Chapters 8 and 17.

This integration illustrates a recurring theme across this book's diagnostic chapters: no single finding, whether a laboratory value, an imaging result, or a physical examination sign, is interpreted in isolation, and the correct diagnostic conclusion consistently emerges from the deliberate synthesis of multiple, complementary data sources rather than from any single decisive test.

THE PLATELET CRISIS DECISION COMPASS — New Thrombocytopenia with Accompanying Cytopenias

The Presentation: A previously well adult presents with new thrombocytopenia (platelet count 62 x10^9/L) accompanied by a new mild anemia and mild leukopenia on the same complete blood count.

Mimic Signature: A primary marrow infiltrative or dysplastic process (myelodysplastic syndrome, acute leukemia, lymphoma involving the marrow); a nutritional deficiency (vitamin B12 or folate) producing multilineage impairment; and a peripheral consumptive process, such as disseminated intravascular coagulation or hypersplenism, secondarily affecting multiple lineages.

The Decision: Obtain peripheral smear review with attention to cell morphology across all three lineages, vitamin B12 and folate levels, and coagulation studies; multilineage cytopenia with abnormal morphology on smear should prompt urgent hematology referral for consideration of bone marrow examination rather than a period of observation.

Trap Logic: Attributing multilineage cytopenia to a single presumed cause, such as a mild concurrent viral illness, without pursuing the smear morphology and marrow-directed evaluation this presentation warrants risks delaying diagnosis of a marrow infiltrative process for which early diagnosis meaningfully affects outcome.

Crisis Anchor: New thrombocytopenia accompanied by unexplained anemia or leukopenia is evaluated with smear review and, when morphology is abnormal, urgent hematology referral for marrow examination — not attributed to a single presumed benign cause without this evaluation.

Figure 8.1: Mechanistic Differential Diagnosis Algorithm for Adult Thrombocytopenia

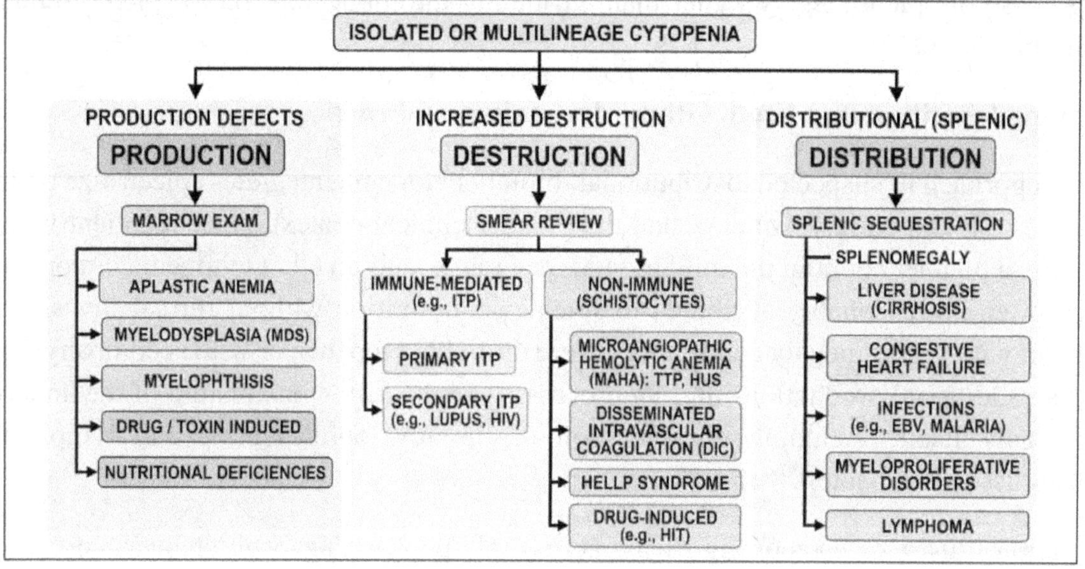

Bone Marrow Examination: Indications and Interpretation

Indications for Bone Marrow Examination in Thrombocytopenia

Bone marrow examination, comprising aspirate and core biopsy, is indicated in the evaluation of thrombocytopenia when the clinical and laboratory findings developed in this chapter suggest a production-limited or infiltrative process, including unexplained multilineage cytopenia, abnormal peripheral smear morphology such as blasts, dysplastic features, or an abnormal white cell differential, or thrombocytopenia in a patient with an otherwise unexplained systemic illness in whom a marrow infiltrative process, including lymphoma or metastatic malignancy, remains a diagnostic consideration after initial evaluation. Marrow examination is generally not required in a patient with isolated thrombocytopenia, a normal smear apart from the reduced platelet count, and a clinical presentation and platelet indices consistent with a straightforward destructive process such as typical immune thrombocytopenia, discussed in Chapter 9, since the marrow in this presentation is characteristically normal or shows only the expected megakaryocytic hyperplasia and adds limited diagnostic value beyond what the clinical and laboratory picture already establishes.

Age is an additional relevant consideration in this decision, since an older adult presenting with new thrombocytopenia carries a somewhat higher pretest probability of an underlying marrow-based process, including myelodysplastic syndrome, than a younger adult with an otherwise typical immune thrombocytopenia presentation, and some hematology guidelines recommend a lower threshold for marrow examination in older patients even when the presentation otherwise appears typical for a peripheral destructive process, a nuance discussed further in the age-specific considerations developed in Chapter 9.

Interpreting Megakaryocyte Number and Morphology

Megakaryocyte assessment on bone marrow examination provides the most direct diagnostic information relevant to the mechanistic framework developed in this chapter: increased or normal megakaryocyte number with normal maturation supports a peripheral destructive process, since the marrow is appropriately responding to peripheral platelet loss by increasing production, while decreased megakaryocyte number supports a primary production defect, and abnormal megakaryocyte morphology, including small, hypolobated megakaryocytes, raises specific concern for myelodysplastic syndrome, discussed further in the context of clonal hematopoiesis in Chapter 17.

This megakaryocyte-focused interpretation directly extends the mechanistic principle established earlier in this chapter from the peripheral blood into the marrow itself, and a marrow examination report that addresses megakaryocyte number, morphology, and maturation specifically, rather than providing only a general overall impression, provides the clinician with the specific information needed to confirm or reconsider the mechanistic hypothesis developed from the peripheral clinical and laboratory evaluation.

Communicating the Rationale and Risks of Marrow Examination to Patients

Bone marrow examination is frequently a source of patient anxiety, and clear communication of the specific rationale for the procedure in an individual patient's case, extending the transparent communication principles developed in Chapter 5, meaningfully improves the patient experience; explaining that the procedure is being pursued to look specifically for a marrow-based explanation for the cytopenia, rather than because a serious diagnosis such as leukemia is presumed likely, helps calibrate patient expectations appropriately without either minimizing legitimate diagnostic uncertainty or unnecessarily alarming a patient whose pretest probability of a serious underlying process may in fact be low.

Discussion of the procedure's risks, predominantly localized bleeding and discomfort at the biopsy site, and the specific precautions taken in a thrombocytopenic patient, including local pressure and, in more severe thrombocytopenia, sometimes platelet transfusion support around the time of the procedure as discussed further in Chapter 19, should be included in this preprocedural conversation, along with a realistic timeline for when results will be available and how they will be communicated.

Algorithmic Approach to New-Onset Thrombocytopenia

Step One: Confirm and Characterize

The algorithmic approach developed in this section begins by applying the confirmatory principles developed in Chapter 6, excluding pseudothrombocytopenia and confirming the platelet count is genuinely abnormal, and by applying the structured clinical evaluation developed in Chapter 5, obtaining the bleeding history, examination findings, and any relevant trend data available from prior records. This first step establishes whether the presentation is genuinely new or represents a previously undocumented chronic finding, a distinction that substantially affects the urgency, though not necessarily the ultimate content, of the subsequent evaluation.

Confirmation and characterization at this first step also includes a focused medication and exposure history directed at the specific etiologies developed in Chapters 10 and 11, since a temporally associated new medication or heparin exposure can substantially redirect the subsequent evaluation toward a specific, testable hypothesis rather than the broader differential diagnosis that would otherwise apply to an unexplained presentation.

Step Two: Localize the Mechanism

The second algorithmic step applies the mechanistic localization framework developed earlier in this chapter, integrating the complete blood count differential, platelet indices, peripheral smear morphology, and, where relevant, splenic imaging, to determine whether the presentation favors decreased production, increased destruction, distributional sequestration, or a combination of these mechanisms. This step directly determines the subsequent testing pathway: a presentation favoring destruction with no other concerning features proceeds toward the immune thrombocytopenia-focused evaluation of Chapter 9, a presentation favoring production proceeds toward bone marrow examination as developed in this chapter, and a presentation with schistocytes proceeds immediately and urgently toward the thrombotic microangiopathy evaluation of Chapter 12 regardless of other findings.

This mechanistic localization step is the analytical core of the entire algorithm, and the diagnostic accuracy of everything that follows depends substantially on the rigor with which this step is performed, reinforcing why the detailed interpretive framework developed in the preceding sections of this chapter deserves careful, deliberate application rather than a cursory glance at the platelet count alone.

Step Three: Confirm the Specific Diagnosis and Initiate Management

The third algorithmic step applies the disease-specific diagnostic criteria developed in the chapters that follow to confirm a specific diagnosis within the mechanistic category identified in step two, recognizing that immune thrombocytopenia, discussed in Chapter 9, remains substantially a diagnosis of exclusion requiring the more specific etiologies developed throughout Part III to be reasonably excluded before it is accepted as the final diagnosis. Once a specific diagnosis, or a confident provisional diagnosis, is reached, management proceeds according to the disease-specific guidance developed in the relevant subsequent chapter, with the urgency of treatment initiation calibrated to the bleeding risk assessment developed in Chapter 5 rather than to the platelet count number in isolation.

This three-step algorithm, though presented sequentially, is applied iteratively in practice, since findings at a later step occasionally prompt reconsideration of the mechanistic localization established at step two, and the algorithm should be understood as an organizing framework for systematic clinical reasoning rather than a rigid, one-directional checklist that precludes reconsideration as new information becomes available during the evaluation.

Thrombocytopenia in the Hospitalized Patient

The Distinct Epidemiology of Hospital-Acquired Thrombocytopenia

Thrombocytopenia developing during hospitalization carries a substantially different differential diagnosis than thrombocytopenia presenting in the ambulatory outpatient setting, reflecting the concentration of specific etiologies in the hospitalized population: sepsis and critical illness-associated thrombocytopenia, discussed fully in Chapter 14, drug-induced thrombocytopenia from the expanded medication exposure of hospitalization, discussed in Chapter 10, heparin-induced thrombocytopenia specifically related to anticoagulant exposure common in hospitalized patients, discussed in Chapter 11, and dilutional thrombocytopenia from large-volume fluid resuscitation or massive transfusion, a distinctly hospital-associated mechanism not typically encountered in the ambulatory evaluation developed earlier in this chapter.

Recognizing this distinct epidemiologic context should directly inform the differential diagnosis constructed for a hospitalized patient, prioritizing these hospital-associated etiologies earlier in the evaluation than would be appropriate for an ambulatory patient with an otherwise similar platelet count, while still applying the same underlying mechanistic framework developed throughout this chapter to organize and direct the specific evaluation pursued.

Timing Relative to Admission and Specific Exposures

The temporal relationship between platelet count decline and specific hospital exposures, including new medications, procedures, and the onset of any new organ dysfunction or infection, provides substantial diagnostic direction in the hospitalized setting, and maintaining a chronologic timeline of platelet count alongside a timeline of relevant medication starts, procedures, and clinical events, ideally displayed together in the medical record, substantially aids the identification of a likely causative exposure. Heparin-induced thrombocytopenia, discussed in detail in Chapter 11, has a particularly characteristic temporal pattern, typically manifesting five to ten days after heparin initiation in a heparin-naive patient, that specifically depends on this kind of careful timeline construction for accurate recognition.

This timeline-based approach extends the tempo and trajectory principle developed earlier in this chapter into the specific, exposure-dense context of hospitalization, where the density of potential causative exposures makes careful temporal correlation particularly valuable for narrowing an otherwise broad differential diagnosis to the specific etiology most likely responsible for a given patient's presentation.

Multidisciplinary Coordination in the Hospitalized Patient

Thrombocytopenia in a hospitalized patient frequently requires coordination across multiple services, including the primary admitting team, hematology, and, when a specific etiology such as heparin-induced thrombocytopenia or thrombotic microangiopathy is suspected, urgent subspecialty involvement to guide time-sensitive management decisions including anticoagulation modification, discussed further in Chapters 11 and 12. Establishing clear communication about the working differential diagnosis, the specific tests pending, and the anticipated timeline for results across this multidisciplinary team reduces both diagnostic delay and the risk of conflicting or duplicated management decisions from different services managing the same patient.

This coordination challenge is compounded by the acuity and complexity typical of hospitalized patients with new thrombocytopenia, many of whom have multiple, simultaneously active medical issues that can each independently contribute to or complicate the thrombocytopenia evaluation, reinforcing the value of early, structured hematology involvement, guided by the mechanistic framework developed throughout this chapter, in complex hospitalized presentations rather than a fragmented, sequential evaluation pursued independently by each individual consulting service.

THE PLATELET CRISIS DECISION COMPASS — Sequencing the Evaluation of New Thrombocytopenia in a Hospitalized Patient

---

The Presentation: A patient hospitalized for pneumonia and started on prophylactic heparin six days ago develops a new platelet count decline from 240 to 95 x10^9/L.

Mimic Signature: Heparin-induced thrombocytopenia given the characteristic five-to-ten-day timing; sepsis-associated thrombocytopenia from the underlying pneumonia and any evolving critical illness; and a drug reaction to a recently started antibiotic or other new hospital medication.

The Decision: Calculate a formal heparin-induced thrombocytopenia pretest probability score using the timing, magnitude of platelet decline, and absence of alternative explanation; obtain smear review and a focused review of all new medications and clinical trajectory since admission; do not discontinue heparin reflexively without this structured assessment, but treat an intermediate or high pretest probability score as warranting urgent alternative anticoagulation pending confirmatory testing, per the approach developed in Chapter 11.

Trap Logic: Attributing hospital-acquired thrombocytopenia reflexively to 'sepsis' without constructing the specific exposure timeline this chapter emphasizes risks missing a time-sensitive, specifically treatable diagnosis such as heparin-induced thrombocytopenia, for which continued heparin exposure carries substantial thrombotic risk.

Crisis Anchor: New thrombocytopenia in a hospitalized patient is evaluated against a specific exposure and procedure timeline, with heparin-induced thrombocytopenia pretest probability formally assessed whenever heparin exposure and compatible timing are present.

Chronic and Recurrent Thrombocytopenia: A Longitudinal Approach

Defining and Recognizing Chronic Thrombocytopenia

Thrombocytopenia persisting beyond twelve months is generally classified as chronic, a threshold most extensively characterized in the context of immune thrombocytopenia discussed in Chapter 9 but applicable as an organizing concept across the broader differential diagnosis developed in this chapter, and recognizing that a patient's thrombocytopenia has entered a chronic phase should prompt a shift in evaluation and management philosophy from acute diagnostic urgency toward longitudinal disease characterization and monitoring, appropriate to the more indolent trajectory chronic thrombocytopenia typically implies. This shift does not eliminate the need for periodic reassessment, since a chronic, previously stable process can still evolve, but it does appropriately deprioritize repeated urgent re-evaluation of a pattern that has already been thoroughly characterized.

Chronic thrombocytopenia should be periodically reassessed for a change in trajectory or the emergence of new findings, extending the trend-based reasoning developed throughout this chapter into the specific longitudinal management context, and a chronic, stable thrombocytopenia diagnosis established years earlier should be reconsidered if the patient develops new symptoms, a substantial further decline in platelet count, or new accompanying laboratory abnormalities, rather than assumed to remain permanently and definitively explained by the original diagnosis without any capacity for reassessment.

Recurrent or Fluctuating Thrombocytopenia

A distinct pattern of recurrent or cyclically fluctuating thrombocytopenia, in which the platelet count repeatedly declines and recovers over a period of weeks to months, raises specific diagnostic considerations distinct from either a stable chronic pattern or a single acute episode, including cyclic thrombocytopenia, a rare condition believed to reflect an oscillating immune or marrow regulatory process, and thrombocytopenia related to a recurrent or intermittent exposure, such as periodic alcohol use producing transient marrow suppression or an intermittently used medication with recognized thrombocytopenic potential.

Careful longitudinal platelet count charting, correlated with a detailed timeline of potential recurrent exposures including medication use, alcohol consumption, and any recurrent illness pattern, is essential to correctly characterizing this fluctuating presentation, and referral to a hematologist with specific experience in these less common recurrent patterns is generally warranted once a straightforward, single explanatory cause has been reasonably excluded through this careful longitudinal evaluation.

Balancing Monitoring Frequency With Patient Burden

Establishing an appropriate long-term monitoring frequency for a patient with chronic thrombocytopenia requires balancing the clinical value of ongoing surveillance against the burden repeated laboratory testing and clinic visits impose on the patient, and this balance should be explicitly discussed with the patient, incorporating their own preferences and the specific stability of their individual pattern, rather than applying a uniform, one-size-fits-all monitoring schedule to every patient with chronic thrombocytopenia regardless of the demonstrated stability or volatility of their individual disease course.

This individualized approach to long-term monitoring closes the loop on the diagnostic framework developed throughout this chapter, extending the same patient-centered, communication-forward philosophy introduced in Chapter 5 into the long-term management phase that follows an initial diagnostic evaluation, and it sets the stage for the disease-specific management approaches developed throughout the remainder of Part III, each of which incorporates its own specific guidance on appropriate longitudinal monitoring for the particular condition addressed.

Congenital and Inherited Thrombocytopenia in the Adult Differential

Recognizing an Inherited Pattern Presenting in Adulthood

Although the inherited thrombocytopenia syndromes catalogued in Chapter 15 are frequently identified in childhood, a meaningful subset of patients with a mild inherited platelet production or survival defect are not recognized until adulthood, often after an incidental low platelet count prompts evaluation, and the mechanistic framework developed throughout this chapter should explicitly incorporate this possibility rather than assuming that any newly identified adult thrombocytopenia necessarily reflects an acquired process. A careful review of prior platelet counts, when available, family history extending the principles from Chapter 5, and a request for old records or family member testing when a mild, lifelong, previously unrecognized pattern is suspected, together help distinguish a genuinely new acquired process from a longstanding, only recently identified inherited one.

This distinction carries direct management implications, since an inherited thrombocytopenia syndrome generally does not respond to and does not require the immune-directed therapies appropriate to immune thrombocytopenia, and misclassifying an inherited pattern as an acquired immune process risks both ineffective treatment and unwarranted patient anxiety about an active, evolving disease process when the true underlying pattern is instead a stable, lifelong trait.

Distinguishing Features on Routine Evaluation

Several features raise suspicion for an inherited pattern within the adult diagnostic evaluation developed in this chapter: a platelet count that has remained essentially stable across every available prior measurement, giant or unusually small platelets on smear review as discussed in Chapter 6, a bleeding phenotype that is disproportionately mild relative to the platelet count, and, when specifically asked, a family history of similarly mild, lifelong low platelet counts that family members themselves may never have formally investigated. Genetic testing, discussed in the platelet function context in Chapter 7 and applicable analogously to production-related inherited disorders, provides definitive confirmation when this pattern is suspected and when a specific diagnosis would meaningfully affect management, surveillance, or family counseling.

Even when genetic confirmation is not pursued, simply recognizing and documenting a probable inherited pattern, following the longitudinal documentation principle developed in Chapters 5 and 6, prevents unnecessary repeated evaluation at future encounters and provides the patient with a clear, reassuring explanation for a finding that might otherwise generate ongoing diagnostic uncertainty and repeated, low-yield testing over subsequent years.

Coordinating Genetics and Hematology Involvement

When an inherited thrombocytopenia syndrome is confirmed or strongly suspected in an adult, coordinated involvement of both hematology and genetics, extending the pediatric coordination principle developed in Chapter 5, ensures appropriate surveillance for the syndrome-specific complications catalogued in Chapter 15, some of which, including an increased risk of hematologic malignancy in specific inherited syndromes, carry meaningful long-term management implications beyond the thrombocytopenia itself. Family counseling and, where appropriate, cascade testing of first-degree relatives should be offered, since other family members may carry the same variant with a similarly mild, previously unrecognized phenotype that would benefit from the same diagnostic clarity.

This adult recognition pathway for inherited thrombocytopenia illustrates a broader principle relevant to the mechanistic framework developed throughout this chapter: the three fundamental categories of decreased production, increased destruction, and distributional sequestration each contain both acquired and inherited variants, and a complete differential diagnosis at every stage of this chapter's algorithm should remain open to an inherited explanation, particularly when the temporal and morphologic clues discussed in this section are present.

Special Populations in the Thrombocytopenia Evaluation

Pregnancy-Associated Thrombocytopenia

Thrombocytopenia identified during pregnancy requires immediate application of the pregnancy-specific framework introduced in Chapter 5 and developed fully in Chapter 13, since gestational thrombocytopenia, the benign and by far most common cause of thrombocytopenia first identified in pregnancy, must be distinguished promptly from the hypertensive and thrombotic microangiopathic syndromes of pregnancy, which share overlapping laboratory features but carry substantially different maternal and fetal risk. The mechanistic framework developed in this chapter applies to pregnancy with specific modification, since the destructive mechanism most relevant to severe pregnancy-associated thrombocytopenia often involves a pregnancy-specific microangiopathic process rather than the immune thrombocytopenia pathway that predominates in the non-pregnant destructive category.

Any pregnant patient with thrombocytopenia accompanied by hypertension, proteinuria, or laboratory evidence of hemolysis or hepatic dysfunction should be evaluated urgently rather than through the routine outpatient pathway otherwise appropriate to mild, isolated gestational thrombocytopenia, reflecting the time-sensitive nature of the pregnancy-specific syndromes this combination of findings suggests, a triage principle developed fully in Chapter 13.

Thrombocytopenia in Older Adults

Older adults presenting with new thrombocytopenia carry a shifted pretest probability distribution relative to younger adults, with clonal hematopoietic processes including myelodysplastic syndrome and myeloproliferative neoplasm-associated cytopenia, discussed in Chapter 17, comprising a larger proportion of the differential diagnosis than in a younger population, while classic immune thrombocytopenia, though still occurring in older adults, represents a comparatively smaller proportion of new thrombocytopenia presentations in this age group than it does in younger adults. This shifted pretest probability supports the lower threshold for bone marrow examination in older patients introduced earlier in this chapter and reinforces the value of careful smear review and attention to accompanying cytopenias in every older adult presenting with new thrombocytopenia.

Polypharmacy, common in older adults, additionally increases the likelihood that a temporally associated new or changed medication contributes to a new thrombocytopenia presentation, and the medication reconciliation and exposure history developed in Chapter 5 deserves particular thoroughness in this population, where multiple concurrent medications, any of which could plausibly contribute to the presentation discussed in Chapter 10, are common.

Thrombocytopenia in Immunocompromised Patients

Patients with human immunodeficiency virus infection, those receiving immunosuppressive therapy following solid organ or hematopoietic stem cell transplantation, and those with other causes of significant immunocompromise present a distinct differential diagnosis for thrombocytopenia, incorporating both an increased risk of the opportunistic infections and secondary marrow suppression associated with their underlying condition or its treatment, and, in the case of human immunodeficiency virus specifically, a well-characterized association with an immune thrombocytopenia-like process that improves substantially with effective antiretroviral therapy. Medication-related marrow suppression from antiretroviral agents, immunosuppressive regimens, and prophylactic antimicrobial agents commonly used in this population adds further complexity to the medication-focused evaluation developed in Chapter 10.

Close coordination with the infectious disease, transplant, or other subspecialty team managing the patient's underlying immunocompromising condition is essential in this population, since the differential diagnosis, appropriate testing sequence, and management approach for thrombocytopenia in an immunocompromised patient frequently depends on disease- and treatment-specific considerations that fall outside the scope of a purely hematologic evaluation conducted in isolation from this broader clinical context.

When to Refer and How to Sequence Subspecialty Involvement

Findings That Warrant Immediate Hematology Referral

Building on the referral triage principles introduced in Chapter 5, several findings specific to the thrombocytopenia evaluation developed in this chapter warrant immediate, same-day hematology involvement rather than routine outpatient referral: schistocytes on peripheral smear, a platelet count below approximately 20 to 30 x10^9/L regardless of symptoms, multilineage cytopenia with abnormal cell morphology, and any presentation in which the mechanistic framework developed in this chapter cannot be confidently applied due to a genuinely atypical or rapidly evolving clinical picture. These findings share a common feature: each represents a scenario in which diagnostic delay carries meaningful risk of clinical deterioration or missed time-sensitive intervention, justifying the resource intensity of urgent subspecialty involvement.

Conversely, mild, isolated, incidentally discovered thrombocytopenia with a reassuring smear and no concerning accompanying findings can generally proceed through the confirmatory and initial evaluation steps developed in this chapter and Chapter 6 in the primary care or general internal medicine setting before hematology referral is considered, reserving subspecialty consultation for cases in which this initial evaluation itself proves abnormal, inconclusive, or fails to identify a clear explanation.

Structuring an Effective Referral

An effective hematology referral for thrombocytopenia includes the specific elements this chapter has developed as diagnostically essential: the platelet count trend over time, smear findings if already obtained, relevant medication and exposure history, any accompanying cytopenia, and the referring clinician's own working assessment of which mechanistic category the presentation appears to favor, providing the consulting hematologist a structured starting point rather than requiring the entire evaluation to be reconstructed from an undifferentiated referral question. This structured referral approach reduces both the time to diagnosis and the burden of duplicated testing, since a hematologist receiving a well-characterized referral can proceed directly to the most diagnostically relevant next steps rather than repeating foundational evaluation already completed by the referring clinician.

Institutions increasingly develop structured referral templates or electronic order sets specifically for thrombocytopenia evaluation, incorporating the key elements developed throughout this chapter as required or prompted fields, a systems-level intervention that parallels the institutional reflex-building discussion introduced in Chapter 6 and that measurably improves referral quality and reduces diagnostic delay across an entire health system rather than depending on individual clinician thoroughness alone.

Shared Management Between Primary Care and Hematology

For many patients with chronic, stable thrombocytopenia of an established, benign etiology, ongoing management can reasonably be shared between hematology and primary care, with hematology establishing the initial diagnosis and monitoring plan and primary care assuming responsibility for routine surveillance testing, escalating back to hematology only if the trend changes or new symptoms develop, an arrangement that reduces the burden of specialist visits for a stable, well-characterized chronic condition while preserving ready access to subspecialty expertise if the clinical picture evolves. Clear documentation of this shared care arrangement, including explicit criteria for when primary care should re-escalate to hematology, extends the longitudinal documentation and communication principles developed throughout this chapter into a durable, actionable long-term care plan.

This chapter has developed the complete diagnostic architecture for adult thrombocytopenia: a mechanistic framework for localizing the underlying process, integration of the clinical and laboratory tools from Chapters 5 through 7, clear indications for bone marrow examination, a stepwise algorithm adaptable to the outpatient, hospitalized, and chronic longitudinal settings, and explicit referral and coordination guidance. The disease-specific chapters that follow, beginning with immune thrombocytopenia in Chapter 9, now apply this architecture to the individual conditions that populate each branch of the diagnostic tree this chapter has constructed.

CLINICAL CASE: A 67-year-old woman is referred to hematology after three consecutive complete blood counts over four months show a platelet count declining from 165 to 98 to 71 x10^9/L, accompanied by a mild, progressive normocytic anemia not previously present. Applying the mechanistic framework developed in this chapter, the combination of multilineage cytopenia and a progressive, rather than abrupt, decline favors a production-limited process over an acute destructive one, prompting peripheral smear review, which reveals occasional teardrop-shaped red cells and rare circulating immature myeloid precursors, findings that further support marrow infiltration or dysplasia over a straightforward peripheral destructive process. Given her age, the multilineage and progressive nature of the cytopenia, and the concerning smear findings, bone marrow aspirate and biopsy are pursued rather than an empiric trial of immune thrombocytopenia-directed therapy, and the marrow reveals hypercellularity with dysplastic megakaryocytes showing hypolobated nuclei, multilineage dysplasia, and five percent myeloblasts, establishing a diagnosis of myelodysplastic syndrome, addressed further in the context of clonal hematopoiesis in Chapter 17. This case illustrates the central lesson of this chapter's mechanistic framework: the pattern of multilineage involvement, progressive rather than abrupt tempo, and specific smear morphology together correctly directed the evaluation toward marrow examination rather than the immune thrombocytopenia-focused pathway that an isolated platelet count alone, considered without this mechanistic framework, might otherwise have suggested as the first diagnostic hypothesis.

THE PLATELET CRISIS DECISION COMPASS — Mechanistic Diagnosis and Triage

Compass Recap: Multilineage Cytopenia: New thrombocytopenia accompanied by unexplained anemia or leukopenia is evaluated with smear review and, when morphology is abnormal, urgent hematology referral for marrow examination — not attributed to a single presumed benign cause without this evaluation.

Compass Recap: Hospital-Acquired Thrombocytopenia: New thrombocytopenia in a hospitalized patient is evaluated against a specific exposure and procedure timeline, with heparin-induced thrombocytopenia pretest probability formally assessed whenever heparin exposure and compatible timing are present.

Chapter Anchor: Thrombocytopenia is localized to decreased production, increased destruction, or distributional sequestration using the complete blood count, platelet indices, smear morphology, and clinical tempo before a specific disease-level diagnosis is pursued — mechanistic localization, not the platelet count alone, directs the entire subsequent evaluation.

Summary and Key Concepts

Thrombocytopenia is organized mechanistically into decreased production, increased destruction, and distributional (splenic) sequestration, with many clinically important conditions involving overlapping mechanisms.

Elevated mean platelet volume and immature platelet fraction, isolated thrombocytopenia, and abrupt onset favor increased destruction; low indices, multilineage cytopenia, and gradual decline favor decreased production.

Splenic sequestration, confirmed by imaging showing splenomegaly, produces a typically milder bleeding phenotype and reflects redistribution rather than reduced total body platelet mass or production.

Bone marrow examination is indicated for multilineage cytopenia, abnormal smear morphology, or an unexplained systemic illness suggesting marrow infiltration — not routinely required for isolated thrombocytopenia with a typical destructive presentation.

Hospital-acquired thrombocytopenia carries a distinct differential (sepsis, drug-induced, heparin-induced, dilutional) requiring careful correlation with the timeline of admission, medications, and procedures.

Chronic thrombocytopenia (persisting beyond 12 months) shifts management toward longitudinal monitoring calibrated to individual stability, while recurrent or fluctuating patterns warrant hematology referral once straightforward causes are excluded.

CHAPTER 9: IMMUNE THROMBOCYTOPENIA

Learning Objectives

1. Define immune thrombocytopenia and apply current classification terminology (newly diagnosed, persistent, chronic; primary versus secondary).
2. Explain the dual antibody-mediated destructive and impaired production mechanisms underlying immune thrombocytopenia.
3. Apply the diagnostic criteria for immune thrombocytopenia as a diagnosis of exclusion, distinguishing it from the broader thrombocytopenia differential developed in Chapter 8.
4. Identify the secondary conditions associated with immune thrombocytopenia and recognize when secondary evaluation is warranted.
5. Select appropriate first-line, second-line, and refractory management strategies based on bleeding severity and disease chronicity.
6. Describe the role of splenectomy and its modern alternatives in refractory immune thrombocytopenia.

Chapter Outline

This chapter develops immune thrombocytopenia as the prototypical destructive thrombocytopenia within the mechanistic framework established in Chapter 8, addressing its epidemiology and classification, the dual mechanisms of antibody-mediated destruction and impaired compensatory production, clinical presentation across age groups, diagnostic criteria as a diagnosis of exclusion, secondary associations, and the full management spectrum from first-line corticosteroid therapy through refractory disease management including splenectomy. Two Platelet Crisis Decision Compass instances address recognition of an immune thrombocytopenia presentation requiring urgent first-line treatment and the correct sequencing of second-line therapy in refractory disease.

Immune thrombocytopenia remains, despite decades of research, substantially a clinical diagnosis of exclusion, and the diagnostic rigor developed in Chapters 5 through 8 finds its most direct application in this chapter, since establishing this diagnosis correctly, having reasonably excluded the secondary and alternative causes catalogued throughout Part III, is the essential prerequisite to selecting appropriate, evidence-based management.

Definition, Classification, and Epidemiology

Current Diagnostic Terminology

Immune thrombocytopenia is defined as an isolated platelet count below 100 x10^9/L in the absence of another identifiable cause, reflecting antibody-mediated platelet destruction, and current international consensus terminology classifies the condition by duration into newly diagnosed immune thrombocytopenia, spanning the first three months from diagnosis; persistent immune thrombocytopenia, spanning three to twelve months without spontaneous remission; and chronic immune thrombocytopenia, persisting beyond twelve months, a terminology framework that replaced the older acute-versus-chronic dichotomy specifically to better capture the variable and often unpredictable natural history the condition follows.

The condition is additionally classified as primary, when occurring in isolation without an identifiable secondary cause, or secondary, when occurring in association with another underlying condition, discussed in detail later in this chapter, and this primary-secondary distinction carries direct management implications, since secondary immune thrombocytopenia often responds best to treatment directed at the underlying associated condition alongside or instead of the standard primary immune thrombocytopenia therapies discussed later in this chapter.

Epidemiology and Age-Specific Patterns

Immune thrombocytopenia demonstrates a distinctly bimodal age distribution, with one peak in early childhood, where the condition frequently follows a preceding viral illness and typically follows a self-limited course resolving within weeks to months, and a second, broader peak in adulthood, where the condition more frequently follows a chronic course requiring longer-term management, a distinction with direct implications for the natural history discussion and management planning developed later in this chapter. Adult immune thrombocytopenia shows a modest female predominance, particularly in the young to middle adult age range, while the pediatric presentation shows a more equal sex distribution, patterns that parallel, though do not fully mirror, the epidemiology of other autoimmune conditions.

Overall incidence estimates for immune thrombocytopenia vary across populations and case-finding methodology, but the condition is generally recognized as an uncommon but not rare cause of thrombocytopenia, consistent with its position within the broader differential diagnosis developed in Chapter 8 as one of several destructive processes requiring careful exclusion of alternative explanations rather than automatic default diagnosis whenever isolated thrombocytopenia is encountered.

Natural History Across the Classification Spectrum

The natural history of immune thrombocytopenia varies substantially between the pediatric and adult presentations discussed above and even within adult presentations, with a meaningful proportion of adults achieving spontaneous or treatment-associated remission within the first year while others progress to a chronic course requiring ongoing management, and no single clinical or laboratory feature at presentation reliably predicts which trajectory an individual patient will follow, a diagnostic and prognostic uncertainty that should be communicated transparently to patients using the communication framework developed in Chapter 5.

This unpredictable natural history directly informs the management philosophy developed throughout the remainder of this chapter, favoring an approach that treats bleeding risk and quality of life at each point in the disease course rather than pursuing an aggressive, uniformly applied treatment strategy predicated on an assumption of chronic, unremitting disease that may not, in fact, apply to a given individual patient.

Pathophysiology: Antibody-Mediated Destruction and Impaired Production

Autoantibody-Mediated Platelet Clearance

The central pathophysiologic mechanism of immune thrombocytopenia involves autoantibodies, most commonly directed against the platelet glycoprotein IIb/IIIa complex or the glycoprotein Ib-IX-V complex developed mechanistically in Chapter 2, that opsonize circulating platelets and target them for accelerated clearance by tissue macrophages, predominantly within the spleen, through Fc receptor-mediated phagocytosis. This mechanism directly explains both the isolated nature of the thrombocytopenia, since the autoantibodies target platelet-specific surface antigens rather than antigens shared with other blood cell lineages, and the historical rationale for splenectomy, discussed later in this chapter, as a treatment directed at the primary site of antibody-mediated platelet destruction.

Complement-mediated platelet destruction and direct antibody-mediated platelet activation and clearance through mechanisms distinct from classical Fc receptor phagocytosis have additionally been identified as contributing pathways in a subset of patients, contributing to the biological heterogeneity that likely underlies the variable treatment response and natural history discussed throughout this chapter, and ongoing research into these alternative destructive pathways has informed the development of some of the second-line therapies discussed later in this chapter.

Impaired Compensatory Megakaryopoiesis

Beyond accelerated peripheral destruction, immune thrombocytopenia additionally involves impaired compensatory platelet production, since the same autoantibodies implicated in peripheral platelet destruction can also target megakaryocytes within the bone marrow, impairing their maturation and platelet release through mechanisms including complement-mediated megakaryocyte injury and antibody-mediated inhibition of proplatelet formation, the process developed mechanistically in Chapter 1. This impaired production mechanism explains why endogenous thrombopoietin levels in immune thrombocytopenia are frequently only modestly elevated, in contrast to the more dramatically elevated thrombopoietin levels seen in primary marrow failure states such as aplastic anemia, since an appropriately responsive marrow would be expected to more substantially upregulate thrombopoietin-driven production in response to peripheral platelet loss.

This dual mechanism of destruction and impaired production directly explains the therapeutic rationale for thrombopoietin receptor agonists, discussed as second-line therapy later in this chapter, which pharmacologically overcome this relative production deficit by providing supraphysiologic thrombopoietin receptor stimulation, and understanding this dual mechanism provides the conceptual foundation for the full spectrum of management approaches developed throughout the remainder of this chapter.

T-Cell Dysregulation and the Broader Immune Context

Beyond the antibody-mediated mechanisms discussed above, immune thrombocytopenia involves broader immune dysregulation, including altered T-helper cell subset balance, impaired regulatory T-cell function, and cytotoxic T-cell-mediated platelet and megakaryocyte injury operating in parallel with, and in some patients independent of, the antibody-mediated mechanisms discussed above. This broader immune dysregulation helps explain the therapeutic effect of immunosuppressive agents beyond those specifically targeting antibody production, and it reflects the condition's positioning within the broader spectrum of autoimmune disease, sharing pathophysiologic features with other antibody-mediated and T-cell-mediated autoimmune conditions.

This evolving mechanistic understanding continues to inform the development of novel therapeutic agents targeting specific nodes within this immune dysregulation network, and clinicians managing immune thrombocytopenia should expect the therapeutic landscape to continue evolving as this pathophysiologic understanding matures further, a point developed further in the discussion of emerging platelet-directed therapies in Chapter 20.

Clinical Presentation in Children and Adults

The Pediatric Presentation

Pediatric immune thrombocytopenia characteristically presents with abrupt-onset mucocutaneous bleeding, including petechiae, purpura, and epistaxis, often following a viral illness by one to four weeks, in an otherwise well-appearing child with an isolated, sometimes severely low platelet count and an unremarkable physical examination beyond the bleeding manifestations themselves, a presentation directly consistent with the destructive mechanism localization developed in Chapter 8. The majority of affected children experience a self-limited course with spontaneous resolution within weeks to a few months, though a minority progress to the persistent or chronic classification introduced earlier in this chapter, and current pediatric hematology guidelines generally favor observation over active treatment in a well-appearing child with mild bleeding symptoms, reserving active treatment for more significant bleeding or specific risk factors discussed later in this chapter.

Serious bleeding complications, most notably intracranial hemorrhage, are rare in pediatric immune thrombocytopenia even at very low platelet counts, though not entirely absent, and this favorable risk profile, combined with the generally self-limited natural history in this age group, supports the observation-favoring management philosophy that distinguishes pediatric from adult immune thrombocytopenia management in a manner discussed further later in this chapter.

The Adult Presentation

Adult immune thrombocytopenia more frequently presents with an insidious rather than abrupt onset, is less consistently preceded by an identifiable triggering illness, and more frequently follows a chronic rather than self-limited course, patterns that together shift the adult management approach toward a somewhat lower threshold for active treatment compared with the pediatric presentation, particularly in an adult with a platelet count low enough to carry meaningful bleeding risk. Bleeding manifestations in adults follow the same mucocutaneous pattern developed in Chapter 5, including petechiae, easy bruising, epistaxis, gingival bleeding, and, in women, heavy menstrual bleeding, with the specific bleeding phenotype and the structured bleeding assessment tool score, rather than the platelet count number in isolation, appropriately guiding treatment urgency as developed throughout Chapter 5.

A meaningful proportion of adult immune thrombocytopenia is identified incidentally on routine complete blood count in an asymptomatic patient, directly paralleling the incidental thrombocytopenia discussion developed in Chapter 5, and this asymptomatic presentation should not be assumed to carry a more favorable natural history than a symptomatic presentation at a similar platelet count, reinforcing the principle, developed throughout this book, that absence of current symptoms does not equate to absence of meaningful underlying risk.

Fatigue and Quality of Life Beyond Bleeding

Beyond the bleeding manifestations that have historically dominated clinical attention, patients with immune thrombocytopenia frequently report substantial fatigue disproportionate to their degree of anemia or overall disease severity, a symptom increasingly recognized as an intrinsic feature of the condition rather than solely a secondary consequence of bleeding-related anemia or treatment side effects, and validated quality-of-life instruments specific to immune thrombocytopenia have been developed and increasingly incorporated into both clinical trials and routine clinical assessment to systematically capture this dimension of the disease burden.

Incorporating fatigue and broader quality-of-life assessment into routine clinical evaluation, alongside the bleeding-focused assessment developed in Chapter 5, provides a more complete picture of disease impact and treatment benefit, particularly relevant when counseling a patient about the risks and benefits of escalating therapy for a platelet count that, while below the normal reference range, may not itself carry substantial imminent bleeding risk at the specific level under consideration.

Diagnostic Criteria and the Exclusion of Secondary Causes

Immune Thrombocytopenia as a Diagnosis of Exclusion

No single laboratory test definitively confirms immune thrombocytopenia, and the diagnosis is established by reasonably excluding the alternative causes of isolated thrombocytopenia developed throughout Chapter 8, including pseudothrombocytopenia, medication effect, and other destructive, production-limited, or distributional processes, in a patient whose presentation is otherwise consistent with the clinical and laboratory pattern developed in this chapter. Antiplatelet antibody testing, though available at some centers, has limited sensitivity and specificity for immune thrombocytopenia and is not routinely recommended as part of the standard diagnostic evaluation, reflecting the test's inability to reliably distinguish immune thrombocytopenia from other causes of thrombocytopenia in most clinical circumstances.

The exclusionary evaluation required before confidently establishing an immune thrombocytopenia diagnosis directly applies the mechanistic and algorithmic framework developed in Chapter 8: confirming isolated thrombocytopenia without accompanying cytopenia, unremarkable peripheral smear apart from the reduced platelet count and, characteristically, larger platelets reflecting the compensatory production response discussed earlier in this chapter, and no clinical or laboratory finding suggesting one of the specific alternative causes catalogued throughout the remainder of Part III of this book.

Baseline Testing Recommended at Diagnosis

Current guidelines recommend a defined baseline evaluation at the time immune thrombocytopenia is first diagnosed, including complete blood count with differential and smear review, testing for hepatitis B and C and human immunodeficiency virus given their recognized association with secondary immune thrombocytopenia discussed later in this chapter, quantitative immunoglobulin levels to screen for an underlying immunodeficiency, and, in the appropriate clinical context, testing for Helicobacter pylori infection given the demonstrated association between its eradication and platelet count improvement in some populations. Additional testing, including antinuclear antibody testing, direct antiglobulin testing, and thyroid function testing, is reasonable in selected patients based on the clinical presentation but is not universally required in every newly diagnosed patient.

This baseline evaluation should be completed promptly at diagnosis rather than deferred, since identifying a secondary cause at the outset directly informs the management approach discussed later in this chapter, and a diagnosis of primary immune thrombocytopenia established without this baseline evaluation should be considered provisional, subject to revision if a secondary cause is subsequently identified through more complete evaluation or through the emergence of new clinical findings over time.

Diagnostic Reassessment Over Time

Because immune thrombocytopenia is a diagnosis of exclusion rather than one confirmed by a definitive positive test, periodic diagnostic reassessment is warranted, particularly in a patient whose clinical course deviates from the expected pattern, including an unexpectedly poor response to standard first-line therapy, discussed later in this chapter, or the emergence of new clinical findings suggesting a secondary cause not apparent at initial presentation. This ongoing diagnostic vigilance directly extends the trend-based and longitudinal reasoning developed throughout Chapters 6 through 8 into the specific context of a condition whose initial diagnosis inherently carries some degree of residual uncertainty.

This principle should be communicated to patients as part of the transparent uncertainty discussion developed in Chapter 5, framing the diagnosis of immune thrombocytopenia as the most likely explanation based on currently available evidence rather than an absolutely certain, permanently fixed conclusion, an important nuance for a chronic condition that may require years of ongoing management and periodic clinical reassessment.

THE PLATELET CRISIS DECISION COMPASS — Determining Urgency of First-Line Treatment in Newly Diagnosed Immune Thrombocytopenia

---

The Presentation: A 34-year-old woman is newly diagnosed with immune thrombocytopenia, platelet count 8 x10^9/L, with scattered petechiae and mild gingival bleeding but no wet purpura, retinal hemorrhage, or major bleeding.

Mimic Signature: Immune thrombocytopenia warranting urgent first-line treatment given the severity of the platelet count; a technical or preanalytic error requiring the confirmatory approach from Chapter 6 before accepting the count as genuine; and an alternative destructive process, such as early thrombotic microangiopathy, that would change the treatment approach entirely.

The Decision: Confirm the count via smear review, excluding clumping and confirming the absence of schistocytes; in the absence of wet purpura or major bleeding, initiate first-line corticosteroid therapy urgently, generally within the same or next clinical day given the severity of the platelet count, without necessarily requiring hospitalization if close follow-up can be reliably arranged.

Trap Logic: Delaying first-line treatment for a platelet count this severe because the patient currently lacks major bleeding conflates current symptom absence with future risk, when a count this low carries substantial risk of a bleeding complication developing before treatment can take effect if initiation is delayed.

Crisis Anchor: A confirmed platelet count below approximately 20-30 x10^9/L in newly diagnosed immune thrombocytopenia warrants prompt first-line treatment initiation, regardless of whether major bleeding is yet present.

Secondary Immune Thrombocytopenia: Associated Conditions

Autoimmune and Rheumatologic Associations

Immune thrombocytopenia occurs with increased frequency in association with systemic lupus erythematosus and other autoimmune conditions, in which the same underlying immune dysregulation that produces the primary rheumatologic disease can independently target platelets through the mechanisms developed earlier in this chapter, and immune thrombocytopenia occasionally precedes the more classic clinical manifestations of an underlying autoimmune condition by months to years, making thrombocytopenia in some patients the first clinical clue to an evolving systemic autoimmune process. This association supports the baseline testing recommendations discussed earlier in this chapter and supports maintaining ongoing clinical vigilance for the emergence of additional autoimmune features in a patient initially diagnosed with apparently primary immune thrombocytopenia.

Evans syndrome, the combination of immune thrombocytopenia with autoimmune hemolytic anemia occurring together, represents a specific and clinically important variant of this autoimmune association, requiring recognition of the combined cytopenia pattern through the direct antiglobulin testing and hemolysis workup discussed in the baseline testing section above, and management of Evans syndrome often requires an integrated approach addressing both cytopenias simultaneously rather than treating each in isolation.

Infectious Associations

Human immunodeficiency virus and hepatitis C virus infection are each independently associated with immune thrombocytopenia through mechanisms including direct viral effects on megakaryocytes and cross-reactive antibody-mediated platelet destruction, and thrombocytopenia in a patient with either infection frequently improves substantially with effective antiviral therapy directed at the underlying infection, making identification of these infections through the baseline testing discussed earlier in this chapter directly actionable rather than merely an epidemiologic association of academic interest. Helicobacter pylori infection, discussed briefly above, shows a geographically variable association with immune thrombocytopenia, with eradication therapy producing platelet count improvement in a meaningful proportion of infected patients in some populations, though this association and treatment benefit appears less pronounced in populations with lower background Helicobacter pylori prevalence.

Common variable immunodeficiency and other primary immunodeficiency syndromes are additionally associated with immune thrombocytopenia, identified through the quantitative immunoglobulin testing included in the baseline evaluation discussed earlier in this chapter, and recognizing this association is clinically important both because it redirects management toward addressing the underlying immunodeficiency and because it has implications for infection risk assessment and immunization planning that extend well beyond the thrombocytopenia itself.

Lymphoproliferative and Drug-Related Associations

Chronic lymphocytic leukemia and other lymphoproliferative disorders are associated with secondary immune thrombocytopenia through an autoimmune mechanism distinct from direct marrow infiltration by the malignant clone, meaning a patient with known chronic lymphocytic leukemia who develops new thrombocytopenia requires the same mechanistic evaluation developed in Chapter 8 to distinguish this autoimmune secondary immune thrombocytopenia from direct marrow infiltration, since the two processes carry different management implications despite occurring in the same underlying disease context. Certain medications, discussed in detail in Chapter 10, can produce a clinical and laboratory picture closely resembling primary immune thrombocytopenia, reinforcing why the thorough medication history developed in Chapter 5 remains essential even when the overall clinical picture otherwise appears consistent with primary immune thrombocytopenia.

Recognizing these varied secondary associations reinforces why the baseline evaluation discussed earlier in this chapter should be pursued systematically at diagnosis rather than selectively based on an incomplete initial impression, since several of these associated conditions, once identified, meaningfully change both the immediate management approach and the long-term monitoring plan appropriate to the individual patient.

First-Line Management: Corticosteroids and Immunoglobulin

Corticosteroid Therapy

Corticosteroids remain the standard first-line therapy for immune thrombocytopenia requiring active treatment, acting through multiple mechanisms including reduced Fc receptor-mediated macrophage clearance of antibody-coated platelets, reduced autoantibody production, and direct effects on megakaryocyte maturation, with a typical response, meaning a rise in platelet count sufficient to substantially reduce bleeding risk, observed within days to a few weeks in the majority of patients. Prolonged high-dose corticosteroid therapy carries substantial and well-characterized toxicity, including hyperglycemia, weight gain, mood disturbance, osteoporosis, and increased infection risk, and current guidelines favor a defined, relatively brief corticosteroid course with a structured taper over prolonged, indefinite corticosteroid maintenance, reserving longer-term disease control for the second-line agents discussed later in this chapter when a sustained corticosteroid-free remission is not achieved.

A substantial proportion of patients who achieve an initial corticosteroid response subsequently relapse as the corticosteroid is tapered, and this relapse pattern should be anticipated and discussed with the patient at the outset of treatment rather than presented as an unexpected treatment failure, framing corticosteroid therapy accurately as an effective means of achieving initial disease control rather than a guaranteed path to durable, treatment-free remission for every patient.

Intravenous Immunoglobulin

Intravenous immunoglobulin produces a more rapid platelet count rise than corticosteroids alone, typically within one to three days, through mechanisms including Fc receptor blockade on splenic macrophages that competitively inhibits antibody-coated platelet clearance, making it the preferred first-line agent when a rapid platelet count response is clinically necessary, including active significant bleeding, an urgent procedure requiring prompt platelet count improvement, or severe thrombocytopenia with wet purpura or other high-risk bleeding stigmata discussed in Chapter 5. The platelet count response to intravenous immunoglobulin, while rapid, is typically transient, generally lasting several weeks, making it most useful as a bridging strategy to achieve rapid, temporary platelet count improvement rather than as a durable, standalone long-term management strategy.

Anti-D immunoglobulin represents an alternative to intravenous immunoglobulin in Rh-positive, non-splenectomized patients, working through a distinct mechanism involving preferential splenic macrophage clearance of anti-D-coated red cells that competitively spares antibody-coated platelets, though its use carries specific precautions, including risk of clinically significant hemolysis, that require careful patient selection and monitoring, and its availability and specific indications vary by region and current supply.

Combining and Sequencing First-Line Therapies

The choice between corticosteroid monotherapy, intravenous immunoglobulin, or a combination of both as initial therapy is guided primarily by the urgency of the required platelet count response, directly applying the bleeding risk assessment framework developed in Chapter 5: a patient with mild bleeding symptoms and a platelet count carrying modest but not urgent bleeding risk can reasonably begin with corticosteroid monotherapy alone, while a patient with active significant bleeding or an urgent procedural need benefits from the addition of intravenous immunoglobulin to achieve the more rapid response this agent provides, often used together with corticosteroids to combine the rapid onset of immunoglobulin with the more sustained effect of corticosteroid therapy.

This individualized, bleeding-risk-calibrated approach to first-line therapy selection exemplifies the broader clinical philosophy developed throughout this book: treatment intensity and urgency are matched to the specific patient's bleeding risk and clinical circumstances, developed through the structured evaluation framework established in Chapter 5, rather than applied uniformly based on the platelet count number alone without regard for the broader clinical context.

Second-Line and Refractory Management

Thrombopoietin Receptor Agonists

Thrombopoietin receptor agonists, which stimulate megakaryopoiesis through the thrombopoietin receptor pathway developed mechanistically in Chapter 1, directly address the impaired production component of immune thrombocytopenia pathophysiology discussed earlier in this chapter and have become a mainstay of second-line therapy for patients requiring ongoing treatment beyond the first-line agents discussed above. These agents typically require several days to weeks to produce a meaningful platelet count response, are generally continued long-term to maintain response since platelet counts characteristically decline again after discontinuation, and require ongoing monitoring for specific class-associated considerations including a theoretical concern regarding marrow reticulin fibrosis with long-term use, discussed further in the long-term monitoring section of this chapter.

A meaningful proportion of patients treated with thrombopoietin receptor agonists achieve sustained treatment-free remission after a defined treatment course, an evolving area of clinical research suggesting these agents may have disease-modifying effects beyond their direct platelet count-raising mechanism, though the optimal treatment duration and discontinuation strategy to maximize the likelihood of durable remission remains an active area of ongoing clinical investigation.

Rituximab and Other Immunosuppressive Agents

Rituximab, a monoclonal antibody targeting the CD20 antigen on B lymphocytes, reduces autoantibody production by depleting the B-cell population responsible for generating the antiplatelet antibodies discussed earlier in this chapter, producing a response in a meaningful proportion of treated patients, with a subset achieving durable, sometimes multi-year remission, though response is not universal and typically requires several weeks to manifest, making rituximab generally unsuitable as a sole agent when an urgent platelet count response is required. Other immunosuppressive agents, including azathioprine, mycophenolate mofetil, and cyclosporine, have demonstrated efficacy in a subset of patients with refractory disease and may be considered based on individual patient factors, prior treatment response, and comorbidity profile, though these agents are generally used less frequently than thrombopoietin receptor agonists and rituximab in contemporary practice given the more extensive evidence base supporting these preferred second-line options.

The selection among these second-line options should incorporate patient preference, comorbidity profile, family planning considerations in women of reproductive age, and practical factors including administration route and monitoring requirements, reflecting a shared decision-making approach that extends the patient-centered communication framework developed in Chapter 5 into this more complex, longer-term treatment selection decision.

Emerging and Novel Second-Line Agents

Newer agents targeting Bruton tyrosine kinase, the neonatal Fc receptor, and other specific nodes within the immune dysregulation pathophysiology discussed earlier in this chapter have entered clinical use or late-stage clinical development, offering additional options for patients who have not achieved adequate response with the more established second-line agents discussed above, and this expanding therapeutic landscape is developed further in the discussion of emerging platelet-directed therapies in Chapter 20. Access to these newer agents varies by region, regulatory approval status, and insurance coverage, and clinicians should remain current on the evolving evidence base and approval status for these agents as the field continues to advance.

This expanding array of second-line options has meaningfully improved the ability to individualize treatment for refractory immune thrombocytopenia, moving beyond the historically more limited choice between splenectomy, discussed in the next section, and a narrower set of traditional immunosuppressive agents, toward a broader menu of options that can be more precisely matched to an individual patient's disease characteristics, treatment history, and personal circumstances and preferences.

THE PLATELET CRISIS DECISION COMPASS — Sequencing Second-Line Therapy After First-Line Treatment Failure

The Presentation: A 41-year-old man with immune thrombocytopenia relapses to a platelet count of 15 x10^9/L with recurrent bruising during corticosteroid taper, three months after initial diagnosis.

Mimic Signature: Genuine corticosteroid-dependent primary immune thrombocytopenia requiring second-line therapy; an unrecognized secondary cause not adequately excluded at initial diagnosis, warranting diagnostic reassessment; and a slower-than-expected but still ongoing corticosteroid taper response that has not yet been given adequate time.

The Decision: Confirm the baseline secondary-cause evaluation from earlier in this chapter was completed and remains unrevealing; if the relapse pattern is confirmed and the patient has now met criteria for persistent immune thrombocytopenia, proceed to shared decision-making regarding second-line therapy selection among thrombopoietin receptor agonists, rituximab, and other options based on the patient's specific circumstances and preferences.

Trap Logic: Repeating additional corticosteroid courses indefinitely in a corticosteroid-dependent relapsing pattern, rather than transitioning to a second-line strategy at the appropriate point, exposes the patient to cumulative corticosteroid toxicity without addressing the underlying pattern of dependency this presentation demonstrates.

Crisis Anchor: A corticosteroid-dependent relapse pattern meeting criteria for persistent immune thrombocytopenia prompts transition to second-line therapy selection rather than indefinite repeated corticosteroid courses.

Splenectomy and Its Alternatives

The Rationale and Historical Role of Splenectomy

Splenectomy directly addresses the primary site of antibody-mediated platelet destruction discussed earlier in this chapter and historically represented the standard second-line therapy for refractory immune thrombocytopenia, producing durable remission in a substantial proportion of patients, with response typically evident within days of the procedure given the immediate removal of the primary destructive site rather than the more gradual, pharmacologically mediated response of the medical second-line therapies discussed above. Current guidelines generally favor delaying splenectomy consideration until at least twelve months from diagnosis given the meaningful proportion of patients who achieve spontaneous or medically induced remission during this interval, and given the expanding array of effective medical second-line options discussed above that has reduced, though not eliminated, the role of splenectomy in contemporary practice.

Splenectomy carries procedural risks including bleeding, given the underlying thrombocytopenia, and infection, along with the lifelong risk of overwhelming post-splenectomy infection and the requirement for lifelong immunization against encapsulated organisms and, in some patients, prophylactic antibiotics, considerations that must be weighed against the durability and immediacy of response splenectomy provides when counseling a patient regarding this treatment option.

Predicting Response and Patient Selection

No test reliably predicts which individual patient will respond durably to splenectomy, though radiolabeled platelet sequestration studies, which assess the relative contribution of splenic versus hepatic platelet clearance, have been used at some centers to help inform this decision, with a predominantly splenic clearance pattern associated with a higher likelihood of durable splenectomy response, though this testing is not universally available or routinely required before proceeding with splenectomy in an appropriate candidate. Patient selection for splenectomy should incorporate the durability of response to prior first- and second-line therapies, overall surgical and infection risk, and patient preference regarding the tradeoff between the durability splenectomy offers and the procedural and long-term infection risks it carries relative to the ongoing medical therapy alternatives discussed earlier in this chapter.

This individualized selection process should incorporate the same shared decision-making principles developed for second-line medical therapy selection above, with explicit discussion of the alternative options, their relative durability and risk profiles, and the patient's own values and preferences regarding these tradeoffs, rather than presenting splenectomy as either a uniformly preferred or uniformly disfavored option independent of individual patient circumstances.

Postsplenectomy Management and Long-Term Considerations

Patients undergoing splenectomy require pre-procedural immunization against encapsulated organisms including Streptococcus pneumoniae, Neisseria meningitidis, and Haemophilus influenzae type b, ideally completed at least two weeks before the planned procedure when timing allows, along with patient education regarding the lifelong risk of overwhelming post-splenectomy infection, the importance of prompt medical attention for febrile illness, and, in some patients, a discussion of prophylactic antibiotic strategies, particularly in the immediate postoperative period and in younger patients who carry the highest lifetime infection risk. Some patients who undergo splenectomy nonetheless experience disease relapse over subsequent years, reflecting the presence of accessory splenic tissue or the persistence of hepatic and other extrasplenic platelet clearance mechanisms, and continued longitudinal monitoring remains appropriate even after an initially successful splenectomy.

This postsplenectomy management extends the longitudinal documentation and monitoring principles developed throughout this book, and a patient's postsplenectomy status, immunization history, and any subsequent relapse pattern should be clearly documented and readily accessible to any future clinician managing febrile illness or considering additional immune thrombocytopenia treatment in this patient population.

Immune Thrombocytopenia in Special Populations

Immune Thrombocytopenia in Pregnancy

Immune thrombocytopenia in pregnancy requires the specific diagnostic and management framework developed in Chapter 13, distinguishing it from the more common gestational thrombocytopenia and pregnancy-specific microangiopathic syndromes introduced in Chapters 5 and 8, with treatment decisions incorporating both maternal bleeding risk and considerations specific to delivery planning and neonatal platelet count monitoring given the potential for maternal antiplatelet antibodies to cross the placenta and affect the fetus, a topic developed in full mechanistic and management detail in Chapter 13. Corticosteroids and intravenous immunoglobulin, discussed earlier in this chapter as first-line agents, remain the preferred first-line options in pregnancy given their more established safety profile relative to several of the second-line agents discussed above, many of which carry specific pregnancy-related precautions or insufficient safety data to support routine use during pregnancy.

Coordination between hematology and maternal-fetal medicine is essential throughout pregnancy in a patient with immune thrombocytopenia, extending the multidisciplinary coordination principle developed in Chapter 8 into this specific high-stakes clinical context, with delivery planning incorporating the maternal platelet count trajectory as pregnancy progresses toward term.

Immune Thrombocytopenia in Older Adults

Older adults with immune thrombocytopenia require particular attention to treatment-related toxicity given the higher prevalence of comorbidities including diabetes, osteoporosis, and cardiovascular disease that corticosteroid therapy can meaningfully exacerbate, supporting consideration of a somewhat earlier transition to steroid-sparing second-line therapy in this population when ongoing treatment is required, balanced against the age-related bleeding risk considerations and the broader differential diagnosis discussed in Chapter 8 that appropriately receives heightened consideration in an older adult presenting with new thrombocytopenia. Falls risk, polypharmacy-related bleeding risk from concurrent medications, and functional status should each be incorporated into the individualized bleeding risk assessment and treatment planning for an older adult with immune thrombocytopenia, extending the age-specific considerations introduced in Chapters 5 and 8 into this specific disease management context.

Splenectomy carries somewhat higher procedural risk in older adults, and this consideration should be weighed alongside the durability benefits discussed earlier in this chapter when splenectomy is considered as a treatment option in this population, generally favoring a more conservative threshold for pursuing splenectomy in an older adult relative to a younger patient with a similar treatment-refractory disease course.

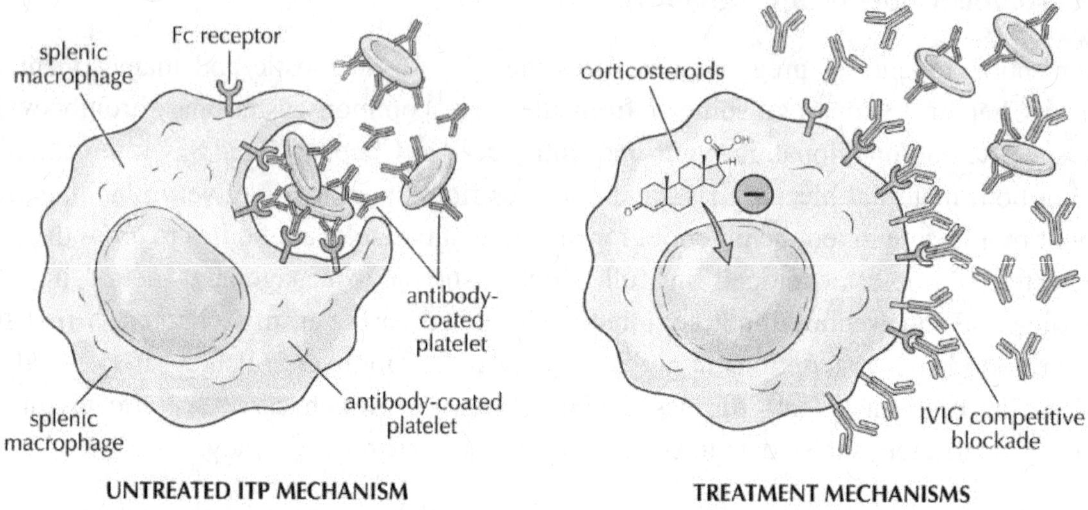

Figure 9.1: Mechanism of Corticosteroid and Intravenous Immunoglobulin Action in Immune Thrombocytopenia

Pediatric-Specific Management Considerations

As introduced earlier in this chapter, the favorable natural history and low serious bleeding risk characteristic of pediatric immune thrombocytopenia support an observation-favoring management approach in a well-appearing child with mild bleeding symptoms, reserving active treatment, generally favoring intravenous immunoglobulin or a brief corticosteroid course over the more prolonged treatment approaches sometimes required in adults, for children with more significant bleeding or specific risk factors including very young age or a lifestyle carrying elevated trauma risk. Splenectomy and the second-line agents discussed earlier in this chapter are generally reserved for the smaller subset of children who progress to chronic disease with clinically significant, treatment-refractory bleeding, reflecting the generally more favorable spontaneous remission rate in this age group compared with adults.

Family education and support are particularly important in pediatric immune thrombocytopenia management, given both the anxiety a new diagnosis in a child characteristically produces and the practical challenges of activity modification and bleeding precaution education for a child, extending the patient and family communication principles developed in Chapter 5 into this specific pediatric management context.

Long-Term Monitoring and Quality of Life

Structuring Long-Term Follow-Up

Patients with chronic immune thrombocytopenia require a structured long-term monitoring plan incorporating periodic platelet count assessment at a frequency calibrated to disease stability and current treatment, following the individualized monitoring philosophy developed in Chapter 8, along with periodic reassessment of bleeding symptoms using the structured bleeding assessment tools introduced in Chapter 5 and ongoing attention to treatment-specific monitoring requirements, including bone marrow reticulin fibrosis surveillance in patients on long-term thrombopoietin receptor agonist therapy and infection risk monitoring in splenectomized or immunosuppressed patients. This structured monitoring plan should be clearly documented and shared between the managing hematologist and the patient's primary care clinician, extending the shared care coordination principle developed in Chapter 8 into the specific long-term management context this chronic condition requires.

Monitoring frequency should be adjusted based on disease stability over time, with a patient in stable, long-standing remission requiring substantially less frequent monitoring than a patient with recently changed therapy or an unstable, fluctuating disease course, again reflecting the balance between clinical value and patient burden developed as a general monitoring principle in Chapter 8.

Integrating Quality of Life Into Ongoing Management

Given the fatigue and broader quality-of-life impact discussed earlier in this chapter, ongoing management should incorporate periodic quality-of-life assessment alongside the platelet count and bleeding-focused monitoring discussed above, recognizing that treatment decisions, including whether to escalate therapy for a stable but persistently low platelet count, should weigh quality-of-life impact and patient preference alongside the objective bleeding risk assessment, rather than pursuing platelet count normalization as an end in itself independent of its actual impact on the patient's wellbeing and daily function. This quality-of-life-integrated approach reflects an evolving shift in immune thrombocytopenia management philosophy, moving from a purely platelet count-driven treatment paradigm toward one that more holistically incorporates the patient's own experience and priorities.

Patient support resources, including connection with patient advocacy organizations and peer support communities specific to immune thrombocytopenia, can provide meaningful additional support beyond what clinical management alone provides, particularly for patients navigating the uncertainty of a chronic, relapsing-remitting disease course, and clinicians should be aware of and able to direct patients toward these resources as part of comprehensive, patient-centered long-term care.

Preparing Patients for a Lifelong Relationship With the Condition

For patients who progress to chronic immune thrombocytopenia, framing the condition as a manageable, monitorable chronic disease, analogous in this respect to other chronic autoimmune conditions, rather than as an acute crisis requiring perpetual anxiety, supports both psychological adjustment and sustained engagement with the long-term monitoring plan developed throughout this section. This framing should be introduced early in the disease course, ideally at the point chronic classification becomes likely or apparent, extending the transparent, forward-looking communication approach developed throughout this book into the specific challenge of helping a patient adjust to a lifelong, though generally manageable, hematologic condition.

This chapter has developed immune thrombocytopenia as the prototypical primary destructive thrombocytopenia within the broader mechanistic framework established in Chapter 8, and the chapters that follow extend this same rigorous, mechanism-based approach to the other important causes of thrombocytopenia this book addresses, beginning with drug-induced thrombocytopenia in Chapter 10, a category whose diagnostic exclusion, as emphasized throughout this chapter, is essential to correctly establishing an immune thrombocytopenia diagnosis in the first place.

CLINICAL CASE: A 52-year-old woman presents with a six-week history of easy bruising and is found to have a platelet count of 22 x10^9/L on complete blood count, confirmed by smear review showing no clumping, giant platelets consistent with a compensatory production response, and no schistocytes or other concerning morphology. Applying the diagnostic framework developed in this chapter, baseline testing is obtained, including hepatitis B and C serologies, human immunodeficiency virus testing, quantitative immunoglobulins, and antinuclear antibody testing, all of which return unremarkable, supporting a diagnosis of primary immune thrombocytopenia. Given her platelet count and moderate bleeding symptoms without wet purpura, she is started on a standard corticosteroid course, achieving a platelet count above 100 x10^9/L within ten days, but experiences a relapse to 18 x10^9/L during the corticosteroid taper at week six, meeting the persistent immune thrombocytopenia classification discussed earlier in this chapter given the ongoing corticosteroid dependency. Following shared decision-making incorporating her strong preference to avoid an indefinite injectable medication given her occupation and travel schedule, she elects treatment with rituximab, achieving a durable platelet count response sustained without further treatment for over eighteen months of follow-up. This case illustrates the complete diagnostic and management arc developed in this chapter: confirmatory laboratory evaluation, systematic secondary cause exclusion, individualized first-line treatment selection calibrated to bleeding severity, and shared decision-making guiding second-line therapy selection once a corticosteroid-dependent relapsing pattern was established.

THE PLATELET CRISIS DECISION COMPASS — Immune Thrombocytopenia Management Sequencing

---

Compass Recap: First-Line Treatment Urgency: A confirmed platelet count below approximately 20-30 x10^9/L in newly diagnosed immune thrombocytopenia warrants prompt first-line treatment initiation, regardless of whether major bleeding is yet present.

Compass Recap: Second-Line Sequencing: A corticosteroid-dependent relapse pattern meeting criteria for persistent immune thrombocytopenia prompts transition to second-line therapy selection rather than indefinite repeated corticosteroid courses.

Chapter Anchor: Immune thrombocytopenia is a diagnosis of exclusion requiring systematic secondary-cause evaluation at diagnosis, with treatment intensity calibrated to bleeding risk rather than platelet count alone, and management individualized across first-line, second-line, and splenectomy options through shared decision-making incorporating disease chronicity, response history, and patient preference.

Summary and Key Concepts

Immune thrombocytopenia is classified by duration (newly diagnosed, persistent, chronic) and by primary versus secondary status, with pediatric disease typically self-limited and adult disease more frequently chronic.

Pathophysiology involves both antibody-mediated peripheral platelet destruction (predominantly splenic, Fc receptor-mediated) and impaired compensatory megakaryopoiesis, providing the mechanistic rationale for both splenectomy and thrombopoietin receptor agonist therapy.

Diagnosis is exclusionary, requiring baseline evaluation for secondary causes (hepatitis B/C, HIV, immunoglobulin levels, H. pylori where relevant) rather than confirmation by a definitive positive test.

First-line therapy (corticosteroids, with or without intravenous immunoglobulin for rapid response) is selected based on bleeding urgency; second-line therapy (thrombopoietin receptor agonists, rituximab, other immunosuppressants) is reserved for persistent or chronic disease.

Splenectomy offers durable remission by removing the primary site of platelet destruction but carries lifelong infection risk and is generally deferred at least 12 months given spontaneous remission rates and expanding medical alternatives.

Special population management (pregnancy, older adults, children) requires distinct treatment thresholds and agent selection, and long-term care integrates quality-of-life assessment alongside platelet count and bleeding monitoring.

CHAPTER 10: DRUG-INDUCED THROMBOCYTOPENIA

Learning Objectives

1. Describe the hapten-dependent and drug-dependent antibody mechanisms underlying most drug-induced thrombocytopenia.
2. Recognize the characteristic timing and clinical pattern of drug-induced thrombocytopenia relative to medication exposure.
3. Identify the medication classes most frequently implicated in drug-induced thrombocytopenia, including their distinct mechanistic and clinical patterns.
4. Apply a structured causality assessment to determine the likelihood that a specific medication is responsible for a patient's thrombocytopenia.
5. Construct an appropriate management plan, including discontinuation strategy and rechallenge considerations.
6. Document a confirmed drug-induced thrombocytopenia episode for effective future clinical reference.

Chapter Outline

This chapter develops drug-induced thrombocytopenia as a distinct, mechanistically defined category within the destructive thrombocytopenia framework established in Chapter 8, addressing the epidemiology and clinical significance of this underrecognized condition, the hapten-dependent and drug-dependent antibody mechanisms that produce it, the specific medication classes and their recognizable patterns, a structured causality assessment approach, and management including discontinuation and rechallenge considerations. Two Platelet Crisis Decision Compass instances address recognition of the characteristic temporal pattern of drug-induced thrombocytopenia and the correct management of an unintentional rechallenge.

Drug-induced thrombocytopenia is substantially underrecognized in clinical practice, in part because its clinical presentation closely resembles immune thrombocytopenia, discussed in Chapter 9, and in part because the causative medication is frequently not among the drugs a clinician would immediately suspect. This chapter equips the reader to systematically consider and evaluate this diagnostic possibility, extending the thorough medication history developed in Chapter 5 into a structured mechanistic and causality framework specific to this condition.

Epidemiology and Clinical Significance

The Scope of the Problem

Drug-induced thrombocytopenia accounts for a meaningful proportion of newly identified thrombocytopenia in both outpatient and hospitalized populations, with estimates varying based on case-finding methodology and population studied, and the condition disproportionately affects older adults and hospitalized patients, populations characterized by the polypharmacy discussed in Chapter 8, which increases both the cumulative medication exposure and the diagnostic complexity of attributing thrombocytopenia to any single specific agent among many concurrent exposures. Underrecognition of this condition carries direct clinical consequences, since a missed diagnosis results in continued exposure to the causative medication, prolonging thrombocytopenia and its associated bleeding risk, and potentially triggering an unnecessary, more invasive evaluation directed at other causes when the straightforward solution of medication discontinuation would resolve the presentation.

Certain medication classes carry substantially higher drug-induced thrombocytopenia risk than others, and awareness of these higher-risk classes, developed throughout this chapter, allows the clinician to maintain appropriately heightened suspicion when evaluating new thrombocytopenia in a patient taking one of these specific agents, directly complementing the systematic medication history developed in Chapter 5 with the mechanistic and epidemiologic knowledge needed to correctly interpret that history.

Distinguishing Drug-Induced Thrombocytopenia From Direct Marrow Toxicity

This chapter addresses immune-mediated drug-induced thrombocytopenia specifically, a peripheral destructive process distinct from the direct, dose-dependent marrow-suppressive thrombocytopenia produced by cytotoxic chemotherapy and certain other medications with recognized, predictable marrow-suppressive effects, discussed within the production-limited mechanistic category developed in Chapter 8. This distinction matters clinically because immune-mediated drug-induced thrombocytopenia is characteristically idiosyncratic, dose-independent, and abrupt in onset, while direct marrow-suppressive thrombocytopenia is characteristically dose-related, predictable, and gradual, patterns that directly parallel the production-versus-destruction tempo distinction developed in Chapter 8.

Recognizing which mechanism applies to a specific suspected medication is essential to correctly anticipating the clinical course and appropriate management, since immune-mediated drug-induced thrombocytopenia typically resolves rapidly, often within one to two weeks, following discontinuation of the causative agent, while marrow-suppressive thrombocytopenia follows a more gradual recovery trajectory tied to marrow regeneration kinetics rather than the rapid antibody clearance dynamics discussed later in this chapter.

Clinical Consequences of Missed or Delayed Recognition

A missed diagnosis of drug-induced thrombocytopenia carries several downstream consequences beyond the immediate bleeding risk of continued thrombocytopenia: unnecessary continuation of an unrecognized causative medication perpetuates risk with each subsequent dose, an incorrect alternative diagnosis, most often immune thrombocytopenia, may lead to inappropriate immunosuppressive treatment carrying its own risks and costs without addressing the true underlying cause, and future inadvertent re-exposure to the same causative medication, without the benefit of prior recognition and documentation, risks a more severe recurrent episode given the anamnestic antibody response discussed later in this chapter.

These consequences underscore why systematic consideration of drug-induced thrombocytopenia, applying the framework developed throughout this chapter, deserves a consistent, deliberate place within the broader thrombocytopenia evaluation established in Chapter 8, rather than being considered only after other, more commonly suspected causes have been exhausted.

Mechanisms of Drug-Induced Platelet Destruction

Overview of Immune-Mediated Mechanisms

Immune-mediated drug-induced thrombocytopenia arises through several distinct but related antibody-mediated mechanisms, each ultimately producing accelerated platelet clearance analogous to the mechanisms developed for immune thrombocytopenia in Chapter 9, but triggered specifically by the presence of the causative drug rather than occurring independently of any external exposure. Understanding these distinct mechanisms, developed in the following subsections and the chapter's subsequent discussion of specific culprit medications, provides the conceptual foundation for recognizing the characteristic clinical patterns, including timing relative to exposure and behavior with rechallenge, that distinguish drug-induced thrombocytopenia from the other destructive processes discussed throughout this book.

This mechanistic understanding also directly informs diagnostic testing strategy, since laboratory confirmation of a drug-dependent antibody, discussed later in this chapter, requires the causative drug to be present in the testing system, a requirement that distinguishes drug-induced thrombocytopenia testing from the antibody testing discussed and generally not recommended for immune thrombocytopenia in Chapter 9.

Hapten-Dependent Mechanisms

In the hapten-dependent mechanism, the causative drug binds covalently to a platelet surface protein, creating a novel drug-protein complex that the immune system recognizes as foreign, generating antibodies directed against this drug-modified platelet surface epitope; these antibodies then bind platelets specifically in the presence of the drug, leading to Fc receptor-mediated clearance analogous to the mechanism developed for immune thrombocytopenia in Chapter 9. This mechanism is classically associated with penicillin and related beta-lactam antibiotics at high doses, though it is a less common cause of clinically significant drug-induced thrombocytopenia in contemporary practice than the drug-dependent antibody mechanism discussed next.

The hapten-dependent mechanism characteristically requires a relatively prolonged or high-dose drug exposure to generate the covalent drug-protein modification needed for antibody formation, distinguishing its typical exposure pattern from the drug-dependent antibody mechanism discussed below, which can occur with more modest cumulative exposure once sensitization has developed.

Drug-Dependent Antibody Mechanisms

The more common and clinically important mechanism involves drug-dependent antibodies that recognize a neoepitope formed by the noncovalent association of the drug with a specific platelet surface glycoprotein, most often glycoprotein IIb/IIIa or glycoprotein Ib-IX-V developed mechanistically in Chapter 2, without requiring covalent drug-protein binding; these antibodies bind platelets only in the presence of the circulating drug and dissociate once the drug is cleared, directly explaining the characteristically rapid platelet count recovery following drug discontinuation discussed earlier in this chapter. This mechanism underlies most of the specific, well-characterized drug-induced thrombocytopenia syndromes discussed later in this chapter, including quinine-associated and glycoprotein IIb/IIIa inhibitor-associated thrombocytopenia.

A related mechanism specific to certain glycoprotein IIb/IIIa inhibitors involves preexisting, naturally occurring antibodies that recognize a conformational change in the glycoprotein IIb/IIIa complex induced by the drug's binding, explaining the distinctive, often severe and abrupt-onset thrombocytopenia that can occur with first exposure to these specific agents, discussed in a dedicated section later in this chapter, without requiring the prior sensitizing exposure that most other drug-dependent antibody mechanisms require.

Common Culprit Medications and Their Recognition Patterns

Antimicrobial Agents

Beyond vancomycin, discussed in a dedicated section later in this chapter given its clinical importance, several other antimicrobial agents carry recognized drug-induced thrombocytopenia risk, including certain sulfonamide antibiotics, rifampin, and, historically, high-dose penicillins through the hapten-dependent mechanism discussed above. The temporal pattern for antimicrobial-associated drug-induced thrombocytopenia typically follows the drug-dependent antibody mechanism timing discussed later in this chapter, with onset most commonly within one to two weeks of a new exposure in a previously unsensitized patient, though prior sensitizing exposure, even remote in time, can produce a substantially more rapid and severe reaction upon reexposure.

Given the frequency with which antimicrobial agents are newly prescribed, particularly in the hospitalized setting discussed in Chapter 8, a systematic review of all recently started antimicrobial agents should be a routine component of the medication history whenever hospital-acquired thrombocytopenia is evaluated, applying the exposure timeline construction principle developed in Chapter 8 specifically to this medication category.

Cardiovascular and Anticoagulant Medications

Beyond heparin, addressed as a distinct and clinically critical entity in Chapter 11 given its specific pathophysiology and thrombotic risk, several other cardiovascular medications carry recognized drug-induced thrombocytopenia association, including certain antiarrhythmic agents structurally or mechanistically related to quinine, discussed in the dedicated section below, and, less commonly, certain antihypertensive agents. Glycoprotein IIb/IIIa inhibitors, discussed in a dedicated section later in this chapter, represent a particularly important cardiovascular medication category given their common use in acute coronary syndrome management and their distinctive capacity to produce severe, abrupt-onset thrombocytopenia even on first exposure.

The cardiovascular medication category illustrates the importance of considering both recently started and long-standing chronic medications when evaluating for drug-induced thrombocytopenia, since some cardiovascular drug-induced thrombocytopenia reactions can occur after months to years of previously well-tolerated use, reflecting either late sensitization or, in some cases, an unrelated intercurrent factor that has newly enabled a previously silent drug-dependent antibody to become clinically manifest.

Analgesic, Anticonvulsant, and Other Common Agents

A broad range of additional medications, including certain nonsteroidal anti-inflammatory drugs, several anticonvulsant agents, and select over-the-counter and herbal supplements, carry documented, though generally less frequent, drug-induced thrombocytopenia association, and this broad potential exposure list reinforces why the directed, specific medication and supplement questioning developed in Chapter 5, rather than a general open-ended medication history, is essential to identifying a potential causative agent that the patient might not otherwise think to report. Herbal and dietary supplements deserve particular attention in this context, since patients frequently do not consider these products medications warranting disclosure, despite several having recognized associations with drug-induced thrombocytopenia through mechanisms analogous to those discussed throughout this chapter.

Given the extensive and continually expanding list of medications with documented drug-induced thrombocytopenia association, clinicians evaluating a patient with new thrombocytopenia and an unclear alternative explanation should consult an updated, maintained reference database of drug-induced thrombocytopenia associations, since the causative medication list continues to grow as new agents are introduced and postmarketing surveillance identifies new associations not apparent at the time of initial drug approval.

THE PLATELET CRISIS DECISION COMPASS — Recognizing the Characteristic Timing Pattern of Drug-Induced Thrombocytopenia

The Presentation: A patient develops an abrupt platelet count drop from 220 to 12 x10^9/L with new petechiae and gum bleeding eight days after starting a new medication for a urinary tract infection, with no other clear explanation.

Mimic Signature: Genuine drug-dependent antibody-mediated thrombocytopenia from the new medication; new-onset primary immune thrombocytopenia coincidentally temporally associated with the medication start; and a superimposed infectious or septic process independently contributing to the thrombocytopenia.

The Decision: Recognize the eight-day interval as classically consistent with drug-dependent antibody sensitization timing; discontinue the suspected medication promptly, obtain smear review to exclude other destructive or production-limited processes, and monitor the platelet count trajectory over the following one to two weeks, during which a rapid recovery strongly supports the drug-induced etiology.

Trap Logic: Continuing a newly started medication because the temporal association 'could be coincidental' while pursuing an extensive alternative workup delays the single intervention, discontinuation, most likely to resolve a severe, high-risk thrombocytopenia.

Crisis Anchor: Abrupt severe thrombocytopenia occurring one to two weeks after a new medication exposure is treated as drug-induced until proven otherwise, with prompt discontinuation of the suspected agent regardless of whether alternative causes have been fully excluded.

Quinine and Quinine-Like Drug-Induced Thrombocytopenia

Quinine as the Prototypical Drug-Dependent Antibody Syndrome

Quinine, historically used for malaria treatment and, in lower doses, for nocturnal leg cramps, though this latter use is now discouraged given its thrombocytopenia risk relative to modest symptomatic benefit, produces one of the best-characterized drug-dependent antibody syndromes in the drug-induced thrombocytopenia literature, with the responsible antibodies binding to a quinine-induced neoepitope on glycoprotein IIb/IIIa or glycoprotein Ib-IX-V through the mechanism developed earlier in this chapter. Quinine-induced thrombocytopenia characteristically presents with abrupt, often severe thrombocytopenia, sometimes accompanied by acute hemolytic anemia or, less commonly, acute kidney injury reflecting a related antibody-mediated mechanism affecting other cell types and tissues, and clinicians should specifically ask about quinine-containing products, including some tonic water preparations and over-the-counter leg cramp remedies, which patients frequently do not consider medications warranting disclosure.

Given quinine's continued presence in some over-the-counter products and beverages despite its declining prescription use, maintaining awareness of quinine as a potential occult exposure remains clinically relevant, and a directed question about tonic water and over-the-counter leg cramp remedy use should be considered part of the comprehensive medication and exposure history whenever unexplained thrombocytopenia is evaluated, extending the supplement-specific questioning discussed earlier in this chapter to this specific, easily overlooked exposure category.

Quinidine and Related Antiarrhythmic Agents

Quinidine, structurally related to quinine and used as an antiarrhythmic agent, produces a mechanistically similar drug-dependent antibody syndrome, and cross-reactivity between quinine and quinidine antibodies has been documented, meaning a patient with a prior quinine-induced thrombocytopenia episode should be considered at elevated risk with quinidine exposure and vice versa, a cross-reactivity consideration directly relevant to the medication selection and avoidance counseling discussed later in this chapter. This cross-reactivity pattern illustrates a broader principle relevant to drug-induced thrombocytopenia counseling: structurally related medications within the same class may carry shared risk even when a specific alternative agent has not itself been directly implicated in a patient's prior episode, warranting caution when considering a structurally similar substitute medication.

This class-level caution should be balanced against the clinical need for effective alternative therapy, and consultation with a specialist familiar with the specific clinical indication, whether antiarrhythmic management or another therapeutic context, alongside hematology input regarding the specific cross-reactivity risk, supports an appropriately individualized decision regarding alternative medication selection following a confirmed quinine-class drug-induced thrombocytopenia episode.

Diagnostic Confirmation of Quinine-Class Reactions

Specialized reference laboratories can perform drug-dependent antibody testing specific to quinine and related compounds, typically using flow cytometric or enzyme-linked immunoassay methods that assess antibody binding to platelets specifically in the presence of the suspected drug, providing laboratory confirmation of the clinical diagnosis when the causative agent remains uncertain or when definitive confirmation would meaningfully affect future medication decisions. This specialized testing is not required to establish a working clinical diagnosis and initiate appropriate management, discussed later in this chapter, but can provide valuable confirmatory or exculpatory information in a complex case involving multiple concurrent medication exposures where clinical judgment alone cannot confidently identify a single causative agent.

Turnaround time for this specialized testing is typically measured in weeks, meaning results generally return well after the acute episode has resolved, and the primary clinical value of this testing lies in informing future medication avoidance counseling and, in ambiguous multi-drug exposure cases, retrospectively clarifying which of several suspected agents was the true causative culprit.

Vancomycin-Induced Thrombocytopenia

Recognition and Clinical Pattern

Vancomycin, among the most commonly used intravenous antibiotics in hospitalized patients, is a well-recognized cause of drug-dependent antibody-mediated thrombocytopenia, with onset typically within one to two weeks of exposure in a previously unsensitized patient, though onset can occur more rapidly with prior sensitizing exposure, and severity ranging from mild to severe, occasionally producing platelet counts low enough to carry substantial bleeding risk. Given vancomycin's widespread hospital use, particularly in the critically ill and postoperative populations discussed in the hospital-acquired thrombocytopenia context in Chapter 8, maintaining specific awareness of vancomycin as a potential causative agent is clinically important in any hospitalized patient receiving this medication who develops new thrombocytopenia without another clear explanation.

Vancomycin-induced thrombocytopenia is frequently underrecognized in the critically ill population specifically because these patients carry numerous alternative potential explanations for thrombocytopenia, including sepsis, disseminated intravascular coagulation, and multiple other concurrent medications, discussed in the broader critical illness context in Chapter 14, making vancomycin easy to overlook amid this complex differential unless specifically and systematically considered.

Confirmatory Testing and the Special Role of Vancomycin-Dependent Antibody Assays

Vancomycin-dependent platelet antibody testing is available at specialized reference laboratories and can provide diagnostic confirmation in cases where the clinical picture is ambiguous, particularly relevant in the critically ill population discussed above where multiple concurrent potential causes complicate clinical attribution, though as with the quinine-class testing discussed earlier in this chapter, this testing typically returns after the acute clinical decision to discontinue or continue vancomycin must already be made based on clinical judgment alone.

Given vancomycin's frequent role as a critical antimicrobial agent for serious infection, the decision to discontinue vancomycin in a patient with suspected drug-induced thrombocytopenia must weigh the infection-related risk of discontinuing an effective antimicrobial agent against the bleeding risk of continued severe thrombocytopenia, a risk-benefit assessment that should generally involve both infectious disease and hematology input when the suspected diagnosis carries significant clinical stakes in either direction.

Alternative Antimicrobial Selection After a Confirmed Episode

Following a confirmed or strongly suspected vancomycin-induced thrombocytopenia episode, alternative antimicrobial selection for the original infectious indication should be guided by infectious disease consultation, since vancomycin frequently serves as first-line therapy for serious gram-positive infections including methicillin-resistant Staphylococcus aureus, and identifying an appropriately effective alternative agent requires balancing the antimicrobial spectrum and efficacy needs of the underlying infection against the confirmed medication allergy or intolerance this episode establishes.

This alternative selection process should be clearly documented in the patient's medical record as a vancomycin-induced thrombocytopenia reaction, distinct from a standard drug allergy, using terminology specific enough that a future clinician encountering this documentation understands both the nature of the prior reaction and the specific rationale for avoiding future vancomycin exposure, extending the documentation principle developed throughout this book into this specific, clinically important medication avoidance context.

Glycoprotein IIb/IIIa Inhibitor-Induced Thrombocytopenia

The Distinctive First-Exposure Risk

Glycoprotein IIb/IIIa inhibitors, used in the management of acute coronary syndrome and during percutaneous coronary intervention, carry a distinctive drug-induced thrombocytopenia risk profile among the medications discussed in this chapter, since, as introduced earlier in this chapter, these agents can produce severe, abrupt-onset thrombocytopenia on first exposure through binding of preexisting naturally occurring antibodies to a drug-induced conformational change in the glycoprotein IIb/IIIa complex, rather than requiring the prior sensitizing exposure that most other drug-dependent antibody mechanisms discussed in this chapter require. This first-exposure risk means glycoprotein IIb/IIIa inhibitor-induced thrombocytopenia can occur within hours of the first dose, a distinctly rapid onset compared with the one-to-two-week typical sensitization interval discussed for other agents throughout this chapter, and this rapid onset carries direct implications for monitoring protocols in patients receiving these agents.

Given this rapid-onset risk, standard clinical protocols for glycoprotein IIb/IIIa inhibitor administration include platelet count monitoring within the first two to four hours of infusion initiation and again within twenty-four hours, allowing early detection of an abrupt platelet count decline before it progresses to severe thrombocytopenia with associated bleeding complications, a monitoring protocol that directly reflects this medication class's distinctive first-exposure risk profile.

Clinical Management of Suspected Glycoprotein IIb/IIIa Inhibitor Reactions

Management of suspected glycoprotein IIb/IIIa inhibitor-induced thrombocytopenia requires prompt discontinuation of the infusion, and given the clinical context in which these agents are typically used, often during or shortly after an acute coronary intervention, this discontinuation decision must be weighed against the ongoing antithrombotic needs of the underlying cardiac indication, a decision that should involve prompt cardiology and hematology coordination given the competing bleeding and thrombotic risks at play in this specific clinical scenario. Platelet transfusion, discussed further in the transfusion medicine context of Chapter 19, may be considered for severe thrombocytopenia with clinically significant bleeding in this setting, recognizing that transfused platelets may be similarly susceptible to the drug-dependent antibody while the causative agent remains present in the circulation, though the half-life of these agents is generally short enough that this limitation resolves relatively quickly following discontinuation.

Recovery from glycoprotein IIb/IIIa inhibitor-induced thrombocytopenia is typically rapid once the agent is discontinued, consistent with the drug-dependent antibody mechanism discussed earlier in this chapter, and platelet counts generally normalize within several days, allowing the clinical team to plan a return to standard antithrombotic management for the underlying cardiac indication once the acute thrombocytopenic episode has resolved.

Implications for Future Cardiac Care

A confirmed glycoprotein IIb/IIIa inhibitor-induced thrombocytopenia episode carries important implications for the patient's future cardiac care, since these agents may be considered again during a future acute coronary syndrome presentation if the prior episode is not clearly documented and readily accessible to the treating team, and clear, prominent documentation of this reaction, extending the documentation principle developed throughout this chapter, is essential given the time-sensitive nature of acute coronary syndrome management, where a treating team may not have time to obtain a detailed medication history before this class of agent might otherwise be considered.

This documentation should specify the particular agent involved, since cross-reactivity among different glycoprotein IIb/IIIa inhibitors is not absolute, and specialist cardiology and hematology input can help determine whether a different agent within this class might be cautiously considered in a future cardiac emergency if clinically necessary, versus whether the entire class should be avoided based on the specific mechanism and severity of the prior reaction.

THE PLATELET CRISIS DECISION COMPASS — Managing an Inadvertent Rechallenge with a Previously Implicated Medication

The Presentation: A patient with a documented history of vancomycin-induced thrombocytopenia two years ago is inadvertently started on vancomycin again during a new hospitalization, and the platelet count begins falling within six hours of the first dose.

Mimic Signature: A more rapid and severe recurrent drug-dependent antibody reaction reflecting anamnestic sensitization from the prior episode; a coincidental new cause of thrombocytopenia unrelated to the rechallenge; and a less severe reaction that may not require immediate discontinuation if the platelet count decline is modest and the clinical need for vancomycin is substantial.

The Decision: Discontinue vancomycin immediately upon recognition of the rechallenge and the falling platelet count, given the anamnestic response risk and the medication's already-documented causative role in this specific patient; do not wait for the platelet count to reach a specific severity threshold before intervening, since prior sensitization predicts a more rapid and potentially more severe course than the original episode.

Trap Logic: Continuing to monitor rather than immediately discontinuing a medication with a documented prior causative history in this specific patient, on the assumption that this episode might follow a milder course, disregards the anamnestic response principle that generally predicts a more rapid and severe reaction upon reexposure to a previously sensitizing drug.

Crisis Anchor: A documented prior drug-induced thrombocytopenia episode with a specific medication is an absolute contraindication to future rechallenge; any inadvertent rechallenge warrants immediate discontinuation upon recognition, not observation pending confirmation of severity.

Diagnostic Approach and Causality Assessment

A Structured Causality Framework

Given the frequent involvement of multiple concurrent medications in patients with suspected drug-induced thrombocytopenia, particularly in the hospitalized setting discussed in Chapter 8, a structured causality assessment framework, adapted from general drug adverse event causality methodology, provides a systematic approach to identifying the most likely causative agent among several candidates. Key elements of this structured assessment include the temporal relationship between drug initiation and thrombocytopenia onset, consistent with the one-to-two-week typical sensitization interval or the more rapid patterns discussed for specific agents earlier in this chapter, the platelet count response following discontinuation, exclusion of alternative explanations using the mechanistic framework developed in Chapter 8, and, where available, prior published literature or reference database documentation supporting the specific suspected agent's association with drug-induced thrombocytopenia.

Applying this structured framework systematically, rather than relying on an intuitive impression of which medication seems most likely responsible, improves diagnostic accuracy in the frequently complex, multi-medication clinical scenarios where drug-induced thrombocytopenia most often requires evaluation, and it produces a more defensible, well-documented causality assessment that better supports the future medication avoidance counseling and documentation discussed throughout this chapter.

The Role of Discontinuation and Rechallenge Response

The platelet count response following discontinuation of the suspected causative agent provides substantial diagnostic weight within the causality assessment framework, with a prompt platelet count recovery, typically within one to two weeks as discussed earlier in this chapter, following discontinuation of a single suspected agent providing strong supportive evidence for that agent's causative role, particularly when no other concurrent medication change or clinical event occurred during the same interval that might independently explain the recovery. Deliberate rechallenge, meaning intentional re-exposure to the suspected causative agent specifically to confirm the diagnosis through observation of a recurrent thrombocytopenic response, is generally not recommended given the risk of precipitating a severe, potentially anamnestic reaction as discussed in the Decision Compass instance above, and this approach should be reserved for the rare circumstance in which definitive causality confirmation is essential and no reasonable therapeutic alternative to the suspected agent exists.

In the more common scenario of multiple concurrent medication changes complicating causality assessment, sequential discontinuation, when clinically feasible and safe, of the medications considered most likely causative based on the structured assessment discussed above, observing the platelet count response after each discontinuation, can help isolate the specific causative agent among several candidates, though this sequential approach must be balanced against the clinical urgency of the presentation and the necessity of each medication for the patient's other active medical conditions.

When Multiple Plausible Candidates Cannot Be Distinguished

In some patients, particularly those with extensive polypharmacy and multiple recent medication changes, the causality assessment framework developed in this section will not definitively isolate a single causative agent, and in this circumstance, a pragmatic approach favoring discontinuation of all reasonably plausible candidate medications, when clinically feasible, followed by careful reintroduction of medications considered clinically essential one at a time with platelet count monitoring, provides both immediate clinical safety and, over time, useful diagnostic information regarding which specific agent, if any, was responsible.

This pragmatic, safety-first approach to diagnostic uncertainty parallels the broader philosophy developed throughout this book regarding the acceptance of diagnostic uncertainty when further evaluation carries diminishing returns, discussed explicitly in the platelet function testing context in Chapter 7, and it should be communicated transparently to the patient using the communication framework developed in Chapter 5, explaining that multiple medications are being cautiously reintroduced specifically to identify which, if any, was responsible for the prior episode.

Management: Discontinuation, Supportive Care, and Rechallenge Considerations

Immediate Management Priorities

The primary management intervention for confirmed or strongly suspected drug-induced thrombocytopenia is prompt discontinuation of the causative agent, and this single intervention, more than any pharmacologic treatment, drives the favorable prognosis and rapid recovery characteristic of this condition when correctly recognized and acted upon promptly, directly paralleling the emphasis on prompt recognition and action developed in the Decision Compass instances throughout this chapter. Supportive care for active bleeding, including platelet transfusion for clinically significant bleeding or a severely low platelet count in a patient at high procedural or bleeding risk, follows the general principles developed in Chapter 19, recognizing that transfused platelets in the setting of ongoing drug exposure carry the same vulnerability to the causative drug-dependent antibody discussed earlier in this chapter until the offending agent has been cleared.

Corticosteroids and intravenous immunoglobulin, the first-line agents for immune thrombocytopenia discussed in Chapter 9, have a less well-established, though sometimes still considered, role in drug-induced thrombocytopenia, and their use is generally reserved for severe, life-threatening bleeding when the more definitive intervention of drug discontinuation alone has not yet produced adequate platelet count recovery, rather than as routine first-line management for every confirmed or suspected drug-induced thrombocytopenia episode.

Anticipated Recovery Trajectory and Monitoring

Following discontinuation of the causative agent, platelet count monitoring should continue at a frequency appropriate to the severity of the presentation, generally daily during the acute recovery phase for a patient with severe thrombocytopenia or significant bleeding, extending to a less frequent outpatient monitoring schedule once a clear, sustained recovery trend has been established, applying the trend-based monitoring principles developed throughout Chapters 6 and 8 to this specific clinical scenario with its characteristically rapid and predictable recovery trajectory. A platelet count that fails to demonstrate the expected recovery trajectory within the typical one-to-two-week window discussed throughout this chapter should prompt diagnostic reconsideration, including reassessment for an alternative or additional concurrent cause of thrombocytopenia not fully addressed by the discontinuation of the initially suspected agent alone.

This monitoring approach exemplifies the trend-based diagnostic confirmation principle that recurs throughout this book: the platelet count trajectory following a specific intervention, in this case medication discontinuation, itself provides diagnostically meaningful information that either supports or challenges the working diagnosis, and clinicians should actively use this trajectory as ongoing diagnostic confirmation rather than passively awaiting recovery without continued diagnostic engagement.

Coordinating Management Across the Care Team

Effective management of drug-induced thrombocytopenia frequently requires coordination among the prescribing clinician for the causative medication's original indication, hematology, and, in specific contexts discussed throughout this chapter, the relevant subspecialty managing the underlying condition the causative medication was treating, including infectious disease for antimicrobial-associated reactions and cardiology for glycoprotein IIb/IIIa inhibitor-associated reactions. This multidisciplinary coordination directly extends the coordination principles developed for hospitalized thrombocytopenia in Chapter 8 into the specific context of balancing medication discontinuation against the ongoing clinical need the discontinued medication was addressing.

Clear communication among this care team regarding the working diagnosis, the plan for alternative therapy where needed, and the anticipated platelet count recovery trajectory reduces the risk of fragmented or conflicting management decisions and ensures that the medication avoidance and documentation priorities discussed throughout this chapter are consistently applied across every clinician involved in the patient's ongoing care.

Prevention and Documentation for Future Care

Medical Record Documentation Standards

Clear, specific, and prominent documentation of a confirmed or strongly suspected drug-induced thrombocytopenia episode is essential to preventing future inadvertent rechallenge, extending the longitudinal documentation principle developed throughout this book into a context where the consequence of inadequate documentation, as illustrated in the Decision Compass instance earlier in this chapter, can be a severe recurrent reaction. This documentation should specify the causative medication using both generic and relevant brand names, the clinical severity and course of the episode, the causality assessment supporting the diagnosis, and, where structurally related medications exist, an explicit note regarding cross-reactivity risk with those related agents, following the class-level caution principle discussed in the quinine-class section of this chapter.

This documentation should be entered as a structured medication allergy or intolerance entry within the electronic health record whenever the record system supports this level of specificity, rather than only as free-text progress note documentation that may not reliably trigger a future prescribing alert, since a structured allergy entry provides an additional systems-level safeguard against inadvertent rechallenge beyond what depends on a future clinician independently reviewing and recalling free-text documentation.

Patient Education and Self-Advocacy

Patient education regarding a confirmed drug-induced thrombocytopenia episode, extending the transparent communication principles developed in Chapter 5, should include clear identification of the specific causative medication, explanation of why future exposure must be avoided, and practical guidance on communicating this history to future healthcare providers, including emergency care providers who may not have ready access to the patient's complete medical record. Providing the patient with a written summary of the episode, including the specific medication name and the nature of the reaction, supports this self-advocacy role and provides a durable, patient-carried record independent of any single health system's electronic record, particularly valuable for a patient who may receive care across multiple different health systems over time.

This patient education and self-advocacy emphasis parallels the medical identification and self-advocacy principles relevant to other serious medication reactions and allergies, and it reflects the broader theme developed throughout this book that effective long-term management extends beyond the acute clinical episode itself to encompass the systems and practices that prevent recurrence over the patient's subsequent lifetime of medical care.

Systems-Level Prevention Strategies

Beyond individual patient documentation, health systems can implement broader systems-level strategies to reduce drug-induced thrombocytopenia risk and improve recognition, including clinical decision support alerts triggered by new thrombocytopenia in a patient recently started on a medication with recognized drug-induced thrombocytopenia association, standardized platelet count monitoring protocols for high-risk medications such as the glycoprotein IIb/IIIa inhibitor monitoring discussed earlier in this chapter, and structured medication reconciliation processes that specifically prompt review of recently started medications whenever new thrombocytopenia is identified in a hospitalized patient.

These systems-level interventions parallel the institutional reflex-building discussion introduced in Chapter 6 for platelet count verification, and their implementation reflects a mature, systematic approach to patient safety that extends beyond reliance on individual clinician vigilance alone, closing this chapter's development of drug-induced thrombocytopenia and setting the stage for Chapter 11's focused treatment of heparin-induced thrombocytopenia, a specific and clinically critical subtype of drug-induced thrombocytopenia distinguished by its associated thrombotic, rather than purely bleeding, risk.

Special Considerations in Oncology and Chemotherapy-Adjacent Contexts

Distinguishing Immune-Mediated Reactions From Cytotoxic Marrow Suppression

Patients receiving cancer treatment present a particularly complex diagnostic context for suspected immune-mediated drug-induced thrombocytopenia, since the expected, dose-dependent marrow-suppressive thrombocytopenia produced by cytotoxic chemotherapy itself, discussed within the production-limited mechanistic framework in Chapter 8, must be distinguished from a superimposed immune-mediated reaction to a non-chemotherapy medication, such as an antimicrobial agent used for a chemotherapy-related infection, using the tempo and pattern principles developed throughout this chapter. A platelet count decline that occurs earlier than expected relative to the chemotherapy cycle timeline, or one whose severity or trajectory does not match the patient's own prior chemotherapy cycles, should prompt consideration of an immune-mediated drug-induced thrombocytopenia superimposed on the expected chemotherapy-related nadir, applying the same medication timeline construction principle developed earlier in this chapter to this specific, more complex clinical context.

This distinction carries direct management implications, since expected chemotherapy-related marrow suppression is managed with supportive care and dose or schedule adjustment for future cycles, discussed further in Chapter 19 regarding transfusion support, while a superimposed immune-mediated reaction to a specific non-chemotherapy agent is managed through the discontinuation-focused approach developed throughout this chapter, and correctly distinguishing between these two processes prevents both under-recognition of a treatable immune-mediated reaction and unnecessary chemotherapy dose reduction attributed incorrectly to the chemotherapy regimen itself.

Targeted Cancer Therapies and Novel Agent Considerations

Beyond traditional cytotoxic chemotherapy, an expanding range of targeted cancer therapies, including certain kinase inhibitors and immune checkpoint inhibitors, carry their own distinct and evolving thrombocytopenia risk profiles, in some cases through immune-mediated mechanisms sharing features with the drug-dependent antibody mechanisms discussed throughout this chapter, and in other cases through direct effects on megakaryocyte function or an immune-related adverse event mechanism more closely resembling secondary immune thrombocytopenia, discussed in the secondary associations section of Chapter 9, than the classic drug-dependent antibody pattern this chapter has primarily emphasized.

Immune checkpoint inhibitor-associated thrombocytopenia in particular often behaves clinically more like immune thrombocytopenia than like the drug-dependent antibody pattern characteristic of the agents discussed earlier in this chapter, including a less predictable relationship to drug clearance and a correspondingly reduced likelihood of rapid resolution with drug discontinuation alone, sometimes requiring the immunosuppressive management approaches discussed in Chapter 9 rather than discontinuation alone.

Given the rapidly evolving landscape of novel cancer therapeutics and their associated thrombocytopenia mechanisms, clinicians managing patients on these newer agents should consult current, regularly updated pharmacovigilance resources and maintain close collaboration with the treating oncology team, since the specific mechanism, expected timeline, and appropriate management approach for thrombocytopenia associated with a specific novel agent may not follow the classic drug-dependent antibody pattern this chapter has primarily developed and may instead require a management approach more closely paralleling the secondary immune thrombocytopenia framework discussed in Chapter 9.

Balancing Cancer Treatment Continuity Against Bleeding Risk

The decision to discontinue, dose-reduce, or continue a cancer therapy associated with suspected drug-induced thrombocytopenia requires careful multidisciplinary weighing of the oncologic consequences of treatment interruption against the bleeding risk of continued thrombocytopenia, a balance that differs meaningfully from the more straightforward discontinuation decision typical of the non-oncologic medications discussed earlier in this chapter, since discontinuing or substantially delaying cancer-directed therapy can carry its own serious, sometimes life-threatening consequences for disease control. This balance should involve explicit discussion with the patient regarding the relative risks of each option, extending the shared decision-making and transparent communication principles developed throughout this book into this specific, high-stakes oncologic context, with the final decision reflecting both the objective risk-benefit assessment and the individual patient's own values and priorities regarding cancer treatment continuity.

Hematology-oncology co-management, with hematology providing specific expertise in the drug-induced thrombocytopenia mechanism and diagnostic approach developed throughout this chapter and oncology providing the disease-specific context regarding treatment alternatives and the consequences of interruption, represents the optimal model for navigating this complex decision, and this collaborative model reflects the broader multidisciplinary coordination theme that has recurred throughout the diagnostic and management chapters of this book.

CLINICAL CASE: A 71-year-old man hospitalized for a complicated skin and soft tissue infection is started on vancomycin, and after nine days of therapy his platelet count, previously stable at 210 x10^9/L throughout the admission, falls abruptly to 14 x10^9/L, accompanied by new petechiae on his lower extremities. Applying the diagnostic framework developed in this chapter, the medical team constructs a timeline of all medication changes over the admission, identifying vancomycin as the medication whose timing most closely matches the classic one-to-two-week drug-dependent antibody sensitization interval, while noting that several other medications had been started earlier in the admission without temporal correlation to the platelet count decline. Peripheral smear review, applying the framework from Chapter 6, excludes clumping and shows no schistocytes or other concerning findings, and given the high pretest probability established by the timing and the absence of a more compelling alternative explanation, vancomycin is discontinued and the patient is transitioned to an alternative antibiotic selected in consultation with infectious disease. The platelet count begins recovering within four days and returns to baseline within twelve days of discontinuation, a trajectory strongly supporting the drug-induced diagnosis per the causality framework developed in this chapter. Vancomycin-dependent antibody testing, sent before discontinuation, subsequently returns positive, providing laboratory confirmation, and the reaction is documented as a structured medication allergy entry with explicit instruction against future vancomycin use, along with a written patient summary provided at discharge. This case illustrates the complete diagnostic and management arc developed in this chapter: systematic timeline construction across multiple concurrent medications, structured causality assessment integrating timing and discontinuation response, prompt intervention without awaiting confirmatory testing, and durable documentation to prevent future inadvertent rechallenge.

THE PLATELET CRISIS DECISION COMPASS — Drug-Induced Thrombocytopenia Recognition and Prevention

---

Compass Recap: Recognizing the Timing Pattern: Abrupt severe thrombocytopenia occurring one to two weeks after a new medication exposure is treated as drug-induced until proven otherwise, with prompt discontinuation of the suspected agent regardless of whether alternative causes have been fully excluded.

Compass Recap: Preventing Rechallenge: A documented prior drug-induced thrombocytopenia episode with a specific medication is an absolute contraindication to future rechallenge; any inadvertent rechallenge warrants immediate discontinuation upon recognition, not observation pending confirmation of severity.

Chapter Anchor: Drug-induced thrombocytopenia is recognized through systematic medication timeline construction against the characteristic drug-dependent antibody sensitization interval, confirmed by prompt platelet count recovery following discontinuation of the causative agent, and prevented from recurrence through structured, durable medical record documentation and patient self-advocacy education.

Summary and Key Concepts

Drug-induced thrombocytopenia is a substantially underrecognized cause of thrombocytopenia, distinct from direct dose-dependent marrow-suppressive drug effects, arising through hapten-dependent or, more commonly, drug-dependent antibody mechanisms.

Characteristic timing is one to two weeks after a new exposure in an unsensitized patient, with prior sensitization producing a more rapid and often more severe reaction upon reexposure.

Quinine and quinidine, vancomycin, and glycoprotein IIb/IIIa inhibitors represent well-characterized culprit medications, each with distinct recognition patterns — glycoprotein IIb/IIIa inhibitors uniquely can cause severe thrombocytopenia on first exposure.

A structured causality assessment integrating exposure timing, discontinuation response, and exclusion of alternative causes should guide diagnosis, particularly given frequent polypharmacy complicating attribution to a single agent.

Prompt discontinuation of the causative agent is the primary and most effective management intervention, typically producing platelet count recovery within one to two weeks.

Durable, structured medical record documentation and patient education are essential to prevent inadvertent future rechallenge, which carries anamnestic risk of a more rapid and severe recurrent reaction.

CHAPTER 11: HEPARIN-INDUCED THROMBOCYTOPENIA

Learning Objectives

1. Explain the platelet factor 4-heparin complex immunogenicity underlying heparin-induced thrombocytopenia pathophysiology.
2. Apply the 4Ts pretest probability score to structure the evaluation of suspected heparin-induced thrombocytopenia.
3. Interpret immunoassay and functional laboratory testing for heparin-induced thrombocytopenia within the context of pretest probability.
4. Recognize the thrombotic complications characteristic of heparin-induced thrombocytopenia and distinguish this condition from other causes of hospital-acquired thrombocytopenia.
5. Select an appropriate alternative anticoagulation strategy for confirmed or strongly suspected heparin-induced thrombocytopenia.
6. Construct a transition plan from alternative anticoagulation to long-term therapy following recovery.

Chapter Outline

This chapter develops heparin-induced thrombocytopenia as a distinct, high-stakes subtype of drug-induced thrombocytopenia, extending Chapter 10's general framework to a condition whose defining feature, in contrast to most other content addressed in this book, is thrombotic rather than purely bleeding risk. It addresses the platelet factor 4-heparin immune mechanism, clinical presentation and timing, the 4Ts pretest probability score, laboratory diagnosis, thrombotic complications, alternative anticoagulation management, special clinical scenarios, and long-term transition planning. Two Platelet Crisis Decision Compass instances address the calculation and application of the 4Ts score and the management of a patient with confirmed heparin-induced thrombocytopenia and thrombosis.

Heparin-induced thrombocytopenia occupies a unique position within this book's broader thrombocytopenia framework: unlike nearly every other condition discussed in Part III, in which the primary clinical concern is bleeding, heparin-induced thrombocytopenia is defined by its associated thrombotic risk, and this inversion of the usual bleeding-focused clinical concern requires the reader to apply a management approach that, at first encounter, can feel counterintuitive relative to the bleeding-focused framework developed throughout the preceding chapters.

Epidemiology and Risk Factors

Incidence and Population Variation

Heparin-induced thrombocytopenia occurs in a small but clinically important minority of patients exposed to heparin, with incidence varying substantially based on the specific heparin preparation used, the clinical population, and the duration of exposure, and unfractionated heparin carries a meaningfully higher risk than low molecular weight heparin, reflecting differences in the platelet factor 4 binding affinity discussed later in this chapter between these two heparin preparations. Surgical patients, particularly those undergoing cardiac and orthopedic surgery, carry higher heparin-induced thrombocytopenia risk than medical patients, reflecting both greater platelet activation from the surgical process itself and, in cardiac surgery specifically, the large heparin doses required for cardiopulmonary bypass, a specific clinical context discussed further later in this chapter.

This population-specific risk variation should directly inform the clinical index of suspicion applied when evaluating new thrombocytopenia in a heparin-exposed patient, with a lower threshold for considering heparin-induced thrombocytopenia in a postoperative cardiac or orthopedic surgical patient receiving unfractionated heparin than in a medical patient receiving prophylactic low molecular weight heparin, though the condition can occur, less commonly, in this lower-risk population as well and should not be entirely dismissed based on risk category alone.

Risk Factors Beyond Heparin Formulation

Beyond the specific heparin preparation and clinical population discussed above, several additional factors influence individual patient risk, including female sex, which carries a modestly elevated risk in most studied populations, and prior heparin exposure, which, as discussed in the drug-induced thrombocytopenia sensitization framework developed in Chapter 10, can influence the timing and severity of a subsequent reaction, though heparin-induced thrombocytopenia differs mechanistically from the classic drug-dependent antibody pattern discussed in that chapter in ways developed further in the pathophysiology section below. Duration of heparin exposure also influences risk, with the classic five-to-ten-day timing discussed later in this chapter reflecting the time typically required for antibody formation with new exposure, though this timing consideration itself becomes a critical diagnostic tool rather than merely a risk factor, as developed in the pretest probability discussion later in this chapter.

Understanding this constellation of risk factors allows the clinician to calibrate clinical suspicion appropriately when evaluating a specific patient, directly feeding into the structured pretest probability assessment that forms the diagnostic core of this chapter, rather than applying a uniform level of suspicion regardless of the specific patient's individual risk profile and heparin exposure context.

The Clinical Stakes of Missed or Delayed Diagnosis

The clinical stakes of a missed or delayed heparin-induced thrombocytopenia diagnosis are substantially higher than for most other conditions discussed in this book, since continued heparin exposure in a patient with unrecognized heparin-induced thrombocytopenia carries a high risk of progression to the thrombotic complications discussed later in this chapter, complications that carry substantial morbidity and mortality risk disproportionate to the platelet count itself. This elevated stakes profile justifies the structured, systematic diagnostic approach developed throughout this chapter and supports a lower threshold for empiric alternative anticoagulation while diagnostic evaluation is pending, discussed further in the management section of this chapter, compared with the more diagnosis-confirmation-first approach appropriate to most other conditions addressed throughout this book.

This distinct risk-benefit calculus, favoring prompt empiric action over awaiting full diagnostic confirmation, represents a deliberate departure from the more measured diagnostic pacing emphasized elsewhere in this book, and understanding why this departure is justified, rooted in the specific thrombotic pathophysiology developed in the next section, is essential to correctly applying this chapter's management recommendations in clinical practice.

Pathophysiology: Platelet Factor 4-Heparin Complex Immunogenicity

Formation of the Immunogenic Complex

Heparin-induced thrombocytopenia arises when heparin binds platelet factor 4, a positively charged chemokine released from platelet alpha granules as developed in Chapter 1, forming a multimolecular complex whose specific molecular configuration creates a neoepitope recognized as foreign by the immune system, generating immunoglobulin G antibodies directed against this platelet factor 4-heparin complex rather than against heparin or platelet factor 4 individually. This mechanism distinguishes heparin-induced thrombocytopenia from the drug-dependent antibody mechanisms discussed in Chapter 10, since the antigenic target is a complex formed between the drug and an endogenous platelet protein rather than a neoepitope on a platelet surface receptor directly modified by the drug itself.

Unfractionated heparin's longer polysaccharide chains form this immunogenic complex more readily than the shorter chains of low molecular weight heparin, directly explaining the differential risk between these two preparations discussed earlier in this chapter, and this same structural principle explains why fondaparinux, a synthetic pentasaccharide too short to effectively bridge platelet factor 4 molecules into an immunogenic complex, carries minimal heparin-induced thrombocytopenia risk and serves as an important alternative anticoagulant discussed later in this chapter.

The Platelet-Activating Consequence of Antibody Binding

Once formed, the platelet factor 4-heparin-immunoglobulin G immune complex binds the platelet Fc gamma receptor IIa developed in Chapter 2, producing platelet activation rather than the phagocytic clearance mechanism characteristic of the immune thrombocytopenia and drug-induced thrombocytopenia mechanisms discussed in Chapters 9 and 10; this activation triggers platelet aggregation, degranulation with further platelet factor 4 release creating a self-amplifying cycle, and generation of platelet-derived microparticles with potent procoagulant activity, directly explaining the paradoxical combination of thrombocytopenia and thrombotic risk that defines this condition and distinguishes it fundamentally from every other condition addressed in Part III of this book.

This platelet-activating mechanism additionally triggers monocyte and endothelial cell activation through analogous immune complex binding, further amplifying the procoagulant state through tissue factor expression and additional prothrombotic pathway activation, illustrating that heparin-induced thrombocytopenia thrombotic risk arises from a multicellular activation process rather than platelet activation alone, a mechanistic breadth that helps explain the severity and diversity of thrombotic complications discussed later in this chapter.

Antibody Formation Timing and the Anamnestic Response

The classic five-to-ten-day timing for heparin-induced thrombocytopenia onset in a heparin-naive patient reflects the time required for de novo antibody formation against the platelet factor 4-heparin complex, directly analogous to the sensitization timing discussed for other drug-dependent antibody mechanisms in Chapter 10, while a patient with heparin exposure within the preceding approximately one hundred days may experience a substantially more rapid onset, sometimes within hours of reexposure, reflecting a preexisting antibody population from the prior exposure, a pattern termed rapid-onset heparin-induced thrombocytopenia that parallels the anamnestic response discussed for other drug-induced thrombocytopenia syndromes in Chapter 10.

Beyond approximately one hundred days from a prior heparin exposure, circulating platelet factor 4-heparin antibody levels typically decline substantially, meaning a patient with more remote prior heparin-induced thrombocytopenia may not necessarily experience the rapid-onset pattern with renewed heparin exposure after this interval, though current management guidance, discussed in the long-term transition section later in this chapter, generally still favors heparin avoidance in a patient with a confirmed prior episode regardless of the interval elapsed, given both the residual uncertainty in this risk stratification and the availability of effective alternative anticoagulants that avoid this uncertainty altogether.

Clinical Presentation and Timing Patterns

The Typical Platelet Count Pattern

Heparin-induced thrombocytopenia characteristically produces a platelet count decline of at least fifty percent from a documented pre-heparin baseline, though the absolute platelet count nadir is frequently only moderately reduced, often remaining above 20 x10^9/L, distinguishing the typical severity pattern from the more severe absolute thrombocytopenia often seen in immune thrombocytopenia discussed in Chapter 9; this relative decline pattern means that a platelet count that remains within the numerically normal reference range can still represent clinically significant heparin-induced thrombocytopenia if it reflects a substantial decline from an elevated pre-heparin baseline, a nuance that requires access to and comparison against a documented baseline count rather than interpretation of the isolated absolute value alone.

This emphasis on relative decline from baseline, rather than absolute platelet count threshold, directly extends the trend-based interpretation principle developed throughout Chapters 6 and 8 into this specific, high-stakes diagnostic context, and it underscores the clinical importance of obtaining and documenting a baseline platelet count before or at the time of heparin initiation whenever feasible, allowing this critical trend comparison to be made accurately when new thrombocytopenia is subsequently identified.

Distinguishing Typical-Onset From Rapid-Onset and Delayed-Onset Presentations

As introduced in the pathophysiology section above, three distinct temporal presentation patterns are recognized: typical-onset heparin-induced thrombocytopenia, occurring five to ten days after heparin initiation in a previously heparin-naive patient; rapid-onset heparin-induced thrombocytopenia, occurring within twenty-four hours of reexposure in a patient with recent prior heparin exposure and preexisting circulating antibody; and delayed-onset heparin-induced thrombocytopenia, a less common but clinically important pattern in which thrombocytopenia and thrombosis develop or worsen after heparin has already been discontinued, reflecting unusually high-titer, persistent antibody activity that continues to activate platelets even without ongoing heparin exposure.

Delayed-onset heparin-induced thrombocytopenia deserves particular clinical attention because it can be easily overlooked, since the temporal disconnect from active heparin administration works against the intuitive timing-based suspicion this chapter otherwise emphasizes, and clinicians should maintain awareness of this pattern in a patient presenting with new thrombocytopenia and thrombosis within several weeks of a discontinued heparin exposure, even when heparin itself is no longer being administered at the time of presentation.

Non-Thrombocytopenic and Atypical Presentations

A small subset of patients with heparin-induced thrombocytopenia present with thrombosis and the characteristic platelet factor 4-heparin antibody without meeting the classic fifty percent platelet count decline threshold, an atypical presentation sometimes termed heparin-induced thrombocytopenia with isolated thrombosis, and awareness of this atypical pattern is clinically relevant when evaluating a heparin-exposed patient with new, otherwise unexplained thrombosis even in the absence of a clearly qualifying platelet count decline. Skin necrosis at heparin injection sites, an uncommon but distinctive dermatologic manifestation reflecting local microvascular thrombosis from the same underlying mechanism, represents another atypical presentation that should prompt heparin-induced thrombocytopenia consideration even when the systemic platelet count decline is comparatively modest.

Recognizing these atypical presentation patterns, alongside the more classic thrombocytopenia-predominant presentation discussed throughout most of this chapter, reinforces the importance of applying the full diagnostic framework developed in this chapter, including the pretest probability scoring discussed next, in any heparin-exposed patient with a clinical picture suggestive of this condition, rather than relying exclusively on platelet count decline as a strict gatekeeping criterion before considering the diagnosis.

Pretest Probability: The 4Ts Score

The Four Components of the 4Ts Score

The 4Ts score, the most widely validated and clinically used pretest probability tool for heparin-induced thrombocytopenia, assigns a score of zero, one, or two points across four categories: the magnitude of Thrombocytopenia, favoring a decline greater than fifty percent to a nadir above 20 x10^9/L; the Timing of platelet count decline relative to heparin exposure, favoring the classic five-to-ten-day or rapid-onset patterns discussed earlier in this chapter; the presence of new Thrombosis or other clinical sequelae including skin necrosis; and the likelihood of oTher causes of thrombocytopenia, applying the broader mechanistic differential diagnosis developed in Chapter 8 to assess whether an alternative, non-heparin explanation is more likely. The summed score, ranging from zero to eight, stratifies patients into low, intermediate, and high pretest probability categories that directly inform both the value of subsequent laboratory testing and the appropriate immediate management approach discussed later in this chapter.

The 4Ts score's principal clinical value lies in its strong negative predictive value at the low-probability category, where the diagnosis of heparin-induced thrombocytopenia can generally be considered excluded without further laboratory testing, allowing clinicians to confidently avoid unnecessary alternative anticoagulation and its associated cost and bleeding risk in patients whose presentation does not genuinely suggest this diagnosis, a diagnostic efficiency benefit directly analogous to the negative predictive value discussion of the bleeding assessment tool developed in Chapter 5.

Applying the Score in Practice

Correct application of the 4Ts score requires deliberate, structured scoring across each of the four categories rather than an intuitive overall gestalt impression, since research has demonstrated that informal, non-structured clinical impression correlates poorly with the validated score and with actual laboratory-confirmed heparin-induced thrombocytopenia status, directly reinforcing the structured-tool-over-intuition principle developed throughout this book, including the bleeding assessment tool discussion in Chapter 5. The scoring exercise should be performed and documented at the time heparin-induced thrombocytopenia is first clinically suspected, providing both immediate diagnostic and management guidance and a durable, auditable record of the clinical reasoning supporting whatever management decision follows.

Institutional adoption of a structured, ideally electronic health record-integrated 4Ts scoring tool, directly paralleling the structured referral template discussion introduced in Chapter 8, improves both the consistency and the documentation quality of this critical diagnostic step, and health systems managing substantial heparin-exposed patient populations should consider implementing such structured tools as a systems-level safeguard against the diagnostic inconsistency that unstructured clinical assessment alone can produce.

Limitations of the 4Ts Score

Despite its strong validation and widespread use, the 4Ts score carries recognized limitations, including modest interobserver reliability, particularly in the scoring of the oTher-causes category, which requires clinical judgment regarding the broader differential diagnosis rather than an objective, easily standardized criterion, and reduced discriminative performance in certain populations, including critically ill patients in whom the broader differential diagnosis for thrombocytopenia developed in Chapter 8 is inherently wider and more difficult to confidently exclude. These limitations support continued clinical judgment alongside, rather than as a complete substitute for, the structured 4Ts score, particularly in atypical or complex clinical presentations where the score's assumptions may not fully apply.

Despite these limitations, the 4Ts score remains the recommended first-step structured assessment for suspected heparin-induced thrombocytopenia across current major guidelines, and its systematic application, understanding both its strengths and limitations, forms the essential first step of the diagnostic and management pathway this chapter develops.

THE PLATELET CRISIS DECISION COMPASS — Applying the 4Ts Score to Guide Immediate Management

---

The Presentation: A patient receiving therapeutic unfractionated heparin for seven days develops a platelet count decline from 260 to 95 x10^9/L, with no new thrombosis identified and several other plausible alternative explanations including recent surgery and a concurrent infection.

Mimic Signature: Genuine heparin-induced thrombocytopenia at intermediate probability given the timing and magnitude of decline; postoperative thrombocytopenia from surgical platelet consumption; and infection-associated thrombocytopenia from the concurrent infectious process, each plausible alternative explanations captured within the oTher-causes 4Ts component.

The Decision: Calculate the formal 4Ts score rather than relying on gestalt impression; an intermediate score in this scenario warrants sending laboratory testing while simultaneously discontinuing heparin and transitioning to an alternative non-heparin anticoagulant pending results, rather than either continuing heparin while awaiting results or assuming the alternative explanations fully account for the presentation without testing.

Trap Logic: Continuing heparin while awaiting laboratory confirmation in a patient with an intermediate or high 4Ts score, on the reasoning that alternative explanations seem equally or more plausible, disregards the asymmetric risk this chapter has emphasized: the consequence of continued heparin exposure in true heparin-induced thrombocytopenia is thrombosis, a risk too severe to accept while awaiting confirmatory testing in an intermediate-or-higher probability patient.

Crisis Anchor: An intermediate or high 4Ts score prompts immediate heparin discontinuation and transition to alternative anticoagulation, with laboratory testing sent concurrently rather than management decisions deferred until results return.

Laboratory Diagnosis: Immunoassay and Functional Testing

Immunoassay Testing

Enzyme-linked immunosorbent assay testing for antibodies against the platelet factor 4-heparin complex is widely available, provides rapid turnaround often within hours, and offers high sensitivity for heparin-induced thrombocytopenia, making a negative result at appropriate optical density thresholds useful for excluding the diagnosis, particularly valuable in a patient with intermediate 4Ts probability where diagnostic clarification meaningfully affects management. This high sensitivity comes at the cost of comparatively lower specificity, since many hospitalized and heparin-exposed patients develop platelet factor 4-heparin antibodies without ever developing the clinical syndrome of heparin-induced thrombocytopenia, meaning a positive immunoassay result alone, particularly at a low-positive optical density, does not definitively confirm clinically significant heparin-induced thrombocytopenia and should be interpreted in conjunction with the 4Ts pretest probability rather than as a standalone diagnostic answer.

The optical density value of a positive immunoassay result carries additional interpretive value beyond a simple positive-negative determination, with higher optical density values correlating with a substantially higher likelihood of a positive confirmatory functional assay, discussed next, and this quantitative interpretation, when combined with the 4Ts score, provides a more refined post-test probability estimate than either the score or the immunoassay result considered in isolation, directly applying the multi-source diagnostic integration principle that has recurred throughout this book.

Functional Testing: The Serotonin Release Assay and Alternatives

The serotonin release assay, the reference standard functional test for heparin-induced thrombocytopenia, assesses whether patient serum, in the presence of heparin, activates donor platelets sufficient to trigger serotonin release, directly confirming the platelet-activating functional consequence of the antibody discussed in the pathophysiology section of this chapter, rather than merely detecting antibody presence as the immunoassay does. This functional confirmation provides substantially higher specificity than immunoassay testing alone, since it specifically identifies platelet-activating antibodies rather than the broader population of platelet factor 4-heparin antibodies detected by immunoassay, but the serotonin release assay requires specialized reference laboratory performance and radioactive material handling, resulting in turnaround times typically measured in days, limiting its utility for the immediate management decisions this chapter has emphasized must often proceed before confirmatory testing returns.

The heparin-induced platelet activation assay and other functional testing alternatives to the serotonin release assay provide comparable functional confirmation through alternative platelet activation readouts, with varying availability across different reference laboratories, and clinicians should be familiar with which specific functional assay their institution's reference laboratory performs and its expected turnaround time when planning the diagnostic and management sequence for a specific patient.

Integrating Immunoassay and Functional Testing With Clinical Probability

The most reliable diagnostic conclusion in suspected heparin-induced thrombocytopenia emerges from integrating the 4Ts pretest probability, the immunoassay result and its optical density value, and, when available, functional testing confirmation, following a Bayesian diagnostic reasoning approach in which each successive test result refines the probability estimate established by the preceding assessment, directly extending the multi-source integration principle developed throughout this book into this specific, algorithmically well-characterized diagnostic context. A low 4Ts score with a negative immunoassay essentially excludes the diagnosis without further testing, a high 4Ts score with a strongly positive immunoassay supports proceeding with alternative anticoagulation management even before functional testing returns, and the more genuinely ambiguous combinations, such as an intermediate 4Ts score with a weakly positive immunoassay, most benefit from functional testing to resolve the diagnostic uncertainty when clinically feasible.

This integrated, staged diagnostic approach allows the clinician to make timely management decisions at each stage of the evaluation, discussed in detail in the management section of this chapter, without either delaying necessary alternative anticoagulation while awaiting the slowest available confirmatory test or committing a patient to potentially unnecessary alternative anticoagulation, with its own bleeding risk and cost implications, based on an isolated, low-specificity positive immunoassay result alone.

Thrombotic Complications and Their Recognition

Venous Thrombotic Manifestations

Venous thromboembolism, including deep vein thrombosis and pulmonary embolism, represents the most common thrombotic manifestation of heparin-induced thrombocytopenia, occurring in a substantial proportion of untreated or inadequately treated patients, and clinicians managing a patient with confirmed or strongly suspected heparin-induced thrombocytopenia should maintain a low threshold for imaging evaluation of any new limb swelling, respiratory symptoms, or other findings suggestive of venous thromboembolism, recognizing that this population carries substantially elevated baseline thrombotic risk beyond what the platelet count decline alone would suggest. Warfarin-induced venous limb gangrene, a specific and severe complication that can occur if warfarin is initiated without adequate alternative anticoagulation overlap during the acute heparin-induced thrombocytopenia phase, discussed further in the management section of this chapter, reflects the paradoxical transient hypercoagulable state that warfarin's early effect on protein C can produce in this specific clinical context, underscoring why the specific anticoagulation transition sequencing developed later in this chapter is not merely a procedural detail but a clinically critical safety consideration.

Cerebral venous sinus thrombosis and other atypical site venous thrombosis, while less common than the more typical deep vein thrombosis and pulmonary embolism presentations, occur with sufficient frequency in heparin-induced thrombocytopenia that unusual neurologic symptoms or other atypical thrombotic presentations in a patient with confirmed or suspected heparin-induced thrombocytopenia should prompt appropriately directed evaluation rather than being dismissed as unrelated to the underlying hematologic process.

Arterial Thrombotic Manifestations

Arterial thrombosis, including limb ischemia, stroke, and myocardial infarction, occurs less frequently than venous thromboembolism in heparin-induced thrombocytopenia but carries substantial morbidity when it occurs, and patients with preexisting atherosclerotic vascular disease appear to carry elevated arterial thrombotic risk in the setting of heparin-induced thrombocytopenia, reflecting the interaction between the underlying vascular pathology and the platelet-activating, procoagulant state this condition produces. Acute limb ischemia from arterial thrombosis represents a surgical and hematologic emergency requiring immediate multidisciplinary evaluation and intervention, and recognition of this possibility in a heparin-exposed patient with new limb pain, pallor, or pulselessness should prompt urgent vascular surgery involvement alongside the hematologic management discussed throughout this chapter.

The relative predominance of venous over arterial thrombosis in heparin-induced thrombocytopenia should inform the surveillance and evaluation priorities applied to a confirmed or strongly suspected patient, while maintaining appropriate vigilance for the less common but clinically severe arterial manifestations discussed in this subsection, particularly in patients with preexisting vascular risk factors that elevate this specific complication's likelihood.

Recognizing Thrombosis as a Diagnostic and Prognostic Signal

The presence of thrombosis at the time heparin-induced thrombocytopenia is first identified carries both diagnostic weight, contributing directly to the 4Ts score discussed earlier in this chapter, and prognostic significance, since heparin-induced thrombocytopenia with thrombosis, sometimes termed heparin-induced thrombocytopenia and thrombosis syndrome, carries meaningfully higher morbidity and requires more intensive anticoagulation management, discussed in the management section of this chapter, than isolated heparin-induced thrombocytopenia without clinically apparent thrombosis. Given that thrombosis can develop or become clinically apparent after the initial thrombocytopenia is first identified, ongoing surveillance for new thrombotic symptoms should continue throughout the acute management phase discussed in this chapter, rather than being limited to a single assessment at the time of initial diagnostic evaluation.

This ongoing surveillance imperative reflects the evolving, dynamic nature of heparin-induced thrombocytopenia as a disease process rather than a single point-in-time diagnostic event, and it directly informs the duration and intensity of the alternative anticoagulation management discussed in the following section, which must be maintained until the acute hypercoagulable phase of this condition has adequately resolved.

Management: Alternative Anticoagulation Strategies

Immediate Discontinuation of All Heparin Exposure

Management of confirmed or strongly suspected heparin-induced thrombocytopenia begins with immediate discontinuation of all heparin exposure, including not only therapeutic and prophylactic dosing but also the less obvious sources of heparin exposure, including heparin-coated catheters and heparin flushes used to maintain intravenous line patency, sources that are easily overlooked but can perpetuate antibody-mediated platelet activation if not identified and discontinued alongside the more obvious therapeutic heparin administration. A systematic medication reconciliation specifically searching for these less obvious heparin sources, extending the thorough medication history principle developed throughout this book, should be performed whenever heparin-induced thrombocytopenia management is initiated, ensuring complete heparin discontinuation rather than an incomplete discontinuation that leaves the underlying immune-mediated process ongoing.

Low molecular weight heparin should also be avoided given its cross-reactivity with the platelet factor 4-heparin antibody discussed in the pathophysiology section of this chapter, meaning that switching from unfractionated to low molecular weight heparin does not constitute adequate management of confirmed or strongly suspected heparin-induced thrombocytopenia and instead requires transition to one of the genuinely alternative, non-heparin anticoagulant classes discussed in the following subsections.

Direct Thrombin Inhibitors and Factor Xa Inhibitors

Parenteral direct thrombin inhibitors, including argatroban and bivalirudin, represent well-established alternative anticoagulants for the acute management of confirmed or strongly suspected heparin-induced thrombocytopenia, working through direct thrombin inhibition independent of the platelet factor 4-heparin mechanism this chapter has developed, with argatroban requiring specific dose adjustment in hepatic impairment given its hepatic clearance and bivalirudin requiring dose adjustment in renal impairment given its renal clearance, considerations that should directly inform agent selection based on a specific patient's organ function. Fondaparinux, the synthetic pentasaccharide introduced in the pathophysiology section of this chapter, provides an alternative parenteral option with minimal cross-reactivity risk, though its use in acute heparin-induced thrombocytopenia management carries a less extensive evidence base than the direct thrombin inhibitors and is generally favored for patients transitioning toward long-term management once the acute, high-risk phase has begun to stabilize.

Direct oral factor Xa inhibitors, including apixaban and rivaroxaban, have an expanding evidence base supporting their use in heparin-induced thrombocytopenia management, particularly once a patient has stabilized sufficiently to tolerate oral anticoagulation, offering practical advantages including oral administration and, for some agents, reduced monitoring requirements relative to the parenteral options discussed above, though their role in the most acute, hemodynamically unstable phase of heparin-induced thrombocytopenia management remains less established than the parenteral direct thrombin inhibitor options.

Platelet Transfusion and Warfarin Avoidance in the Acute Phase

Prophylactic platelet transfusion is generally avoided in heparin-induced thrombocytopenia, in contrast to the transfusion approach appropriate to several of the destructive thrombocytopenia conditions discussed elsewhere in this book, since transfused platelets can theoretically fuel further platelet activation and thrombosis through the same mechanism discussed in the pathophysiology section of this chapter, and platelet transfusion in this condition is generally reserved for active, clinically significant bleeding rather than used prophylactically based on platelet count alone, a management approach directly contrasting with the transfusion thresholds discussed for other thrombocytopenic conditions in Chapter 19. Warfarin should not be initiated during the acute, thrombocytopenic phase of heparin-induced thrombocytopenia management, given the venous limb gangrene risk discussed in the thrombotic complications section of this chapter, and warfarin initiation should be deferred until the platelet count has substantially recovered, typically to at least 150 x10^9/L, and then only with adequate overlap with a therapeutic non-heparin, non-warfarin anticoagulant, a specific transition sequence developed further in the long-term transition section of this chapter.

This combination of platelet transfusion avoidance and careful warfarin transition timing exemplifies the counterintuitive nature of heparin-induced thrombocytopenia management relative to the bleeding-focused management philosophy developed throughout most of this book, and clinicians and care teams less familiar with this specific condition should be explicitly reminded of these distinct management principles to avoid inadvertently applying the more generally applicable thrombocytopenia management approaches developed elsewhere in this book to this specific, mechanistically distinct condition.

THE PLATELET CRISIS DECISION COMPASS — Managing Confirmed Heparin-Induced Thrombocytopenia with Thrombosis

The Presentation: A patient with a high 4Ts score and strongly positive immunoassay develops acute lower extremity deep vein thrombosis, with platelet count 45 x10^9/L.

Mimic Signature: Heparin-induced thrombocytopenia and thrombosis syndrome requiring immediate therapeutic non-heparin anticoagulation; a coincidental venous thromboembolism from an unrelated risk factor that might otherwise be managed with standard heparin-based therapy; and a bleeding-risk concern from the thrombocytopenia that might inappropriately prompt anticoagulation withholding.

The Decision: Initiate therapeutic-dose non-heparin anticoagulation (a direct thrombin inhibitor or fondaparinux) immediately despite the thrombocytopenia, since the thrombotic risk in confirmed heparin-induced thrombocytopenia and thrombosis syndrome substantially outweighs the bleeding risk from the platelet count alone; do not withhold or reduce to prophylactic-dose anticoagulation based on the platelet count.

Trap Logic: Withholding or reducing anticoagulation intensity because the platelet count appears to indicate bleeding risk applies the wrong mental model to this condition — heparin-induced thrombocytopenia thrombocytopenia does not reflect the bleeding-prone state typical of the destructive thrombocytopenias discussed elsewhere in this book, and under-anticoagulating in this setting substantially increases, rather than decreases, patient risk.

Crisis Anchor: Confirmed heparin-induced thrombocytopenia with thrombosis is treated with full therapeutic-dose non-heparin anticoagulation regardless of platelet count severity — thrombocytopenia in this specific condition is not a reason to withhold or reduce anticoagulation intensity.

Special Clinical Scenarios

Cardiac Surgery and Cardiopulmonary Bypass

Cardiac surgery requiring cardiopulmonary bypass presents a distinct management challenge for patients with confirmed or recent heparin-induced thrombocytopenia, since cardiopulmonary bypass has historically depended on high-dose unfractionated heparin for the procedure itself, and alternative strategies including bivalirudin-based anticoagulation for the surgical procedure, or, when feasible, delaying elective surgery until circulating platelet factor 4-heparin antibodies have declined sufficiently to allow brief, deliberate intraoperative heparin use followed by immediate postoperative avoidance, each represent recognized approaches requiring specialized cardiac anesthesia and cardiac surgery expertise beyond the general hematologic management this chapter has primarily developed. This scenario represents one of the most complex clinical situations addressed in this book, requiring close, deliberate coordination among hematology, cardiac surgery, and cardiac anesthesia well in advance of any planned procedure, extending the perioperative coordination principles developed in Chapters 5 and 7 into this specific, high-complexity clinical context.

Given this complexity, any patient with a history of heparin-induced thrombocytopenia requiring future cardiac surgery should have this history clearly documented and flagged well before the surgical date, allowing adequate time for the specialized planning and, where relevant, antibody titer reassessment this scenario requires, directly extending the documentation and advance-planning principles developed throughout Chapters 5 through 10 into this specific, high-stakes procedural context.

Renal Replacement Therapy and Extracorporeal Circuits

Patients requiring renal replacement therapy or other extracorporeal circuits, including extracorporeal membrane oxygenation, present a similar anticoagulation challenge to the cardiac surgery scenario discussed above, since these circuits typically require continuous anticoagulation to prevent circuit thrombosis, and heparin has historically been the preferred agent for this purpose given its short half-life and reversibility, properties less readily matched by the alternative anticoagulants discussed earlier in this chapter. Citrate-based regional anticoagulation, which avoids systemic heparin exposure entirely by anticoagulating only the extracorporeal circuit itself through calcium chelation, has become an increasingly favored strategy for renal replacement therapy in patients with confirmed or suspected heparin-induced thrombocytopenia, avoiding the systemic bleeding risk of therapeutic-dose alternative anticoagulation that would otherwise be required to prevent circuit thrombosis using a non-heparin systemic agent.

When citrate-based regional anticoagulation is not available or not tolerated, systemic direct thrombin inhibitor anticoagulation, using the agents discussed in the management section of this chapter with dosing specifically adjusted for the extracorporeal circuit context, represents the primary alternative, again requiring specialized expertise, typically from a nephrology or critical care team experienced in this specific anticoagulation context, working in coordination with the hematologic management this chapter has developed.

Pediatric and Pregnancy Considerations

Heparin-induced thrombocytopenia occurs less frequently in children than in adults, reflecting both generally lower heparin exposure in this population and possibly age-related differences in immune response, but the diagnostic and management principles developed throughout this chapter apply with appropriate pediatric dosing adjustment when the condition does occur, extending the pediatric-specific considerations developed throughout Chapters 5 through 8 into this specific condition. Heparin-induced thrombocytopenia in pregnancy requires particular attention to the placental transfer and fetal safety profile of the alternative anticoagulants discussed in this chapter, with fondaparinux and, in some circumstances, direct thrombin inhibitors preferred over agents with less established pregnancy safety data, and management should involve close coordination between hematology and maternal-fetal medicine, directly extending the pregnancy coordination principles developed in Chapters 8 and 9 into this specific, anticoagulation-focused clinical context.

These special population considerations reinforce a theme that has recurred throughout this book: the core diagnostic and management framework developed for the general adult population requires thoughtful, evidence-informed adaptation when applied to pediatric, pregnant, and other special populations, and clinicians should seek subspecialty input specific to these populations rather than directly extrapolating general adult management guidance without this population-specific consideration.

Transitioning to Long-Term Anticoagulation

Determining the Appropriate Duration of Alternative Anticoagulation

For a patient with heparin-induced thrombocytopenia without clinically apparent thrombosis, alternative anticoagulation is generally continued until the platelet count has recovered to a stable baseline, typically for a total duration of several weeks, reflecting the time required for the acute antibody-mediated process to resolve, while a patient with heparin-induced thrombocytopenia and thrombosis syndrome generally requires a more extended anticoagulation duration analogous to standard venous thromboembolism treatment duration guidance, typically a minimum of three months, given the confirmed thrombotic event this population has experienced. This duration determination should be individualized based on the specific thrombotic burden, ongoing risk factors, and platelet count recovery trajectory, following the individualized management philosophy that has recurred throughout this book's disease-specific management chapters.

Platelet count recovery trajectory should be monitored throughout this anticoagulation period using the trend-based principles developed in Chapters 6 and 8, with a platelet count that fails to demonstrate the expected recovery pattern prompting diagnostic reconsideration, analogous to the recovery trajectory monitoring principle developed for drug-induced thrombocytopenia more broadly in Chapter 10.

The Warfarin Transition Sequence

When warfarin represents the intended long-term anticoagulant, transition from the acute alternative agent to warfarin must follow a specific, carefully timed sequence to avoid the venous limb gangrene risk discussed in the thrombotic complications section of this chapter: warfarin initiation should be deferred until the platelet count has substantially recovered, generally to at least 150 x10^9/L, warfarin should be started at a low, non-loading dose rather than an aggressive initiation regimen, and the non-heparin alternative anticoagulant should be continued with adequate overlap, generally until the international normalized ratio has been within the therapeutic range for at least two consecutive days and a minimum overlap duration has been satisfied, mirroring the general principle of anticoagulant bridging while avoiding heparin-class agents throughout the entire transition.

This specific transition sequence should be clearly documented and communicated across the care team managing the patient's anticoagulation, given the serious consequences of transition sequence errors discussed earlier in this chapter, and structured order sets or clinical pathways specifically addressing this transition, analogous to the structured tools discussed elsewhere in this chapter and book, can reduce the risk of an inadvertent transition sequence error in a busy clinical environment.

Direct Oral Anticoagulants as a Long-Term Alternative to Warfarin

Direct oral anticoagulants, discussed earlier in this chapter as an option for acute-phase management, increasingly serve as the preferred long-term anticoagulation strategy following heparin-induced thrombocytopenia, offering the practical advantage of avoiding the warfarin transition sequence complexity discussed above entirely, along with the more general advantages of oral administration without the routine laboratory monitoring warfarin requires, discussed further in the antithrombotic pharmacology context of Chapter 18. Selection between a direct oral anticoagulant and warfarin for long-term management should incorporate patient preference, renal function, cost and access considerations, and any specific comorbidity or medication interaction profile that might favor one approach over the other, following the individualized, shared decision-making approach developed throughout this book's management chapters.

This chapter has developed heparin-induced thrombocytopenia as a distinct and clinically critical entity within the broader thrombocytopenia framework established in this book, characterized by its inverted, thrombosis-predominant risk profile relative to the bleeding-focused concerns addressed elsewhere in Part III. The chapters that follow return to more classically bleeding-focused thrombocytopenic conditions, beginning with the thrombotic microangiopathies in Chapter 12, a category that, notably, shares some pathophysiologic and management complexity with the condition this chapter has developed despite important underlying mechanistic differences.

CLINICAL CASE: A 68-year-old man undergoes coronary artery bypass grafting and receives high-dose unfractionated heparin intraoperatively followed by postoperative prophylactic low molecular weight heparin. On postoperative day seven, his platelet count, which had recovered appropriately from the expected postoperative nadir by day three, unexpectedly declines from 210 to 88 x10^9/L, and he develops new left calf swelling. Applying the framework developed in this chapter, the team calculates a formal 4Ts score, scoring two points for the magnitude and pattern of thrombocytopenia, two points for the classic timing relative to the initial intraoperative heparin exposure, two points for the new thrombosis, and one point for oTher causes given the recent surgery as a competing but less compelling explanation, yielding a high total score of seven. Following the management principle developed in this chapter, all heparin products, including line flushes, are discontinued immediately, and the patient is transitioned to therapeutic-dose argatroban while platelet factor 4-heparin immunoassay testing is sent, which returns strongly positive the same day, and lower extremity ultrasound confirms an acute deep vein thrombosis. Given the confirmed heparin-induced thrombocytopenia and thrombosis syndrome, argatroban is continued at therapeutic intensity, and platelet transfusion is specifically avoided despite the moderate thrombocytopenia, consistent with the mechanistic rationale developed in this chapter. The platelet count recovers to above 150 x10^9/L by day fourteen, at which point transition to a direct oral anticoagulant is initiated for a planned minimum three-month treatment duration, and the episode is documented prominently in the medical record with explicit instruction against future heparin exposure. This case illustrates the complete diagnostic and management arc developed in this chapter: structured 4Ts scoring driving immediate empiric action, laboratory confirmation obtained concurrently rather than before treatment, thrombosis-appropriate anticoagulation intensity maintained despite thrombocytopenia, and careful transition planning to durable long-term anticoagulation.

THE PLATELET CRISIS DECISION COMPASS — Heparin-Induced Thrombocytopenia Recognition and Management

---

Compass Recap: Structured Probability Assessment: An intermediate or high 4Ts score prompts immediate heparin discontinuation and transition to alternative anticoagulation, with laboratory testing sent concurrently rather than management decisions deferred until results return.

Compass Recap: Thrombosis-Appropriate Intensity: Confirmed heparin-induced thrombocytopenia with thrombosis is treated with full therapeutic-dose non-heparin anticoagulation regardless of platelet count severity — thrombocytopenia in this specific condition is not a reason to withhold or reduce anticoagulation intensity.

Chapter Anchor: Heparin-induced thrombocytopenia inverts the usual bleeding-focused thrombocytopenia paradigm: structured 4Ts scoring drives prompt empiric heparin discontinuation and alternative anticoagulation before laboratory confirmation returns, platelet transfusion is avoided outside active bleeding, and warfarin is deferred until platelet count recovery to prevent venous limb gangrene.

Summary and Key Concepts

Heparin-induced thrombocytopenia arises from IgG antibodies against the platelet factor 4-heparin complex, which activate platelets via Fc gamma receptor IIa, producing a paradoxical combination of thrombocytopenia and thrombotic risk.

Typical onset is five to ten days after heparin initiation in a heparin-naive patient; rapid-onset (within hours) occurs with recent prior exposure; delayed-onset can develop after heparin discontinuation.

The 4Ts score (Thrombocytopenia magnitude, Timing, Thrombosis, oTher causes) provides validated pretest probability with strong negative predictive value at the low-probability category, and should be calculated formally rather than by clinical gestalt.

Immunoassay testing offers high sensitivity but modest specificity; functional testing (serotonin release assay or equivalent) provides confirmatory specificity but slower turnaround — both are interpreted together with the 4Ts score.

Management requires immediate discontinuation of all heparin sources (including flushes and low molecular weight heparin) and transition to a non-heparin anticoagulant (direct thrombin inhibitor, fondaparinux, or direct oral anticoagulant) at therapeutic intensity when thrombosis is present, regardless of platelet count.

Platelet transfusion is avoided outside active bleeding, and warfarin is deferred until platelet count recovery (generally ≥150 x10^9/L) with adequate overlap to prevent venous limb gangrene.

CHAPTER 12: THROMBOTIC MICROANGIOPATHIES: TTP, SHIGA TOXIN-ASSOCIATED HUS, AND ATYPICAL HUS

Learning Objectives

1. Define thrombotic microangiopathy and recognize the shared clinical and laboratory features across its constituent diagnoses.
2. Explain the ADAMTS13 deficiency mechanism underlying thrombotic thrombocytopenic purpura and its diagnostic and therapeutic implications.
3. Distinguish thrombotic thrombocytopenic purpura, Shiga toxin-associated hemolytic uremic syndrome, and atypical hemolytic uremic syndrome using clinical, laboratory, and mechanistic features.
4. Recognize thrombotic microangiopathy as a hematologic emergency requiring same-day evaluation and treatment initiation.
5. Apply the current management approach for thrombotic thrombocytopenic purpura, including plasma exchange and caplacizumab.
6. Apply the current management approach for atypical hemolytic uremic syndrome, including complement inhibitor therapy.

Chapter Outline

This chapter develops the thrombotic microangiopathies as the most acutely life-threatening thrombocytopenic emergencies addressed in this book, building on the schistocyte recognition introduced in Chapters 6 and 8 and representing the single finding that most urgently redirects the diagnostic algorithm developed throughout Part III. It addresses the classification and shared features of thrombotic microangiopathy, the ADAMTS13-deficiency mechanism of thrombotic thrombocytopenic purpura, Shiga toxin-associated and atypical hemolytic uremic syndrome, the diagnostic approach distinguishing these entities, and their distinct management pathways including plasma exchange, caplacizumab, and complement inhibitor therapy. Two Platelet Crisis Decision Compass instances address the recognition of thrombotic microangiopathy as requiring same-day plasma exchange initiation and the distinction between thrombotic thrombocytopenic purpura and atypical hemolytic uremic syndrome when ADAMTS13 results are pending.

No condition addressed in this book carries a more time-sensitive diagnostic and treatment imperative than thrombotic thrombocytopenic purpura, historically fatal in the substantial majority of untreated patients but now associated with survival in most patients who receive prompt, appropriate treatment, a transformation entirely dependent on rapid recognition and treatment initiation, often before definitive laboratory confirmation is available. This chapter equips the reader to recognize this presentation immediately and to initiate the treatment sequence this urgency demands.

Overview and Classification of Thrombotic Microangiopathy

The Shared Pathophysiologic Signature

Thrombotic microangiopathy describes a shared clinical and pathophysiologic pattern, rather than a single disease, characterized by microvascular platelet-rich thrombus formation causing mechanical red cell fragmentation, producing the combination of thrombocytopenia and microangiopathic hemolytic anemia that defines this category and distinguishes it from every other condition discussed in this book. This shared downstream pattern arises from several distinct upstream mechanisms, developed throughout this chapter, including severe ADAMTS13 deficiency in thrombotic thrombocytopenic purpura, Shiga toxin-mediated endothelial injury in Shiga toxin-associated hemolytic uremic syndrome, and uncontrolled complement activation in atypical hemolytic uremic syndrome, each converging on the same fundamental microvascular thrombotic process despite their mechanistic diversity.

Recognizing thrombotic microangiopathy as a shared clinical syndrome, rather than immediately committing to one specific underlying diagnosis, is the essential first step in evaluation, since the immediate treatment priority, discussed later in this chapter, often must begin before the specific underlying mechanism has been definitively established, directly paralleling the empiric treatment-before-confirmation principle developed for heparin-induced thrombocytopenia in Chapter 11 but applied here to an even more immediately life-threatening presentation.

Schistocytes as the Defining Diagnostic Clue

Schistocytes on peripheral smear, introduced as an urgent red flag finding throughout Chapters 6 and 8, represent the defining morphologic signature of thrombotic microangiopathy, reflecting the mechanical red cell fragmentation that occurs as red cells pass through microvascular channels partially occluded by platelet-rich thrombi, and the identification of schistocytes accompanying thrombocytopenia should immediately trigger the urgent evaluation pathway developed throughout this chapter, superseding the more routine outpatient evaluation timelines discussed for most other conditions in this book. The degree of schistocytosis, generally quantified as a percentage of red cells on smear review, correlates imprecisely but meaningfully with disease severity, and even a modest schistocyte percentage in the appropriate clinical context should prompt the urgent evaluation this chapter develops rather than being dismissed as an insignificant or borderline finding.

This chapter's emphasis on immediate action upon schistocyte recognition reflects the singular time-sensitivity of thrombotic microangiopathy relative to every other thrombocytopenic condition addressed in this book, and clinicians should treat this specific morphologic finding, combined with thrombocytopenia, as an unambiguous trigger for the emergency evaluation and treatment pathway this chapter develops, without awaiting additional confirmatory findings before initiating this urgent response.

Distinguishing Primary Thrombotic Microangiopathy From Secondary Mimics

Beyond the primary thrombotic microangiopathy syndromes that form the primary focus of this chapter, a similar clinical and laboratory picture can arise secondary to malignant hypertension, disseminated malignancy, certain medications including some chemotherapeutic and immunosuppressive agents, and disseminated intravascular coagulation discussed further in Chapter 14, each producing microangiopathic hemolytic anemia and thrombocytopenia through mechanisms distinct from the primary conditions this chapter emphasizes. Distinguishing primary from secondary thrombotic microangiopathy requires careful attention to the broader clinical context, including blood pressure, evidence of an underlying malignancy or systemic illness, and coagulation studies, since secondary thrombotic microangiopathy management focuses on the underlying precipitating condition rather than the specific plasma exchange and complement-directed therapies developed later in this chapter for the primary syndromes.

Despite this important distinction, the immediate initial evaluation and treatment urgency this chapter emphasizes should apply broadly to any patient presenting with the schistocyte-thrombocytopenia combination, since distinguishing primary from secondary thrombotic microangiopathy, and further distinguishing among the primary syndromes themselves, frequently requires time and testing that should not delay the emergency initial management this presentation demands.

Thrombotic Thrombocytopenic Purpura: ADAMTS13 Deficiency

The Physiologic Role of ADAMTS13

ADAMTS13, the plasma metalloprotease introduced mechanistically in Chapter 3, normally cleaves ultra-large von Willebrand factor multimers released from endothelial Weibel-Palade bodies into smaller, less thrombogenic forms, and this cleavage function is essential to preventing the spontaneous platelet aggregation that ultra-large multimers, with their exceptionally high avidity for platelet glycoprotein Ib, would otherwise readily trigger even under normal, non-pathologic shear conditions. Severe ADAMTS13 deficiency, generally defined as activity below ten percent of normal, removes this critical regulatory check, allowing ultra-large von Willebrand factor multimers to persist in circulation and spontaneously recruit and activate platelets, generating the platelet-rich microvascular thrombi that define thrombotic thrombocytopenic purpura and produce the mechanical red cell fragmentation discussed earlier in this chapter.

This ADAMTS13-deficiency mechanism directly explains the therapeutic rationale for plasma exchange, discussed in the management section of this chapter, which simultaneously removes the pathologic antibody responsible for most acquired ADAMTS13 deficiency and replenishes functional ADAMTS13 through the replacement plasma, addressing both sides of the underlying pathophysiologic deficit in a single therapeutic intervention.

Acquired Autoimmune Thrombotic Thrombocytopenic Purpura

The substantial majority of thrombotic thrombocytopenic purpura cases are acquired, arising from an autoantibody, typically immunoglobulin G, directed against ADAMTS13, that either directly inhibits its proteolytic activity or accelerates its clearance from circulation, producing the severe functional deficiency discussed above despite normal or near-normal ADAMTS13 gene function and protein synthesis. This autoimmune mechanism explains why immunosuppressive therapy, discussed alongside plasma exchange in the management section of this chapter, has become an increasingly central component of contemporary thrombotic thrombocytopenic purpura treatment, directly addressing the underlying antibody-producing process rather than only the downstream ADAMTS13 deficiency and its consequences.

Acquired thrombotic thrombocytopenic purpura can occur in isolation or in association with several precipitating factors and underlying conditions, including pregnancy, discussed further in the pregnancy-specific context of Chapter 13, certain infections, and, in a manner analogous to the secondary immune thrombocytopenia associations discussed in Chapter 9, underlying autoimmune conditions including systemic lupus erythematosus, reinforcing the value of a directed evaluation for these associated conditions once the acute thrombotic thrombocytopenic purpura episode has been stabilized.

Congenital Thrombotic Thrombocytopenic Purpura

A minority of thrombotic thrombocytopenic purpura cases, termed congenital or hereditary thrombotic thrombocytopenic purpura, arise from biallelic pathogenic variants in the ADAMTS13 gene itself, producing severe ADAMTS13 deficiency through an inherited rather than autoimmune mechanism, and this congenital form should be specifically suspected in a patient with recurrent thrombotic microangiopathy episodes, an onset in childhood, or a family history suggestive of an inherited pattern, distinguishing it from the more common acquired autoimmune form discussed above. Congenital thrombotic thrombocytopenic purpura frequently first manifests or substantially worsens during pregnancy, given the physiologic decline in ADAMTS13 activity that occurs even in unaffected individuals during normal pregnancy, and unmasking of previously unrecognized congenital thrombotic thrombocytopenic purpura during pregnancy represents an important, though uncommon, diagnostic consideration developed further in Chapter 13.

Distinguishing congenital from acquired thrombotic thrombocytopenic purpura carries direct management implications, since congenital thrombotic thrombocytopenic purpura does not respond to the immunosuppressive therapies effective in the autoimmune form and instead requires periodic plasma infusion, rather than plasma exchange, to replenish ADAMTS13 without the antibody-removal component that plasma exchange provides, a distinction developed further in the management section of this chapter.

Clinical Presentation and the Classic Pentad

The Historical Pentad and Its Contemporary Relevance

The classically described thrombotic thrombocytopenic purpura pentad, comprising thrombocytopenia, microangiopathic hemolytic anemia, neurologic symptoms, renal dysfunction, and fever, is now understood to represent a comparatively late or severe presentation, and current clinical practice recognizes that the combination of thrombocytopenia and microangiopathic hemolytic anemia alone, without the full pentad, is sufficient to trigger the urgent evaluation and treatment pathway this chapter develops, reflecting the substantial improvement in outcomes achieved by treating earlier in the disease course before the full pentad has necessarily developed. This shift away from requiring the full pentad before initiating treatment represents one of the most clinically important evolutions in thrombotic thrombocytopenic purpura management over recent decades, and clinicians trained on the historical pentad framework should specifically recognize that awaiting its full development before treatment initiation reflects outdated practice inconsistent with current, evidence-based, outcome-improving management.

Neurologic symptoms, when present, are notably protean and can range from mild headache and confusion to seizure, focal neurologic deficit, or coma, reflecting the diffuse microvascular thrombotic process affecting the cerebral microcirculation, and this neurologic variability means that thrombotic thrombocytopenic purpura should remain a diagnostic consideration in any patient with thrombocytopenia, microangiopathic hemolytic anemia, and neurologic symptoms of any severity or specific character, rather than only in the presence of a specific, classically described neurologic presentation.

Renal and Cardiac Involvement

Renal involvement in thrombotic thrombocytopenic purpura is typically less severe than in the hemolytic uremic syndrome variants discussed later in this chapter, though meaningful renal dysfunction can occur, and the relative severity of renal involvement, developed further in the diagnostic distinction section of this chapter, provides one of several clinical clues helping to distinguish thrombotic thrombocytopenic purpura from the hemolytic uremic syndrome variants, though this distinction should never be relied upon in isolation given meaningful clinical overlap between these conditions. Cardiac involvement, including microvascular thrombosis affecting the coronary microcirculation, can produce troponin elevation, arrhythmia, and, in severe cases, cardiogenic shock, and cardiac biomarker assessment should be considered as part of the initial evaluation given both its prognostic value and its relevance to monitoring during the acute treatment phase discussed later in this chapter.

This multi-organ involvement pattern, potentially affecting the neurologic, renal, and cardiac systems simultaneously through the same underlying microvascular thrombotic process, underscores why thrombotic thrombocytopenic purpura evaluation and management often requires multidisciplinary coordination extending well beyond hematology alone, a coordination imperative developed further in the management section of this chapter.

The Fluctuating, Relapsing Nature of Acute Presentation

Thrombotic thrombocytopenic purpura symptoms can fluctuate substantially over hours, with a patient's neurologic status in particular sometimes improving and then acutely deteriorating as the underlying microvascular thrombotic process waxes and wanes before definitive treatment achieves control, and this fluctuating pattern should not be misinterpreted as reassuring or as evidence against the diagnosis, since apparent clinical improvement without treatment does not indicate resolution of the underlying process and should not delay the urgent evaluation and treatment pathway this chapter develops. This fluctuating pattern also has direct implications for ongoing monitoring during treatment, discussed in the management section of this chapter, since clinical status alone, without concurrent laboratory trend monitoring, may not reliably indicate whether treatment is achieving the intended therapeutic effect.

Recognizing this fluctuating natural history reinforces the urgency this chapter has emphasized throughout: any patient presenting with thrombocytopenia and microangiopathic hemolytic anemia, regardless of the apparent severity or stability of their current clinical status, warrants the same urgent evaluation pathway, since clinical stability at a single point in time does not reliably predict the trajectory of this dynamic, rapidly evolving condition.

Diagnostic Evaluation and ADAMTS13 Testing

Confirming Microangiopathic Hemolytic Anemia

The initial laboratory evaluation for suspected thrombotic microangiopathy, applying and extending the smear review principles developed in Chapter 6, confirms microangiopathic hemolytic anemia through the combination of schistocytes on smear, elevated lactate dehydrogenase, low haptoglobin, indirect hyperbilirubinemia, and a negative direct antiglobulin test, this last finding specifically distinguishing microangiopathic hemolysis from the antibody-mediated hemolysis of autoimmune hemolytic anemia, a distinction that carries direct diagnostic weight given the very different management implications of these two hemolytic processes. This confirmatory hemolysis panel should be obtained immediately alongside the complete blood count and smear review whenever thrombotic microangiopathy is suspected, and results should be available rapidly enough to inform the same-day treatment decision this chapter's urgency demands.

Coagulation studies, including prothrombin time, activated partial thromboplastin time, and fibrinogen, are generally normal or near-normal in primary thrombotic microangiopathy, in contrast to the deranged coagulation studies characteristic of disseminated intravascular coagulation discussed in Chapter 14, and this distinction provides additional diagnostic clarification when the broader differential diagnosis for thrombocytopenia with hemolysis and organ dysfunction remains uncertain at initial presentation.

The PLASMIC Score and Clinical Probability Assessment

The PLASMIC score, a validated clinical prediction tool analogous in principle to the 4Ts score developed for heparin-induced thrombocytopenia in Chapter 11, incorporates readily available clinical and laboratory features, including platelet count, evidence of hemolysis, absence of active malignancy or transplant history, mean corpuscular volume, international normalized ratio, and creatinine, to stratify patients into low, intermediate, and high probability categories for severe ADAMTS13 deficiency, providing a bedside tool to guide the urgency of empiric plasma exchange initiation while definitive ADAMTS13 testing remains pending. A high PLASMIC score supports immediate empiric plasma exchange initiation without awaiting ADAMTS13 results, directly applying the empiric-treatment-before-confirmation principle this chapter has emphasized throughout, while a low score should prompt reconsideration of alternative diagnoses within the broader thrombocytopenia and hemolysis differential this chapter and Chapter 8 together establish.

This structured clinical probability assessment tool exemplifies the same evidence-based, structured-over-intuitive diagnostic philosophy that has recurred throughout this book, providing a validated, reproducible framework for the specific, extraordinarily time-sensitive clinical decision this chapter addresses, where the consequences of diagnostic delay are more severe than in almost any other condition this book discusses.

ADAMTS13 Activity and Inhibitor Testing

Definitive diagnosis of thrombotic thrombocytopenic purpura requires ADAMTS13 activity testing, with severe deficiency, generally below ten percent of normal activity, confirming the diagnosis, and ADAMTS13 inhibitor testing further distinguishes the acquired autoimmune form from the congenital form discussed earlier in this chapter, with inhibitor presence supporting the acquired autoimmune mechanism and its absence in a patient with confirmed severe deficiency supporting consideration of congenital thrombotic thrombocytopenic purpura and prompting the genetic testing discussed earlier in this chapter. ADAMTS13 testing turnaround time varies by laboratory, ranging from same-day rapid testing at some specialized centers to several days at reference laboratories without on-site testing capability, and this turnaround time variability directly informs the PLASMIC score's clinical value as a bridging tool for the empiric treatment decision this chapter has emphasized must often precede definitive ADAMTS13 confirmation.

Given the treatment-altering distinction between thrombotic thrombocytopenic purpura and the hemolytic uremic syndrome variants discussed later in this chapter, ADAMTS13 testing should be sent as part of the initial evaluation for any patient with suspected thrombotic microangiopathy, even when empiric plasma exchange has already been initiated based on clinical probability, since the result meaningfully informs both ongoing management, discussed later in this chapter, and long-term monitoring and relapse prevention planning developed in the final section of this chapter.

THE PLATELET CRISIS DECISION COMPASS — Recognizing Thrombotic Microangiopathy as Requiring Same-Day Treatment

The Presentation: A 38-year-old woman presents with fatigue and mild confusion, and initial laboratory testing reveals a platelet count of 18 x10^9/L, hemoglobin 7.8 g/dL, and schistocytes on peripheral smear.

Mimic Signature: Thrombotic thrombocytopenic purpura requiring immediate plasma exchange; disseminated intravascular coagulation from an unrecognized underlying trigger, distinguished by deranged coagulation studies; and severe immune thrombocytopenia with a coincidental, unrelated anemia, distinguished by the absence of true hemolysis on confirmatory testing.

The Decision: Obtain the confirmatory hemolysis panel (lactate dehydrogenase, haptoglobin, indirect bilirubin, direct antiglobulin test) and coagulation studies immediately; calculate the PLASMIC score using available data; a high-probability score should trigger same-day hematology consultation and plasma exchange initiation without awaiting ADAMTS13 results, which should be sent concurrently.

Trap Logic: Deferring plasma exchange initiation until ADAMTS13 results return, when the clinical and laboratory picture and PLASMIC score already support a high probability of thrombotic thrombocytopenic purpura, exposes the patient to a delay that meaningfully increases mortality risk in a condition where each day of delayed treatment carries measurable additional risk.

Crisis Anchor: Thrombocytopenia with microangiopathic hemolytic anemia (schistocytes, elevated lactate dehydrogenase, low haptoglobin) and a high PLASMIC score triggers same-day plasma exchange initiation, not deferral until ADAMTS13 confirmation returns.

Shiga Toxin-Associated Hemolytic Uremic Syndrome

Pathophysiology and the Role of Shiga Toxin

Shiga toxin-associated hemolytic uremic syndrome arises from infection with Shiga toxin-producing Escherichia coli, most commonly serotype O157:H7, though other Shiga toxin-producing strains can also cause this syndrome, in which the toxin binds a specific glycosphingolipid receptor expressed prominently on renal glomerular and microvascular endothelium, producing direct endothelial injury that triggers the microvascular thrombotic process defining this condition, with the renal predominance of the causative receptor directly explaining the more severe and consistent renal involvement characteristic of this variant relative to thrombotic thrombocytopenic purpura discussed earlier in this chapter. This distinct receptor-mediated mechanism, entirely independent of the ADAMTS13 deficiency discussed for thrombotic thrombocytopenic purpura, explains why plasma exchange, though sometimes still used empirically before diagnostic clarification given the shared initial presentation, does not address the underlying pathophysiology of Shiga toxin-associated hemolytic uremic syndrome and is not considered standard, evidence-based therapy for this specific variant once the diagnosis is confirmed.

The characteristic prodrome of bloody diarrhea preceding the hematologic and renal manifestations by several days provides an important clinical clue distinguishing this variant from thrombotic thrombocytopenic purpura and atypical hemolytic uremic syndrome, discussed later in this chapter, though this prodrome is not universally present or recognized, and its absence should not be used to definitively exclude Shiga toxin-associated hemolytic uremic syndrome without appropriate stool testing, discussed in the following subsection.

Epidemiology and Diagnostic Testing

Shiga toxin-associated hemolytic uremic syndrome predominantly affects children, representing the most common cause of acute kidney injury in the pediatric population in many settings, though it can occur in adults, particularly during outbreak settings involving contaminated food or water sources, and stool culture or polymerase chain reaction-based Shiga toxin testing, obtained as part of the initial evaluation whenever this diagnosis is suspected, particularly in a pediatric patient with an appropriate prodrome, confirms the diagnosis and directly distinguishes this variant from the other thrombotic microangiopathy syndromes discussed in this chapter. This predominantly pediatric epidemiology directly informs the diagnostic prioritization applied when evaluating suspected thrombotic microangiopathy in a child, where Shiga toxin-associated hemolytic uremic syndrome should generally receive higher initial diagnostic priority than in an adult presenting with an analogous clinical picture, though thrombotic thrombocytopenic purpura and atypical hemolytic uremic syndrome remain important considerations across all ages and should not be dismissed in a pediatric patient without appropriate evaluation.

Given the outbreak potential of Shiga toxin-producing organisms, public health reporting and, where relevant, investigation of a potential common source, including contaminated food products, is an important component of Shiga toxin-associated hemolytic uremic syndrome management beyond the individual patient care this chapter primarily addresses, reflecting the broader public health dimension this specific thrombotic microangiopathy variant carries relative to the other conditions discussed in this chapter.

Management and Supportive Care

Management of Shiga toxin-associated hemolytic uremic syndrome centers on supportive care, including careful fluid and electrolyte management, blood pressure control, and, in patients with significant renal impairment, renal replacement therapy, discussed in the special clinical scenarios context of Chapter 11, with antibiotic therapy for the underlying gastrointestinal infection generally avoided given evidence suggesting that antibiotic-induced bacterial lysis may increase Shiga toxin release and worsen the hematologic and renal manifestations of this syndrome, a specific and clinically important management nuance distinguishing this condition from most other infectious processes addressed throughout medicine. Eculizumab, the complement inhibitor discussed in the atypical hemolytic uremic syndrome management context later in this chapter, has been used in severe or refractory Shiga toxin-associated hemolytic uremic syndrome in some clinical circumstances, reflecting emerging evidence that complement activation may contribute to disease severity in a subset of patients beyond the direct Shiga toxin-mediated endothelial injury this section has primarily emphasized, though this remains a less established, evolving area of practice relative to its well-established role in atypical hemolytic uremic syndrome.

The generally more favorable prognosis of Shiga toxin-associated hemolytic uremic syndrome relative to the other thrombotic microangiopathy variants discussed in this chapter, with most pediatric patients achieving full recovery with supportive care alone, should not diminish the urgency of prompt recognition and appropriate supportive management, since a subset of patients, particularly those with more severe presentations, experience significant morbidity including chronic kidney disease, and early, expert nephrology and, where available, hematology involvement optimizes outcomes even in this generally more favorable prognostic category.

Atypical Hemolytic Uremic Syndrome and Complement Dysregulation

Complement Pathway Dysregulation as the Underlying Mechanism

Atypical hemolytic uremic syndrome arises from uncontrolled activation of the alternative complement pathway, most commonly due to pathogenic variants in complement regulatory genes including complement factor H, complement factor I, membrane cofactor protein, or, less commonly, gain-of-function variants in complement component C3 or complement factor B, each producing a loss of the normal regulatory checks that would otherwise constrain complement activation on host endothelial cell surfaces, allowing uncontrolled complement-mediated endothelial injury and the microvascular thrombotic process this chapter has developed throughout. This complement-mediated mechanism, entirely distinct from both the ADAMTS13 deficiency of thrombotic thrombocytopenic purpura and the Shiga toxin-mediated endothelial injury of the syndrome discussed in the preceding section, directly explains the therapeutic rationale for complement inhibitor therapy, discussed in the management section of this chapter, which specifically and effectively addresses this underlying dysregulated complement activation.

Atypical hemolytic uremic syndrome frequently requires a triggering event, including infection, pregnancy, or certain medications, to unmask clinically apparent disease in a genetically predisposed individual, reflecting an incomplete penetrance pattern in which the underlying complement regulatory gene variant creates susceptibility rather than guaranteed disease expression, a pattern that explains why a family history of atypical hemolytic uremic syndrome may be absent even in a patient who ultimately proves to carry a known pathogenic complement regulatory variant.

Clinical Presentation and Renal Predominance

Atypical hemolytic uremic syndrome characteristically presents with renal involvement as prominent as, or more prominent than, that of Shiga toxin-associated hemolytic uremic syndrome discussed earlier in this chapter, often without the preceding bloody diarrheal prodrome characteristic of that condition, and this renal predominance, combined with the absence of a diarrheal prodrome and negative Shiga toxin testing, provides an important though imperfect clinical clue supporting consideration of atypical hemolytic uremic syndrome within the broader thrombotic microangiopathy differential this chapter develops. The condition can present across the age spectrum, in contrast to the predominantly pediatric epidemiology of Shiga toxin-associated hemolytic uremic syndrome, and a triggering event, when identifiable, should be specifically sought and documented, both for its diagnostic value and because it may inform subsequent risk assessment and monitoring following the acute episode.

Extrarenal manifestations, including neurologic, cardiac, and gastrointestinal involvement, can occur in atypical hemolytic uremic syndrome and reflect the same underlying complement-mediated microvascular process affecting organ systems beyond the kidney, a multi-organ involvement pattern that parallels, though arises through a mechanistically distinct pathway from, the multi-organ involvement discussed for thrombotic thrombocytopenic purpura earlier in this chapter.

Genetic and Complement Functional Testing

Diagnostic evaluation for suspected atypical hemolytic uremic syndrome includes complement functional and genetic testing, assessing complement factor H, factor I, and membrane cofactor protein levels and function, along with targeted or broader genetic panel testing for pathogenic variants in the complement regulatory genes discussed earlier in this section, testing that typically requires specialized reference laboratory processing with turnaround times extending well beyond the immediate treatment decision window this chapter has emphasized throughout. Given this testing turnaround limitation, the diagnosis of atypical hemolytic uremic syndrome in the acute setting is substantially a diagnosis of exclusion, established by confirming the absence of severe ADAMTS13 deficiency, discussed earlier in this chapter, and the absence of Shiga toxin infection, discussed in the preceding section, in a patient with a compatible clinical presentation, with genetic and complement functional testing results subsequently confirming and further characterizing the diagnosis, often well after empiric treatment has already been initiated.

This exclusionary diagnostic approach, applying the same clinical reasoning framework this chapter has developed for distinguishing among the thrombotic microangiopathy variants more broadly, underscores why the structured diagnostic distinction developed in the following section of this chapter deserves careful, systematic application whenever a patient's presentation does not clearly and immediately localize to one specific thrombotic microangiopathy variant based on the more rapidly available clinical and laboratory features this chapter has discussed.

Distinguishing TTP, STEC-HUS, and Complement-Mediated TMA

A Structured Comparative Framework

Bringing together the distinct features developed throughout this chapter, a structured comparative framework aids the clinician in rapidly generating an initial working diagnosis while definitive confirmatory testing remains pending: severe ADAMTS13 deficiency confirms thrombotic thrombocytopenic purpura and should prompt immediate continuation or initiation of plasma exchange if not already started; positive Shiga toxin testing with a compatible diarrheal prodrome, particularly in a pediatric patient, supports Shiga toxin-associated hemolytic uremic syndrome and the specific supportive management approach discussed earlier in this chapter; and the combination of preserved ADAMTS13 activity, negative Shiga toxin testing, and a compatible clinical presentation, particularly with prominent renal involvement, supports atypical hemolytic uremic syndrome and the complement-directed therapy discussed in the management section of this chapter.

This structured comparative framework should be applied iteratively as results become available over the course of the initial evaluation, recognizing that empiric plasma exchange, given its relative safety and its specific efficacy in thrombotic thrombocytopenic purpura, is frequently initiated before this full distinguishing evaluation is complete, and the framework's primary function is to guide the ongoing refinement and, where necessary, redirection of therapy as each additional diagnostic result becomes available rather than to delay initial treatment until every distinguishing feature has been fully characterized.

The Value and Limits of Renal Function in Distinguishing These Conditions

Renal function severity, while generally more pronounced in the hemolytic uremic syndrome variants than in thrombotic thrombocytopenic purpura as discussed throughout this chapter, shows substantial overlap across these conditions and should never be used as a sole distinguishing criterion, since a subset of thrombotic thrombocytopenic purpura patients present with significant renal impairment, and conversely some atypical hemolytic uremic syndrome patients present with comparatively preserved renal function early in their disease course, particularly before the underlying complement dysregulation has produced its full clinical impact. This overlap reinforces why the definitive, mechanism-specific testing discussed throughout this chapter, rather than clinical pattern recognition alone, ultimately drives the confirmed diagnosis and long-term management plan, even though clinical pattern recognition appropriately guides the immediate empiric treatment decisions this chapter has emphasized throughout.

This limitation of clinical pattern recognition alone exemplifies a theme that has recurred throughout this book: structured clinical assessment tools and pattern recognition frameworks provide essential guidance for time-sensitive initial decisions, but they are appropriately superseded by definitive mechanism-specific testing once that testing becomes available, and clinicians should remain prepared to revise an initial working diagnosis as this more definitive information emerges over the course of a patient's evaluation and treatment course.

Multidisciplinary Coordination Across the Diagnostic Uncertainty Period

Given the diagnostic uncertainty that frequently persists during the initial days of thrombotic microangiopathy evaluation, coordinated hematology, nephrology, and, in pediatric patients, pediatric nephrology or pediatric hematology involvement from the outset of evaluation, extending the multidisciplinary coordination principles developed throughout Chapters 8 and 11, ensures that the evolving diagnostic picture is interpreted by clinicians with the specific expertise needed to correctly apply the distinguishing framework this chapter has developed. This early multidisciplinary involvement additionally facilitates the specific treatment interventions discussed in the following sections of this chapter, including plasma exchange access and complement inhibitor therapy, both of which typically require specialized resources and expertise not uniformly available in every clinical setting.

Transfer to a center with these specialized resources, when not locally available, should be considered early in the evaluation of suspected thrombotic microangiopathy given the time-sensitive treatment imperative this chapter has emphasized throughout, and this transfer decision should not be delayed pending complete diagnostic clarification, since the specific treatment resources required may be needed urgently regardless of which specific thrombotic microangiopathy variant is ultimately confirmed.

Management of Thrombotic Thrombocytopenic Purpura

Therapeutic Plasma Exchange

Therapeutic plasma exchange, the cornerstone of acquired thrombotic thrombocytopenic purpura management, removes the pathologic anti-ADAMTS13 antibody discussed earlier in this chapter while simultaneously replenishing functional ADAMTS13 through the replacement plasma, and this dual mechanism directly explains why plasma exchange, rather than simple plasma infusion or plasmapheresis without replacement, represents standard, evidence-based first-line therapy, with daily plasma exchange sessions generally continued until platelet count and hemolysis markers have normalized and remained stable for at least two consecutive days, reflecting the need for sustained biochemical remission rather than a single favorable laboratory value before treatment de-escalation. Plasma exchange should be initiated as urgently as institutional resources allow once thrombotic thrombocytopenic purpura is suspected with sufficient clinical probability, ideally within hours of presentation, directly reflecting the urgency this chapter has emphasized throughout, and delay in accessing plasma exchange capability, whether due to resource limitations or diagnostic uncertainty, should prompt consideration of transfer to a center with more immediate access when locally unavailable.

Plasma exchange carries its own procedural risks, including central venous catheter-related complications and citrate-related electrolyte disturbances, that require careful monitoring throughout the treatment course, and these procedural considerations, while important, should not be used to justify delaying or withholding plasma exchange in a patient with a sufficiently high clinical probability of thrombotic thrombocytopenic purpura, given the substantially greater risk of untreated or delayed-treatment disease relative to these generally manageable procedural risks.

Caplacizumab and Immunosuppressive Therapy

Caplacizumab, a nanobody that blocks the interaction between ultra-large von Willebrand factor multimers and platelet glycoprotein Ib, directly addressing the final common pathway of platelet recruitment discussed in the pathophysiology section of this chapter, has become an important adjunct to plasma exchange in acquired thrombotic thrombocytopenic purpura management, producing more rapid platelet count normalization and reducing the risk of disease exacerbation during the treatment course, though its use requires careful attention to bleeding risk given its direct antiplatelet mechanism, and current guidelines generally recommend its use alongside, rather than as a substitute for, plasma exchange and immunosuppressive therapy. Immunosuppressive therapy, most commonly corticosteroids initiated alongside plasma exchange and, increasingly, rituximab either as part of initial therapy for severe presentations or reserved for refractory or relapsing disease, directly addresses the underlying autoantibody production discussed earlier in this chapter, and the trend toward earlier, more aggressive immunosuppressive therapy reflects accumulating evidence that this approach reduces both acute treatment duration and long-term relapse risk relative to plasma exchange alone.

The combination of plasma exchange, caplacizumab, and immunosuppressive therapy represents the current standard of care for acquired thrombotic thrombocytopenic purpura at most specialized centers, reflecting a multi-mechanism therapeutic approach that simultaneously addresses antibody removal and replacement of the deficient enzyme through plasma exchange, blockade of the final common pathophysiologic pathway through caplacizumab, and suppression of ongoing antibody production through immunosuppressive therapy, together achieving the substantially improved outcomes that distinguish contemporary thrombotic thrombocytopenic purpura management from the historical, largely fatal natural history this condition once carried.

Management of Congenital Thrombotic Thrombocytopenic Purpura

Congenital thrombotic thrombocytopenic purpura, discussed earlier in this chapter, is managed with periodic prophylactic or on-demand plasma infusion rather than plasma exchange, since the therapeutic goal is simply ADAMTS13 replacement rather than antibody removal, a mechanistically distinct treatment approach reflecting the mechanistically distinct underlying pathophysiology this congenital form represents. Recombinant ADAMTS13 replacement therapy, an emerging treatment approach specifically developed for congenital thrombotic thrombocytopenic purpura, offers the potential for more precise, targeted enzyme replacement without the volume and infectious risk considerations inherent to plasma-derived products, and clinicians managing patients with confirmed congenital thrombotic thrombocytopenic purpura should remain aware of this evolving therapeutic landscape as availability expands.

Pregnancy planning in a patient with confirmed congenital thrombotic thrombocytopenic purpura requires particular attention, given the physiologic ADAMTS13 decline during normal pregnancy discussed earlier in this chapter, with prophylactic plasma infusion throughout pregnancy generally recommended to prevent the disease exacerbation that pregnancy characteristically precipitates in this population, a management consideration developed further in the pregnancy-specific context of Chapter 13.

THE PLATELET CRISIS DECISION COMPASS — Distinguishing TTP from Atypical HUS While ADAMTS13 Results Are Pending

The Presentation: A 45-year-old man presents with thrombocytopenia, microangiopathic hemolytic anemia, and acute kidney injury requiring dialysis, with no preceding diarrheal illness; ADAMTS13 activity results are pending and expected to take three days.

Mimic Signature: Thrombotic thrombocytopenic purpura with atypically prominent renal involvement; atypical hemolytic uremic syndrome given the renal predominance and absent diarrheal prodrome; and Shiga toxin-associated hemolytic uremic syndrome despite the atypical absence of prodrome, requiring stool testing to fully exclude.

The Decision: Initiate empiric plasma exchange immediately given the inability to exclude thrombotic thrombocytopenic purpura before ADAMTS13 results return, while simultaneously sending Shiga toxin stool testing and complement functional/genetic testing; if ADAMTS13 activity subsequently returns preserved (not severely deficient) and Shiga toxin testing is negative, transition management toward the complement-directed atypical hemolytic uremic syndrome pathway discussed later in this chapter.

Trap Logic: Withholding plasma exchange while awaiting ADAMTS13 results because the renal predominance and absent prodrome seem to favor atypical hemolytic uremic syndrome over thrombotic thrombocytopenic purpura risks withholding effective therapy from a patient who, in fact, has thrombotic thrombocytopenic purpura with an atypical presentation — clinical pattern alone cannot reliably exclude thrombotic thrombocytopenic purpura before ADAMTS13 confirmation.

Crisis Anchor: Empiric plasma exchange is initiated for any patient meeting thrombotic microangiopathy criteria regardless of which specific variant clinical pattern initially suggests, continuing until ADAMTS13 results definitively exclude severe deficiency and allow transition to variant-specific therapy.

Management of Atypical HUS: Complement Inhibition

Terminal Complement Inhibitor Therapy

Eculizumab and ravulizumab, monoclonal antibodies that block terminal complement pathway activation by targeting complement component C5, directly address the underlying complement dysregulation mechanism discussed earlier in this chapter and have transformed atypical hemolytic uremic syndrome from a condition with historically poor renal and overall outcomes into one with substantially improved prognosis when this targeted therapy is initiated promptly, mirroring the transformation plasma exchange and its adjuncts have achieved for thrombotic thrombocytopenic purpura discussed earlier in this chapter. These agents are generally continued long-term given the ongoing underlying complement regulatory defect this condition reflects, though evolving evidence and clinical experience increasingly support consideration of treatment discontinuation in carefully selected, stable patients after a defined treatment period, a decision requiring specialized nephrology and hematology expertise and careful ongoing monitoring given the relapse risk this discontinuation decision carries.

Given the mechanism of terminal complement blockade these agents provide, patients require specific pre-treatment vaccination against Neisseria meningitidis and other encapsulated organisms, directly paralleling the splenectomy-related infection risk and vaccination requirements discussed in Chapter 9, along with ongoing vigilance for meningococcal and other invasive infection given the impaired complement-mediated host defense this therapy produces, considerations that should be explicitly discussed with the patient as part of the informed treatment decision this therapy requires.

Timing of Complement Inhibitor Initiation Relative to Diagnostic Confirmation

Given the substantial cost and specific infection risk considerations associated with complement inhibitor therapy, current practice generally favors initiating this therapy once thrombotic thrombocytopenic purpura and Shiga toxin-associated hemolytic uremic syndrome have been reasonably excluded through the exclusionary diagnostic approach discussed earlier in this chapter, rather than as an immediate empiric therapy alongside plasma exchange in every patient with suspected thrombotic microangiopathy, reflecting a somewhat different treatment initiation threshold than the immediate empiric plasma exchange approach this chapter has emphasized for suspected thrombotic thrombocytopenic purpura. This distinction reflects both the different risk-benefit profile of complement inhibitor therapy relative to plasma exchange and the more immediately available diagnostic tools, including ADAMTS13 and Shiga toxin testing, that can reasonably exclude the alternative diagnoses before complement inhibitor therapy is initiated, in contrast to the more prolonged turnaround time for the complement functional and genetic testing that would definitively confirm atypical hemolytic uremic syndrome itself.

This nuanced treatment initiation timing, distinct from the immediate empiric approach this chapter has emphasized for plasma exchange, should be applied with close nephrology and hematology coordination, recognizing that a patient with a strongly compatible clinical presentation and reasonably excluded alternative diagnoses should not experience unnecessary treatment delay while awaiting the more prolonged definitive genetic confirmation this condition ultimately requires.

Renal Support and Long-Term Renal Outcomes

Renal replacement therapy, discussed in the special clinical scenarios context of Chapter 11, is frequently required during the acute phase of atypical hemolytic uremic syndrome given the prominent renal involvement this condition characteristically produces, and the citrate-based regional anticoagulation approach discussed in that chapter is generally preferred when renal replacement therapy is required in this population, avoiding the systemic anticoagulation considerations that would otherwise complicate management in a patient already receiving complement inhibitor therapy and its associated monitoring requirements. Long-term renal outcomes in atypical hemolytic uremic syndrome have improved substantially with prompt complement inhibitor therapy relative to the historical natural history, though a subset of patients, particularly those with delayed diagnosis or treatment initiation, progress to chronic kidney disease or end-stage renal disease requiring ongoing nephrology management well beyond the acute episode this chapter has primarily addressed.

This improved but still imperfect long-term renal outcome profile reinforces the urgency of prompt recognition and treatment initiation this chapter has emphasized throughout, and it underscores why the diagnostic distinction framework developed earlier in this chapter, applied promptly and systematically, carries direct, measurable consequences for a patient's long-term renal function and overall prognosis.

Long-Term Monitoring and Relapse Prevention

Relapse Risk in Acquired Thrombotic Thrombocytopenic Purpura

Patients with acquired thrombotic thrombocytopenic purpura carry meaningful long-term relapse risk, with ADAMTS13 activity level at clinical remission serving as an important prognostic marker, since persistently low ADAMTS13 activity despite clinical and hematologic remission predicts substantially higher relapse risk than a patient who has achieved both clinical remission and normalized ADAMTS13 activity, directly informing the intensity and duration of the long-term monitoring plan developed in this final section of this chapter. Periodic ADAMTS13 activity monitoring following recovery from an acute episode, at a frequency informed by the specific risk factors and remission depth discussed above, allows identification of a subclinical relapse, characterized by declining ADAMTS13 activity before clinically apparent thrombocytopenia and hemolysis develop, potentially allowing preemptive treatment, most often with rituximab, to prevent a full clinical relapse from developing.

This subclinical relapse detection and preemptive treatment strategy represents an evolving area of clinical practice, and clinicians managing patients with a history of acquired thrombotic thrombocytopenic purpura should coordinate with a hematologist experienced in this condition to establish an appropriate individualized long-term monitoring plan, extending the individualized, trend-based monitoring philosophy developed throughout Chapters 6 through 9 into this specific, high-relapse-risk condition.

Long-Term Follow-Up in Atypical Hemolytic Uremic Syndrome

Patients with atypical hemolytic uremic syndrome, particularly those who have discontinued long-term complement inhibitor therapy following the extended stability period discussed earlier in this chapter, require ongoing monitoring for disease relapse, including periodic complete blood count, renal function assessment, and patient education regarding the specific symptoms that should prompt immediate medical attention given the relapse risk this discontinuation decision carries. Genetic counseling for the patient and, where appropriate, family members, given the underlying complement regulatory gene variants discussed earlier in this chapter, provides important information regarding the risk of disease expression in relatives who may carry the same genetic predisposition, extending the family counseling principles developed for inherited platelet disorders in Chapters 7 and 15 into this specific complement-mediated disease context.

This genetic counseling should address the incomplete penetrance pattern discussed earlier in this chapter, helping family members understand that carrying a pathogenic complement regulatory variant confers susceptibility rather than certainty of disease development, an important nuance for accurate risk communication that avoids both false reassurance and undue anxiety among family members undergoing this genetic evaluation.

Psychological Support and Patient Education Following a Life-Threatening Episode

Given the acute, life-threatening nature of the thrombotic microangiopathy episode this chapter has developed throughout, patients recovering from thrombotic thrombocytopenic purpura or atypical hemolytic uremic syndrome frequently benefit from psychological support addressing the trauma of a sudden, severe, and potentially fatal illness, extending the quality-of-life and psychological wellbeing considerations developed for chronic immune thrombocytopenia in Chapter 9 into this acute, though potentially recurrent, condition. Patient education regarding relapse warning signs, the ongoing monitoring plan established for their specific condition and treatment history, and clear guidance on when and how to seek urgent care should symptoms recur, extending the transparent communication and self-advocacy principles developed throughout this book, equips patients to participate actively in the long-term surveillance that meaningfully improves outcomes in these relapsing-prone conditions.

This chapter has developed the thrombotic microangiopathies as the most acutely life-threatening emergencies within this book's broader thrombocytopenia framework, requiring recognition and treatment initiation that, more than any other condition this book addresses, cannot wait for complete diagnostic certainty. The chapters that follow return to conditions with somewhat less immediate time pressure, beginning with thrombocytopenia in pregnancy in Chapter 13, a context that, notably, intersects directly with several of the conditions this chapter has developed, including both congenital thrombotic thrombocytopenic purpura and atypical hemolytic uremic syndrome.

CLINICAL CASE: A 29-year-old woman presents to the emergency department with three days of progressive fatigue and new-onset confusion. Initial laboratory testing reveals platelet count 9 x10^9/L, hemoglobin 6.9 g/dL, lactate dehydrogenase markedly elevated, haptoglobin undetectable, and peripheral smear showing numerous schistocytes with no evidence of platelet clumping. Coagulation studies, including prothrombin time and activated partial thromboplastin time, are normal, and the direct antiglobulin test is negative, together confirming microangiopathic hemolytic anemia rather than an alternative hemolytic or consumptive process. Applying the framework developed in this chapter, the PLASMIC score is calculated and returns in the high-probability range, prompting immediate hematology consultation and same-day initiation of therapeutic plasma exchange without awaiting ADAMTS13 results, which are sent concurrently along with Shiga toxin stool testing given the diagnostic uncertainty appropriately maintained at this early stage. Caplacizumab and corticosteroid therapy are initiated alongside the first plasma exchange session, following the multi-mechanism management approach developed in this chapter, and ADAMTS13 activity subsequently returns at less than five percent with a positive inhibitor, confirming acquired autoimmune thrombotic thrombocytopenic purpura and supporting continuation of the current treatment approach. The patient's neurologic status improves progressively over the following three days as platelet count and hemolysis markers normalize, and rituximab is added given the severity of her initial presentation and the evidence supporting earlier, more aggressive immunosuppression discussed in this chapter. She is discharged after achieving sustained biochemical remission, with a structured long-term monitoring plan including periodic ADAMTS13 activity assessment to detect subclinical relapse. This case illustrates the complete diagnostic and management arc developed in this chapter: immediate recognition of the schistocyte-thrombocytopenia combination, structured probability assessment driving same-day treatment before definitive confirmation, multi-mechanism therapy reflecting current evidence-based practice, and structured long-term relapse monitoring.

THE PLATELET CRISIS DECISION COMPASS — Thrombotic Microangiopathy Recognition and Treatment Sequencing

Compass Recap: Same-Day Treatment Trigger: Thrombocytopenia with microangiopathic hemolytic anemia (schistocytes, elevated lactate dehydrogenase, low haptoglobin) and a high PLASMIC score triggers same-day plasma exchange initiation, not deferral until ADAMTS13 confirmation returns.

Compass Recap: Empiric Treatment Pending Distinction: Empiric plasma exchange is initiated for any patient meeting thrombotic microangiopathy criteria regardless of which specific variant clinical pattern initially suggests, continuing until ADAMTS13 results definitively exclude severe deficiency and allow transition to variant-specific therapy.

Chapter Anchor: Thrombotic microangiopathy — thrombocytopenia plus microangiopathic hemolytic anemia — is a hematologic emergency treated empirically before definitive mechanism-specific confirmation, with ADAMTS13 severe deficiency directing plasma exchange-based therapy, Shiga toxin positivity directing supportive care alone, and exclusion of both directing complement inhibitor therapy for atypical hemolytic uremic syndrome.

Summary and Key Concepts

Thrombotic microangiopathy is a shared clinical syndrome (thrombocytopenia plus microangiopathic hemolytic anemia with schistocytes) arising from distinct mechanisms: severe ADAMTS13 deficiency (TTP), Shiga toxin-mediated endothelial injury (STEC-HUS), or complement dysregulation (atypical HUS).

The classic pentad is no longer required for TTP diagnosis or treatment initiation; thrombocytopenia and microangiopathic hemolytic anemia alone warrant urgent evaluation and empiric treatment.

The PLASMIC score provides validated bedside pretest probability for severe ADAMTS13 deficiency, supporting same-day empiric plasma exchange initiation before definitive ADAMTS13 confirmation.

Shiga toxin-associated HUS, predominantly pediatric, presents with a diarrheal prodrome and is managed with supportive care alone (antibiotics avoided; plasma exchange not indicated); atypical HUS presents with prominent renal involvement without prodrome and requires complement inhibitor therapy (eculizumab/ravulizumab).

TTP management combines therapeutic plasma exchange, caplacizumab, and immunosuppressive therapy (corticosteroids, increasingly rituximab), reflecting a multi-mechanism approach that has transformed historically fatal outcomes.

Long-term monitoring includes ADAMTS13 activity trending to detect subclinical TTP relapse and genetic counseling for atypical HUS given its complement regulatory gene basis and incomplete penetrance.

CHAPTER 13: THROMBOCYTOPENIA IN PREGNANCY AND THE NEONATE

Learning Objectives

1. Describe the physiologic platelet count changes that occur during normal pregnancy and distinguish gestational thrombocytopenia from pathologic causes.
2. Recognize the clinical and laboratory features distinguishing preeclampsia, HELLP syndrome, and pregnancy-associated thrombotic microangiopathy.
3. Apply the diagnostic and management framework for immune thrombocytopenia in pregnancy, including delivery planning considerations.
4. Explain the pathophysiology and management of neonatal alloimmune thrombocytopenia.
5. Construct a differential diagnosis and evaluation approach for neonatal thrombocytopenia.
6. Coordinate delivery planning and anesthesia considerations for a pregnant patient with thrombocytopenia of any etiology.

Chapter Outline

This chapter develops thrombocytopenia across the maternal-fetal dyad, addressing the physiologic platelet changes of normal pregnancy, gestational thrombocytopenia, the pregnancy-specific hypertensive and microangiopathic syndromes, immune thrombocytopenia in pregnancy, delivery and anesthesia planning, and the distinct evaluation of neonatal thrombocytopenia including neonatal alloimmune thrombocytopenia. Two Platelet Crisis Decision Compass instances address the urgent distinction between benign gestational thrombocytopenia and a pregnancy-specific emergency, and the recognition of neonatal alloimmune thrombocytopenia risk in a subsequent pregnancy.

Pregnancy introduces physiologic and pathophysiologic considerations that intersect with nearly every category of thrombocytopenia addressed throughout this book, from the benign physiologic decline discussed early in this chapter to the pregnancy-specific presentations of thrombotic microangiopathy introduced in Chapter 12, and this chapter integrates and extends the frameworks developed throughout Part III into this specific, time-pressured clinical context in which both maternal and fetal wellbeing depend on prompt, accurate diagnosis.

Physiologic Platelet Changes in Normal Pregnancy

Mechanisms of the Physiologic Decline

Platelet count declines modestly during normal pregnancy, particularly in the third trimester, through a combination of hemodilution from the physiologic plasma volume expansion characteristic of pregnancy, increased platelet consumption at the low-pressure uteroplacental circulation, and accelerated platelet clearance, together producing a physiologic nadir that remains, in the substantial majority of pregnant individuals, within or only modestly below the standard non-pregnant reference range discussed in

Chapter 6. This physiologic decline typically does not produce clinically significant thrombocytopenia, and understanding its expected magnitude and timing provides the essential baseline against which pathologic thrombocytopenia in pregnancy, discussed throughout the remainder of this chapter, must be distinguished.

The physiologic mechanisms underlying this decline directly parallel, though in an exaggerated and pregnancy-specific form, the splenic sequestration and hemodilutional mechanisms discussed within the broader distributional thrombocytopenia framework developed in Chapter 8, reinforcing that pregnancy represents a physiologic state that shifts, rather than replaces, the mechanistic framework this book has developed throughout, requiring pregnancy-specific calibration rather than an entirely separate diagnostic approach.

Expected Magnitude and Reference Range Considerations

Population studies of platelet count across normal pregnancy demonstrate that the great majority of pregnant individuals maintain a platelet count above 150 x10^9/L throughout gestation, with a modest additional subset experiencing a physiologic decline to the 100 to 150 x10^9/L range, particularly in the third trimester, without any pathologic explanation, directly informing the gestational thrombocytopenia diagnostic criteria discussed in the next section of this chapter. Platelet count below 100 x10^9/L during pregnancy substantially exceeds the range attributable to physiologic decline alone and should prompt the systematic evaluation for pathologic causes developed throughout the remainder of this chapter, applying the same confirmation and mechanistic localization principles developed in Chapters 6 and 8 with the pregnancy-specific modifications this chapter provides.

This population-based reference framework directly extends the population-and-physiology-specific reference range principle developed in Chapter 6, reinforcing that a platelet count must be interpreted against the specific physiologic context, in this case gestational age and trimester, rather than against a single universal threshold, to correctly distinguish expected physiologic variation from a finding warranting further evaluation.

Timing and Trajectory Across Gestation

The physiologic platelet count decline discussed in this section typically becomes most apparent in the third trimester, with earlier pregnancy platelet counts generally remaining closer to the non-pregnant baseline, and this trajectory pattern means that thrombocytopenia identified in the first or early second trimester more strongly warrants consideration of a pathologic cause than a similar finding identified for the first time in the third trimester, directly applying the trend and trajectory reasoning developed throughout Chapters 6 and 8 to this pregnancy-specific temporal pattern. A platelet count trend that continues to decline progressively through the third trimester and does not stabilize as delivery approaches similarly warrants closer attention than a stable, modest decline that plateaus at a mildly reduced level, reinforcing the value of serial platelet count monitoring throughout pregnancy in any patient whose count approaches or falls below the reference threshold discussed above.

This gestational-age-specific and trajectory-based interpretation framework provides the essential clinical context for every subsequent section of this chapter, and it should be applied systematically whenever thrombocytopenia is identified at any point during pregnancy, integrating the specific gestational age and platelet count trend into the broader mechanistic and clinical evaluation this chapter develops.

Gestational Thrombocytopenia

Diagnostic Criteria and Clinical Features

Gestational thrombocytopenia, the most common cause of thrombocytopenia identified during pregnancy, is a diagnosis of exclusion characterized by mild thrombocytopenia, generally with a platelet count above 70 $\times 10^9$/L, onset in the late second or third trimester, no prior history of thrombocytopenia outside pregnancy, no associated fetal thrombocytopenia, and spontaneous resolution within one to two months following delivery, features that together distinguish this entirely benign condition from the pathologic causes discussed throughout the remainder of this chapter. This condition carries no increased maternal or fetal bleeding risk and requires no specific intervention beyond routine monitoring, and correctly recognizing gestational thrombocytopenia, applying the diagnostic criteria discussed in this section, avoids the unnecessary anxiety, additional testing, and potential intervention that an incorrect alternative diagnosis might otherwise prompt.

The absence of associated findings, including hypertension, proteinuria, hemolysis, and significant bleeding symptoms, forms an essential component of the gestational thrombocytopenia diagnosis, directly paralleling the exclusionary approach developed for immune thrombocytopenia in Chapter 9, and any accompanying finding beyond isolated mild thrombocytopenia should prompt reconsideration of the pathologic causes developed throughout the remainder of this chapter rather than default acceptance of the more common and reassuring gestational thrombocytopenia diagnosis.

Distinguishing Gestational Thrombocytopenia From Early Immune Thrombocytopenia

Distinguishing gestational thrombocytopenia from immune thrombocytopenia presenting during pregnancy, discussed in detail later in this chapter, can be challenging given overlapping clinical features, and several distinguishing considerations, including platelet count severity, with a count below 70 $\times 10^9$/L favoring immune thrombocytopenia over the milder gestational pattern, onset timing, with first-trimester or early second-trimester onset favoring immune thrombocytopenia over the characteristically later gestational thrombocytopenia onset, and a prior non-pregnant history of thrombocytopenia, which would exclude gestational thrombocytopenia by definition, together inform this distinction, though no single feature definitively separates these conditions in every case. This diagnostic ambiguity, while clinically important to resolve when possible, does not always require aggressive additional testing to definitively distinguish, since the initial management approach for mild, uncomplicated thrombocytopenia of either etiology in a well patient without bleeding symptoms is similar, with the practical distinction becoming most clinically important as the platelet count approaches thresholds relevant to delivery planning, discussed later in this chapter.

This pragmatic approach to diagnostic ambiguity, accepting a degree of uncertainty when it does not immediately alter management, reflects the broader philosophy developed throughout this book regarding the acceptance of diagnostic uncertainty when further evaluation carries diminishing clinical return, while maintaining ongoing vigilance and platelet count monitoring throughout the remainder of pregnancy to detect any evolution that would clarify or redirect the working diagnosis.

Monitoring and Reassurance

Once gestational thrombocytopenia is reasonably diagnosed, ongoing management consists of periodic platelet count monitoring through the remainder of pregnancy, generally at a frequency informed by the specific count and trajectory, along with clear communication to the patient regarding the benign nature of this finding, applying the transparent communication framework developed in Chapter 5 to reassure a patient who may otherwise experience considerable anxiety upon learning of any abnormal laboratory finding during pregnancy. This monitoring should continue through delivery, given the delivery planning considerations discussed later in this chapter that apply regardless of the specific underlying thrombocytopenia etiology, and postpartum platelet count confirmation of the expected resolution discussed earlier in this section provides final retrospective confirmation of the gestational thrombocytopenia diagnosis.

This monitoring-and-reassurance approach exemplifies the broader principle developed throughout this book that not every abnormal finding requires aggressive intervention, and gestational thrombocytopenia represents perhaps the clearest example within this entire book of a finding whose correct management is confident reassurance and routine monitoring rather than escalating evaluation or treatment.

Hypertensive Disorders of Pregnancy: Preeclampsia and HELLP Syndrome

Preeclampsia-Associated Thrombocytopenia

Preeclampsia, defined by new-onset hypertension after twenty weeks gestation accompanied by proteinuria or other evidence of end-organ involvement, produces thrombocytopenia in a meaningful proportion of affected patients through a mechanism involving endothelial dysfunction, increased platelet activation and consumption, and, in severe cases, a component of microangiopathic process overlapping with the thrombotic microangiopathy mechanisms developed in Chapter 12. The severity of thrombocytopenia in preeclampsia generally correlates with overall disease severity, and a declining platelet count in a patient with established preeclampsia should be interpreted as a marker of disease progression warranting reassessment of delivery timing and other management decisions, discussed further in the maternal-fetal medicine collaborative management this condition requires.

Any pregnant patient presenting with new thrombocytopenia should have blood pressure and urine protein assessed as part of the initial evaluation, directly extending the pregnancy-specific triage principle introduced in Chapters 5 and 8, since preeclampsia and its more severe variant HELLP syndrome, discussed next, represent among the most common pathologic causes of thrombocytopenia in pregnancy and require prompt recognition given their potential for rapid progression and serious maternal and fetal consequences.

HELLP Syndrome

HELLP syndrome, an acronym describing Hemolysis, Elevated Liver enzymes, and Low Platelets, represents a severe variant of preeclampsia, though it can occasionally occur without the classic hypertension and proteinuria criteria for preeclampsia being fully met, and its diagnosis requires the combination of microangiopathic hemolysis, applying the same confirmatory laboratory approach developed in Chapter 12, elevated hepatic transaminases reflecting hepatic microvascular involvement, and thrombocytopenia, typically more severe than in preeclampsia without this syndrome. HELLP syndrome carries substantial maternal risk, including hepatic hematoma or rupture in severe cases, disseminated intravascular coagulation discussed further in Chapter 14, and placental abruption, along with significant fetal risk from the underlying placental insufficiency this syndrome reflects, and definitive management requires delivery, generally regardless of gestational age once the diagnosis is confirmed and maternal or fetal status warrants intervention, a management principle distinguishing this condition from the supportive, expectant management appropriate to milder preeclampsia presentations remote from term.

The overlapping laboratory features between HELLP syndrome and the thrombotic microangiopathy syndromes developed in Chapter 12, both producing microangiopathic hemolysis and thrombocytopenia, require careful clinical distinction, discussed further in the differential diagnosis section of this chapter, given the substantially different management approach delivery represents for HELLP syndrome relative to the plasma exchange and complement-directed therapies appropriate to the thrombotic microangiopathy syndromes discussed in Chapter 12.

Monitoring and Management Coordination

Management of preeclampsia and HELLP syndrome requires close coordination between maternal-fetal medicine and, when the platelet count or clinical severity warrants, hematology, extending the multidisciplinary coordination principle developed throughout Chapters 8 through 12 into this specific obstetric emergency context, with corticosteroid therapy sometimes used specifically for fetal lung maturation in anticipation of preterm delivery, distinct from the immunosuppressive corticosteroid use discussed for immune thrombocytopenia in Chapter 9, a distinction important to clarify when discussing treatment rationale with the patient and broader care team. Platelet transfusion, discussed further in the transfusion medicine context of Chapter 19, is generally reserved for active bleeding or in anticipation of cesarean delivery at a specific platelet count threshold, discussed in the delivery planning section of this chapter, rather than used routinely based on the platelet count alone in the absence of bleeding or an imminent procedural indication.

This coordinated management approach reflects the time-sensitive, potentially rapidly progressive nature of preeclampsia and HELLP syndrome, and clinicians managing a pregnant patient with new thrombocytopenia and hypertension should maintain a low threshold for urgent maternal-fetal medicine involvement given the potential for rapid clinical evolution this condition characteristically demonstrates.

Immune Thrombocytopenia in Pregnancy

Diagnostic Considerations Specific to Pregnancy

Immune thrombocytopenia, discussed in full mechanistic and general management detail in Chapter 9, can present for the first time during pregnancy or can represent a preexisting condition that persists or fluctuates through gestation, and the diagnostic distinction from gestational thrombocytopenia, discussed earlier in this chapter, and from the hypertensive and microangiopathic syndromes developed elsewhere in this chapter, follows the general exclusionary diagnostic principles developed in Chapter 9 with the pregnancy-specific alternative diagnoses this chapter adds to that differential. A platelet count below 100 x10^9/L, particularly earlier in pregnancy or accompanied by bleeding symptoms, should prompt consideration of immune thrombocytopenia alongside the pregnancy-specific causes this chapter has developed, applying the same structured bleeding history and examination framework developed in Chapter 5 to the pregnant patient.

This diagnostic evaluation should specifically exclude the pregnancy-specific alternative causes discussed throughout this chapter, including confirming normal blood pressure and the absence of proteinuria to reasonably exclude preeclampsia and HELLP syndrome, and confirming the absence of significant hemolysis to reasonably exclude the thrombotic microangiopathy syndromes discussed in Chapter 12 and later in this chapter, before confidently establishing an immune thrombocytopenia diagnosis in the pregnant patient.

Treatment Selection in Pregnancy

As introduced in Chapter 9, corticosteroids and intravenous immunoglobulin remain the preferred first-line treatments for immune thrombocytopenia requiring active management during pregnancy, given their more established pregnancy safety profile relative to several of the second-line agents discussed in Chapter 9, many of which carry pregnancy-specific precautions or insufficient safety data, and treatment initiation thresholds during pregnancy generally favor a somewhat lower platelet count threshold for intervention than outside pregnancy, given the additional consideration of anticipated delivery and the platelet count thresholds relevant to delivery planning discussed later in this chapter. Splenectomy, discussed as a second-line option in Chapter 9, is generally avoided during pregnancy given both surgical risk considerations specific to the gravid uterus and the availability of effective medical alternatives, and is reserved for the rare circumstance of severe, refractory disease not adequately controlled with medical therapy alone.

This pregnancy-specific treatment selection approach directly extends the individualized, risk-calibrated management philosophy developed throughout Chapter 9 into the specific context of balancing maternal disease control against fetal medication exposure considerations, requiring close collaboration between hematology and maternal-fetal medicine throughout the treatment planning and monitoring process.

Fetal and Neonatal Monitoring Considerations

Maternal antiplatelet antibodies in immune thrombocytopenia can cross the placenta and produce fetal and subsequently neonatal thrombocytopenia, though this fetal transmission is generally less predictable and typically less severe than the neonatal alloimmune thrombocytopenia mechanism discussed later in this chapter, and severe fetal thrombocytopenia from maternal immune thrombocytopenia is comparatively uncommon, meaning that invasive fetal platelet count assessment, which carries its own procedural risks, is generally not recommended as a routine component of management for maternal immune thrombocytopenia in current practice. Neonatal platelet count should be assessed after delivery in an infant born to a mother with immune thrombocytopenia, applying the neonatal evaluation framework developed later in this chapter, with the neonatal platelet count nadir sometimes occurring several days after delivery rather than immediately at birth, a timing consideration relevant to the duration of postpartum neonatal monitoring appropriate in this specific clinical scenario.

This fetal and neonatal monitoring approach reflects a more measured, less invasive surveillance strategy than the alloimmune thrombocytopenia management discussed later in this chapter, reflecting the generally lower and less predictable fetal risk this maternal condition carries, though ongoing clinical vigilance and appropriate neonatal assessment remain important components of comprehensive management for this specific maternal-fetal clinical scenario.

THE PLATELET CRISIS DECISION COMPASS — Distinguishing Benign Gestational Thrombocytopenia from a Pregnancy Emergency

The Presentation: A woman at 34 weeks gestation is found to have a platelet count of 88 x10^9/L on routine prenatal laboratory testing, with no prior thrombocytopenia history.

Mimic Signature: Benign gestational thrombocytopenia given the third-trimester timing and mild severity; early preeclampsia or HELLP syndrome that has not yet manifested its full laboratory picture; and immune thrombocytopenia presenting for the first time during pregnancy.

The Decision: Immediately assess blood pressure, urine protein, and obtain a hepatic panel and hemolysis studies (lactate dehydrogenase, haptoglobin, peripheral smear for schistocytes) at the same visit, applying the pregnancy-specific triage principle from this chapter, before reassuring the patient that this represents benign gestational thrombocytopenia; if all additional findings are unremarkable, gestational thrombocytopenia can be reasonably diagnosed with continued monitoring through delivery.

Trap Logic: Reassuring a pregnant patient that a mildly low platelet count 'is probably just pregnancy' without obtaining the blood pressure, urine protein, and hemolysis assessment this chapter requires risks missing early preeclampsia or HELLP syndrome, both of which can progress rapidly once initially subtle laboratory abnormalities become clinically apparent.

Crisis Anchor: Any new thrombocytopenia identified during pregnancy triggers same-visit assessment of blood pressure, urine protein, and hemolysis markers before a benign gestational thrombocytopenia diagnosis is accepted, regardless of how mild or reassuring the presentation initially appears.

Thrombotic Microangiopathy in Pregnancy

Pregnancy as a Trigger for Thrombotic Thrombocytopenic Purpura

Pregnancy represents a recognized trigger for both new-onset acquired thrombotic thrombocytopenic purpura and unmasking of previously unrecognized congenital thrombotic thrombocytopenic purpura, discussed in Chapter 12, reflecting the physiologic decline in ADAMTS13 activity that occurs even in unaffected individuals during normal pregnancy, which can unmask a marginal congenital deficiency or precipitate an autoimmune episode in a susceptible individual. Distinguishing thrombotic thrombocytopenic purpura from HELLP syndrome during pregnancy represents one of the most diagnostically challenging distinctions in this entire book, given substantial overlap in the microangiopathic hemolysis and thrombocytopenia both conditions produce, and this distinction carries critical management implications, since HELLP syndrome management centers on delivery while thrombotic thrombocytopenic purpura management centers on plasma exchange as developed in Chapter 12, with delivery alone inadequate to address the underlying ADAMTS13 deficiency.

Several distinguishing features aid this critical distinction, including the degree of hepatic transaminase elevation, typically more pronounced in HELLP syndrome, the presence and severity of hypertension and proteinuria, more characteristic of HELLP syndrome, and ADAMTS13 activity testing, applying the same testing framework developed in Chapter 12, though this testing's turnaround time limitation discussed in that chapter applies equally in the pregnancy context, often requiring the same empiric treatment-before-confirmation approach this book has emphasized throughout the thrombotic microangiopathy discussion.

Pregnancy-Associated Atypical Hemolytic Uremic Syndrome

Pregnancy and the postpartum period also represent a recognized trigger for atypical hemolytic uremic syndrome in a genetically predisposed individual, discussed mechanistically in Chapter 12, with postpartum presentation particularly characteristic and sometimes delayed by days to weeks after delivery, a timing pattern that can lead to diagnostic delay if the temporal relationship to the recent pregnancy is not specifically considered in a postpartum patient presenting with new thrombocytopenia and renal dysfunction. This postpartum-predominant timing pattern for atypical hemolytic uremic syndrome contrasts with the more immediately pregnancy-associated timing typical of HELLP syndrome and pregnancy-triggered thrombotic thrombocytopenic purpura, providing an additional temporal clue within the broader distinguishing framework this chapter and Chapter 12 together develop for the pregnancy-associated thrombotic microangiopathy differential.

Given this distinct timing pattern, any patient presenting with thrombocytopenia and renal dysfunction within several weeks postpartum, even after apparent resolution of an antepartum hypertensive or hematologic complication, should have atypical hemolytic uremic syndrome specifically considered within the broader thrombotic microangiopathy differential this chapter and Chapter 12 develop, applying the complement functional and genetic testing discussed in Chapter 12 to confirm this specific, pregnancy-triggered presentation.

Multidisciplinary Management of Pregnancy-Associated Thrombotic Microangiopathy

Given the diagnostic complexity and high clinical stakes this section has developed, any pregnant or postpartum patient with suspected thrombotic microangiopathy warrants immediate multidisciplinary evaluation involving maternal-fetal medicine, hematology, and, when renal involvement is significant, nephrology, extending the multidisciplinary coordination principle developed throughout this book into this specific, exceptionally high-stakes clinical intersection between obstetric and hematologic emergency. This coordinated evaluation should proceed with the same urgency emphasized throughout Chapter 12, recognizing that the diagnostic ambiguity between HELLP syndrome, thrombotic thrombocytopenic purpura, and atypical hemolytic uremic syndrome discussed throughout this section should not delay the empiric treatment interventions, whether expedited delivery for suspected HELLP syndrome or plasma exchange initiation for suspected thrombotic thrombocytopenic purpura, that the working diagnosis at each stage of evaluation supports.

This pregnancy-specific application of the thrombotic microangiopathy framework developed in Chapter 12 illustrates how pregnancy intersects with and complicates nearly every diagnostic category this book has developed, reinforcing why obstetric and hematologic expertise must be combined, rather than applied sequentially or in isolation, whenever a pregnant or postpartum patient presents with thrombocytopenia and any accompanying finding suggestive of these serious underlying processes.

Delivery Planning and Anesthesia Considerations

Platelet Count Thresholds for Neuraxial Anesthesia

Neuraxial anesthesia, including epidural and spinal anesthesia, carries a small but serious risk of epidural hematoma in the setting of significant thrombocytopenia, and current anesthesia society guidance generally supports neuraxial anesthesia at a platelet count above 70 x10^9/L in an otherwise reassuring clinical picture, with more individualized risk-benefit assessment, incorporating the platelet count trend, the underlying etiology, and the presence or absence of any coagulopathy, required at lower platelet counts, directly applying the individualized, trend-informed risk assessment principle developed throughout Chapters 6 and 8 to this specific, time-critical delivery planning decision. This threshold should be considered a general guideline rather than an absolute cutoff, and anesthesia consultation well in advance of the anticipated delivery date, whenever a pregnant patient's platelet count trajectory suggests it may approach this threshold range, allows for coordinated planning rather than a last-minute decision made under the time pressure of active labor.

This advance planning imperative directly extends the perioperative timing principle developed in Chapter 7 into this specific obstetric context, where the timing of delivery is often less flexible than an elective surgical procedure, making early identification of a potentially complicating platelet count trajectory and early anesthesia involvement particularly valuable for optimizing the delivery plan and anesthesia options available to the patient.

Mode of Delivery Considerations

The underlying thrombocytopenia etiology, rather than the platelet count alone, should primarily inform mode of delivery decisions, with maternal thrombocytopenia from most of the causes discussed in this chapter, including gestational thrombocytopenia and immune thrombocytopenia, generally not by itself indicating cesarean delivery, since vaginal delivery does not carry substantially elevated maternal bleeding risk at platelet counts that do not otherwise contraindicate this delivery route, and cesarean delivery introduces its own additional surgical bleeding risk considerations that must be weighed against any anticipated benefit. Fetal or neonatal alloimmune thrombocytopenia risk, discussed later in this chapter, represents an important exception to this general principle, since severe fetal thrombocytopenia from this specific mechanism can carry elevated intracranial hemorrhage risk during the mechanical stress of vaginal delivery, and cesarean delivery is often specifically recommended in this scenario, discussed further in the alloimmune thrombocytopenia section of this chapter.

This etiology-specific approach to mode of delivery decision-making exemplifies the broader principle developed throughout this book that management decisions are calibrated to the specific underlying mechanism and its associated risk profile, rather than applied uniformly based on the platelet count number alone, extending this principle into the specific, time-sensitive context of delivery planning.

Coordinating a Comprehensive Delivery Plan

A comprehensive delivery plan for a pregnant patient with thrombocytopenia should be documented well in advance of the anticipated delivery date, incorporating the anesthesia platelet count threshold discussed above, any specific mode of delivery recommendation based on the underlying etiology, availability of platelet transfusion support if needed, and clear communication among obstetrics, anesthesia, hematology, and, for the neonate, pediatrics or neonatology, extending the structured, documented, multidisciplinary planning principle developed throughout this book into this specific, time-critical clinical event. This plan should be readily accessible to the entire delivery team, ideally through a structured, prominently flagged element of the patient's obstetric record, given that delivery can occur urgently or outside of planned working hours when the full outpatient care team may not be immediately available to provide real-time guidance.

This proactive, documented delivery planning approach reflects the same longitudinal documentation and communication principles that have recurred throughout this book, applied here to a specific, time-bounded clinical event whose successful management depends on advance preparation rather than reactive decision-making under the acute time pressure that active labor and delivery characteristically involve.

Neonatal Alloimmune Thrombocytopenia

Pathophysiology of Fetal and Neonatal Alloimmunization

Neonatal alloimmune thrombocytopenia arises when a mother lacking a specific platelet surface antigen, most commonly human platelet antigen 1a, is exposed to fetal platelets expressing this paternally inherited antigen, generating maternal alloantibodies that cross the placenta and destroy fetal platelets through a mechanism directly analogous to red cell alloimmunization in hemolytic disease of the newborn, but affecting platelets specifically rather than red cells. Unlike red cell alloimmunization, which typically does not affect a first pregnancy given the sensitization timing involved, neonatal alloimmune thrombocytopenia can affect a first pregnancy, since the sensitizing fetal platelet antigen exposure and the causative antibody response can occur early enough in gestation to affect that same pregnancy, a distinction with important implications for antenatal risk stratification discussed later in this section.

This mechanism produces some of the most severe thrombocytopenia discussed anywhere in this book, with intracranial hemorrhage representing the most feared complication, occurring in a meaningful proportion of untreated severe cases and carrying substantial risk of long-term neurologic morbidity, underscoring why this specific condition, though comparatively uncommon, receives dedicated, structured antenatal management attention disproportionate to its population frequency.

Antenatal Risk Stratification in a Subsequent Pregnancy

A prior pregnancy affected by neonatal alloimmune thrombocytopenia substantially elevates the risk of an equally or more severely affected subsequent pregnancy if the father again carries the sensitizing platelet antigen, and structured antenatal management for a subsequent pregnancy in this specific circumstance includes maternal antibody titer monitoring, paternal and fetal antigen genotyping to confirm ongoing risk, and, in specialized centers, intravenous immunoglobulin administration to the mother during pregnancy specifically to reduce fetal platelet destruction, an antenatal intervention distinct from and more intensive than the general immune thrombocytopenia management discussed earlier in this chapter. This structured, intensified antenatal management approach for a subsequent at-risk pregnancy reflects the severity of potential outcomes this condition carries and the demonstrated efficacy of antenatal intervention in reducing this risk, representing one of the clearest examples within this book of antenatal, preemptive intervention meaningfully altering an otherwise high-risk pregnancy trajectory.

Given the specialized nature of this antenatal management, referral to a center with specific maternal-fetal medicine and hematology expertise in neonatal alloimmune thrombocytopenia is generally recommended once a prior affected pregnancy or other risk factor is identified, extending the specialized referral principle developed throughout this book into this specific, comparatively rare but high-stakes clinical scenario.

Neonatal Diagnosis and Acute Management

Diagnosis of neonatal alloimmune thrombocytopenia in an affected infant is confirmed through platelet antigen genotyping of the infant and parents along with maternal antiplatelet antibody testing directed against the specific platelet antigen system implicated, and acute neonatal management for significant thrombocytopenia includes intravenous immunoglobulin and, for severe thrombocytopenia or active bleeding, transfusion of antigen-negative platelets, meaning platelets lacking the specific antigen the maternal antibody targets, since standard random-donor platelets, if they carry the implicated antigen, would be subject to the same antibody-mediated destruction affecting the infant's own platelets. Cranial ultrasound is generally recommended in an affected neonate to assess for intracranial hemorrhage, even in the absence of overt neurologic symptoms, given the clinical importance of this specific complication discussed earlier in this section and the value of early detection in guiding both acute management and long-term neurologic follow-up planning.

This acute neonatal management approach, requiring close coordination between neonatology, hematology, and the blood bank to identify and provide antigen-negative platelet products, exemplifies the specialized, multidisciplinary response this specific condition requires, and clear communication of a confirmed neonatal alloimmune thrombocytopenia diagnosis to the family, including its implications for future pregnancy planning discussed earlier in this section, forms an essential component of comprehensive care for this condition.

THE PLATELET CRISIS DECISION COMPASS — Recognizing Neonatal Alloimmune Thrombocytopenia Risk in a Subsequent Pregnancy

The Presentation: A woman whose first child was born with severe thrombocytopenia and a grade 2 intracranial hemorrhage, later confirmed as neonatal alloimmune thrombocytopenia, presents now pregnant with her second child by the same partner.

Mimic Signature: A subsequent pregnancy at high risk for equally or more severe recurrent neonatal alloimmune thrombocytopenia given the same paternal antigen exposure; a lower-risk scenario if paternal antigen status has changed (different partner) or genotyping reveals the father is heterozygous with a chance of an antigen-negative fetus; and a coincidental, unrelated cause of any thrombocytopenia identified in this new pregnancy.

The Decision: Refer immediately to a center with specialized maternal-fetal medicine and hematology expertise in neonatal alloimmune thrombocytopenia for paternal and fetal antigen genotyping and structured antenatal management, including maternal antibody titer monitoring and consideration of antenatal intravenous immunoglobulin, rather than managing this pregnancy through routine prenatal care alone.

Trap Logic: Treating this pregnancy as routine because the mother herself is asymptomatic and her own platelet count is normal overlooks that neonatal alloimmune thrombocytopenia is a fetal, not maternal, hematologic condition — normal maternal platelet count provides no reassurance regarding fetal risk given the alloimmune, rather than autoimmune, mechanism this condition reflects.

Crisis Anchor: A prior pregnancy affected by neonatal alloimmune thrombocytopenia mandates specialized antenatal referral for any subsequent pregnancy with the same partner, regardless of normal maternal platelet count, given the substantially elevated recurrence risk this history establishes.

Neonatal Thrombocytopenia: Broader Differential and Approach

Early-Onset Versus Late-Onset Neonatal Thrombocytopenia

Neonatal thrombocytopenia, beyond the alloimmune mechanism discussed in the preceding section, is clinically organized by timing of onset, with early-onset thrombocytopenia, appearing within the first seventy-two hours of life, most commonly reflecting placental insufficiency-related conditions including maternal preeclampsia and intrauterine growth restriction, producing a pattern of impaired fetal megakaryopoiesis analogous in mechanism to the chronic hypoxic stress response discussed in other production-limited contexts throughout this book, while late-onset thrombocytopenia, appearing after seventy-two hours of life, more commonly reflects neonatal sepsis or necrotizing enterocolitis, conditions in which the destructive and consumptive mechanisms developed in Chapter 8 predominate. This timing-based organizing framework, directly paralleling the timing-based reasoning developed throughout this book for both drug-induced thrombocytopenia in Chapter 10 and heparin-induced thrombocytopenia in Chapter 11, provides an efficient initial framework for approaching neonatal thrombocytopenia evaluation, narrowing the differential diagnosis substantially based on this single, readily available clinical parameter.

This timing framework should be applied alongside the broader maternal history, including any maternal condition discussed throughout this chapter, and the neonate's own clinical status, including signs of sepsis, birth trauma, or congenital anomaly, together forming a comprehensive initial assessment that, similar to the adult thrombocytopenia algorithm developed in Chapter 8, directs subsequent, more targeted evaluation toward the most likely underlying category rather than an undirected, exhaustive testing approach applied uniformly to every affected neonate.

Congenital and Inherited Causes in the Neonatal Period

Congenital and inherited thrombocytopenia syndromes, developed in full in Chapter 15, can present in the neonatal period, and specific findings including characteristic physical anomalies, discussed in the syndromic examination framework developed in Chapter 5, a family history of thrombocytopenia, or thrombocytopenia that persists or fails to resolve despite treatment or resolution of an initially suspected acquired cause, should prompt consideration of an inherited etiology within the broader neonatal thrombocytopenia differential this section develops. Congenital infection, including cytomegalovirus, toxoplasmosis, rubella, and other TORCH pathogens, represents an additional important consideration in neonatal thrombocytopenia, particularly when accompanied by other suggestive findings including hepatosplenomegaly, growth restriction, or characteristic imaging findings, and directed testing for these congenital infections should be incorporated into the evaluation when this etiology is clinically suspected.

This broader differential diagnosis, incorporating inherited and congenital infectious causes alongside the more common placental insufficiency and sepsis-related causes discussed earlier in this section, reinforces the value of a systematic, comprehensive evaluation approach in the neonate, extending the thoroughness principle developed throughout this book's diagnostic chapters into this specific, vulnerable patient population where diagnostic accuracy carries particularly high stakes given the neonate's limited physiologic reserve.

Coordinating Neonatal and Maternal Evaluation

Given the frequent maternal-fetal interconnection this chapter has developed throughout, evaluation of neonatal thrombocytopenia should routinely incorporate review of the maternal history and, where relevant, maternal platelet count and any pregnancy complications discussed throughout this chapter, since the maternal history frequently provides essential diagnostic context that the neonatal presentation alone would not reveal, directly paralleling the family history value discussed for inherited platelet disorders throughout this book but applied here to the immediately preceding maternal-fetal clinical course rather than a more distant family history. This coordinated maternal-neonatal evaluation approach requires effective communication between the obstetric and neonatal care teams, ideally facilitated by structured handoff documentation specifically addressing any maternal hematologic history relevant to the neonate's evaluation, extending the structured handoff and documentation principles developed throughout this book into this specific, time-critical maternal-to-neonatal information transfer.

This coordinated approach exemplifies the broader theme this chapter has developed throughout: thrombocytopenia in the maternal-fetal dyad cannot be fully understood or managed by considering the mother and infant in isolation from one another, and the most effective evaluation and management integrates information and expertise across both the obstetric and neonatal domains.

Postpartum Considerations and Long-Term Follow-Up

Expected Postpartum Platelet Count Resolution

Following delivery, the platelet count should be monitored to confirm the expected resolution pattern appropriate to the underlying etiology established during pregnancy: gestational thrombocytopenia should resolve within one to two months as discussed earlier in this chapter, preeclampsia and HELLP syndrome-associated thrombocytopenia typically improve within days following delivery, reflecting delivery's role as definitive treatment for these conditions, and immune thrombocytopenia may persist postpartum requiring continued management following the framework developed in Chapter 9. A platelet count that fails to follow the expected postpartum trajectory for the presumed antepartum diagnosis should prompt diagnostic reconsideration, applying the same trend-based diagnostic confirmation principle developed throughout Chapters 6 through 12 to this specific postpartum monitoring context, potentially revealing that the antepartum working diagnosis requires revision.

This postpartum monitoring period also provides an opportunity to complete any diagnostic evaluation that was reasonably deferred during pregnancy given testing limitations or clinical urgency, including definitive ADAMTS13 or complement functional and genetic testing for a patient with suspected pregnancy-associated thrombotic microangiopathy discussed earlier in this chapter, allowing full diagnostic clarification once the acute peripartum period has passed.

Counseling Regarding Future Pregnancies

Once a specific thrombocytopenia diagnosis has been established during a pregnancy, counseling regarding recurrence risk and management implications for future pregnancies should be provided before the patient's next pregnancy, ideally as part of dedicated preconception counseling, extending the transparent, forward-looking communication principle developed throughout this book into this specific reproductive planning context. This counseling should address condition-specific recurrence risk, including the elevated risk of preeclampsia recurrence in a subsequent pregnancy, the neonatal alloimmune thrombocytopenia recurrence risk discussed earlier in this chapter, and the pregnancy-triggered thrombotic microangiopathy risk discussed for patients with an underlying congenital thrombotic thrombocytopenic purpura or complement regulatory gene variant, each requiring the specific antenatal management planning this chapter has developed.

This preconception counseling, when feasible, allows a patient and her care team to proactively plan for a subsequent pregnancy's specific hematologic considerations rather than reactively managing them once pregnancy has already begun, optimizing both the timing of specialized referral and the depth of monitoring and intervention available from the earliest stages of a subsequent pregnancy.

Integrating This Chapter's Framework Into Ongoing Care

This chapter has developed thrombocytopenia across the maternal-fetal dyad as a distinct clinical domain requiring integration of the mechanistic frameworks developed throughout this book with pregnancy- and neonatal-specific physiology, differential diagnosis, and management considerations, extending from the entirely benign physiologic decline discussed at the chapter's outset through the most severe, potentially life-threatening pregnancy-associated emergencies this chapter has addressed. The chapters that follow continue this book's systematic coverage of thrombocytopenia across additional clinical contexts, beginning with thrombocytopenia in critical illness in Chapter 14, a setting that shares meaningful pathophysiologic overlap with several of the severe presentations this chapter has developed, particularly disseminated intravascular coagulation and its relationship to the hypertensive and microangiopathic pregnancy syndromes this chapter has addressed.

The maternal-fetal dyad framework developed throughout this chapter, emphasizing coordinated evaluation, advance planning, and integration across obstetric, hematologic, and neonatal expertise, exemplifies the multidisciplinary, systems-oriented approach that has recurred as a consistent theme throughout this book's diagnostic and management chapters, applied here to one of medicine's most consequential and time-sensitive clinical relationships.

CLINICAL CASE: A 31-year-old woman at 37 weeks gestation with no prior thrombocytopenia history presents with new-onset headache, and evaluation reveals blood pressure 158/102 mmHg, 2+ proteinuria, platelet count 62 x10^9/L, aspartate aminotransferase 340 U/L, alanine aminotransferase 298 U/L, lactate dehydrogenase markedly elevated, and schistocytes present on peripheral smear. Applying the framework developed in this chapter, the constellation of hypertension, proteinuria, hemolysis, elevated liver enzymes, and thrombocytopenia establishes a diagnosis of HELLP syndrome, and given the gestational age and severity of findings, maternal-fetal medicine proceeds with expedited delivery via cesarean section after platelet count and coagulation studies confirm adequate hemostatic parameters for the anesthesia and surgical team's planning. Given the platelet count above the neuraxial anesthesia threshold discussed in this chapter, spinal anesthesia is used for the cesarean delivery, and the neonate, though preterm, is delivered without complication and admitted to the neonatal intensive care unit for routine preterm monitoring given the gestational age alone rather than any specific hematologic concern, since HELLP syndrome does not typically produce neonatal thrombocytopenia through the mechanism this chapter has developed for the alloimmune and immune-mediated maternal conditions discussed earlier in the chapter. The mother's platelet count and hepatic function begin improving within forty-eight hours of delivery, consistent with the expected postpartum resolution pattern for HELLP syndrome discussed in this chapter, and she is counseled before discharge regarding her substantially elevated risk of preeclampsia recurrence in any future pregnancy, with a plan for early, structured maternal-fetal medicine involvement should she become pregnant again. This case illustrates the complete diagnostic and management arc developed in this chapter: prompt recognition of the HELLP syndrome laboratory constellation, delivery as definitive treatment, coordinated anesthesia planning informed by the platelet count threshold this chapter establishes, and forward-looking counseling regarding future pregnancy recurrence risk.

THE PLATELET CRISIS DECISION COMPASS — Maternal-Fetal Thrombocytopenia Recognition and Planning

Compass Recap: Gestational Triage: Any new thrombocytopenia identified during pregnancy triggers same-visit assessment of blood pressure, urine protein, and hemolysis markers before a benign gestational thrombocytopenia diagnosis is accepted, regardless of how mild or reassuring the presentation initially appears.

Compass Recap: Alloimmune Recurrence Risk: A prior pregnancy affected by neonatal alloimmune thrombocytopenia mandates specialized antenatal referral for any subsequent pregnancy with the same partner, regardless of normal maternal platelet count, given the substantially elevated recurrence risk this history establishes.

Chapter Anchor: Thrombocytopenia in pregnancy is triaged by gestational age, trajectory, and accompanying findings (blood pressure, proteinuria, hemolysis) to distinguish benign gestational thrombocytopenia from preeclampsia/HELLP syndrome and pregnancy-associated thrombotic microangiopathy, with delivery planning and neonatal evaluation coordinated across obstetrics, hematology, anesthesia, and neonatology well in advance of delivery.

Summary and Key Concepts

Physiologic platelet decline occurs in normal pregnancy (hemodilution, uteroplacental consumption), typically remaining above 150 x10^9/L; gestational thrombocytopenia (generally >70 x10^9/L, third trimester, resolving postpartum) is the most common pathologic-appearing but benign finding.

Preeclampsia and HELLP syndrome (Hemolysis, Elevated Liver enzymes, Low Platelets) require prompt blood pressure, proteinuria, and hemolysis assessment in any new pregnancy thrombocytopenia, with delivery as definitive treatment.

Pregnancy-associated thrombotic microangiopathy (pregnancy-triggered TTP, postpartum-predominant atypical HUS) overlaps diagnostically with HELLP syndrome but requires plasma exchange or complement inhibitor therapy rather than delivery alone.

Neuraxial anesthesia is generally supported above a platelet count of 70 x10^9/L; mode of delivery is determined primarily by underlying etiology, with alloimmune thrombocytopenia risk favoring cesarean delivery given intracranial hemorrhage risk.

Neonatal alloimmune thrombocytopenia arises from maternal antibodies against paternally-inherited fetal platelet antigens (most commonly HPA-1a), can affect a first pregnancy, and carries substantial intracranial hemorrhage risk requiring structured antenatal management in subsequent at-risk pregnancies.

Neonatal thrombocytopenia is organized by timing (early-onset favoring placental insufficiency; late-onset favoring sepsis/NEC) and requires coordinated maternal-neonatal history review; postpartum counseling should address recurrence risk for future pregnancies.

CHAPTER 14: THROMBOCYTOPENIA IN CRITICAL ILLNESS, SEPSIS, DIC, AND LIVER DISEASE

Learning Objectives

1. Describe the multifactorial pathophysiology of thrombocytopenia in critically ill and septic patients.
2. Apply diagnostic scoring criteria for disseminated intravascular coagulation and distinguish it from other causes of critical illness thrombocytopenia.
3. Explain the mechanisms of thrombocytopenia in advanced liver disease, including impaired thrombopoietin production and splenic sequestration.
4. Construct a systematic approach to new thrombocytopenia in the intensive care unit incorporating the full differential developed throughout this book.
5. Apply appropriate platelet transfusion and supportive management strategies in the critically ill thrombocytopenic patient.
6. Recognize thrombocytopenia as an independent prognostic marker in critical illness.

Chapter Outline

This chapter develops thrombocytopenia in the critically ill patient as a setting of maximal diagnostic complexity, where the mechanistic categories developed throughout this book, decreased production, increased destruction, and distributional sequestration, frequently coexist rather than presenting in the cleaner, more isolated patterns typical of the ambulatory presentations addressed in earlier chapters. It addresses the multifactorial pathophysiology of critical illness and sepsis-associated thrombocytopenia, disseminated intravascular coagulation diagnosis and management, liver disease-associated thrombocytopenia, and a systematic approach integrating this book's full diagnostic framework into the intensive care unit setting. Two Platelet Crisis Decision Compass instances address the recognition of evolving disseminated intravascular coagulation and the distinction between chronic liver disease thrombocytopenia and a superimposed acute process.

The critically ill patient represents the setting in which this book's diagnostic frameworks are most severely tested, since the density of simultaneous potential causes, developed throughout Chapters 8 through 13, is nowhere greater than in the intensive care unit, and this chapter's primary contribution is not a new mechanistic category but rather a structured approach to applying this book's existing framework when multiple mechanisms plausibly operate simultaneously in a single, critically ill patient.

Multifactorial Pathophysiology of Critical Illness Thrombocytopenia

The Convergence of Multiple Mechanisms

Thrombocytopenia in the critically ill patient characteristically arises from the simultaneous operation of multiple mechanisms developed throughout this book, including decreased production from marrow suppression related to critical illness itself, sepsis, or medications; increased destruction and consumption from disseminated intravascular coagulation, discussed later in this chapter, sepsis-associated immune mechanisms, and mechanical destruction from extracorporeal circuits or intra-aortic balloon pumps when present; dilutional thrombocytopenia from large-volume fluid resuscitation and massive transfusion, introduced in Chapter 8; and, in some patients, drug-induced mechanisms from the dense medication exposure characteristic of intensive care, discussed in Chapter 10, and heparin-induced thrombocytopenia given the near-universal anticoagulant prophylaxis this population receives, discussed in Chapter 11. This mechanistic convergence means that the clean, single-mechanism localization approach developed in Chapter 8 for the ambulatory patient often cannot be directly applied without modification in the critically ill patient, requiring instead a systematic assessment of the relative contribution of each plausible mechanism to a given patient's overall presentation.

Recognizing this multifactorial reality from the outset of evaluation, rather than searching for a single unifying diagnosis as might be appropriate in the ambulatory settings addressed in earlier chapters, represents the essential conceptual shift this chapter introduces, and clinicians should approach critical illness thrombocytopenia expecting to identify and address multiple contributing factors rather than a single definitive cause.

Sepsis-Specific Mechanisms

Sepsis produces thrombocytopenia through several distinct pathways operating in parallel, including direct bone marrow suppression from circulating inflammatory cytokines, accelerated platelet consumption at sites of endothelial injury and microthrombosis throughout the septic inflammatory process, platelet activation and clearance through pathogen-associated molecular pattern recognition and subsequent immune-mediated destruction, and, in more severe cases, superimposed disseminated intravascular coagulation discussed in detail later in this chapter. The severity of sepsis-associated thrombocytopenia generally correlates with overall sepsis severity and carries independent prognostic significance, discussed further in the final section of this chapter, reflecting thrombocytopenia's role as a marker of the overall severity of the systemic inflammatory and endothelial injury process sepsis produces rather than merely an isolated laboratory abnormality.

This prognostic significance should inform the clinical urgency and thoroughness applied to evaluating new or worsening thrombocytopenia in a septic patient, since a declining platelet count in this context may signal clinical deterioration warranting reassessment of the overall management plan, extending the trend-based clinical significance principle developed throughout Chapters 6 through 13 into this specific, high-acuity clinical context.

Distinguishing Critical Illness Thrombocytopenia From the Other Causes Developed Throughout This Book

Given the multifactorial mechanisms discussed above, distinguishing straightforward critical illness or sepsis-associated thrombocytopenia from a specific, more discretely treatable superimposed condition, including heparin-induced thrombocytopenia discussed in Chapter 11, drug-induced thrombocytopenia discussed in Chapter 10, or thrombotic microangiopathy discussed in Chapter 12, remains clinically essential despite the general expectation of multifactorial contribution this chapter has emphasized, since several of these superimposed conditions carry specific, time-sensitive treatment implications distinct from the general supportive management appropriate to uncomplicated critical illness thrombocytopenia. This distinction requires the same systematic, structured evaluation this book has developed throughout, including smear review for schistocytes that would suggest thrombotic microangiopathy, formal 4Ts scoring when heparin exposure and compatible timing are present, and careful medication timeline construction as developed in Chapter 10, applied with particular rigor in the critically ill patient given the density of confounding factors this population presents.

This layered diagnostic approach, applying the general critical illness thrombocytopenia framework while simultaneously and systematically screening for the specific, more discretely treatable conditions this book has developed throughout Part III, exemplifies the integrated diagnostic philosophy this chapter introduces, and it prevents the diagnostic complacency that might otherwise result from assuming every critically ill patient's thrombocytopenia simply reflects the expected, multifactorial critical illness pattern without further specific evaluation.

Disseminated Intravascular Coagulation: Diagnosis

Pathophysiology of Disseminated Intravascular Coagulation

Disseminated intravascular coagulation represents a systemic activation of the coagulation cascade, triggered by an underlying condition including sepsis, trauma, obstetric complications discussed in Chapter 13, and malignancy, producing widespread microvascular fibrin deposition that consumes platelets and coagulation factors faster than they can be replenished, while simultaneously triggering a compensatory fibrinolytic response that can produce clinically significant bleeding alongside the underlying thrombotic process, a combined thrombotic-and-hemorrhagic picture that distinguishes disseminated intravascular coagulation from the more purely thrombotic or purely hemorrhagic conditions discussed elsewhere in this book. This dual thrombotic-hemorrhagic pathophysiology directly explains the distinctive combined coagulation abnormality pattern discussed in the diagnostic criteria section below, in which prolonged coagulation times, low fibrinogen, and elevated fibrin degradation products coexist with the thrombocytopenia this chapter's broader discussion addresses.

Unlike the primary hemostatic disorders that form the primary focus of most of this book, disseminated intravascular coagulation is fundamentally a secondary hemostatic and systemic coagulation activation process, applying the primary-versus-secondary hemostatic distinction developed in Chapter 5, and its management, discussed later in this chapter, accordingly centers on treating the underlying trigger rather than the platelet-specific interventions that predominate throughout most of this book's disease-specific management chapters.

Diagnostic Scoring Systems

Several validated scoring systems, most notably the International Society on Thrombosis and Haemostasis overt disseminated intravascular coagulation scoring system, integrate platelet count, prothrombin time prolongation, fibrinogen level, and fibrin degradation product or D-dimer elevation into a composite score that supports or excludes the diagnosis, directly paralleling the structured scoring approach this book has developed for other complex diagnostic scenarios, including the 4Ts score for heparin-induced thrombocytopenia in Chapter 11 and the PLASMIC score for thrombotic thrombocytopenic purpura in Chapter 12. This structured scoring approach should be applied whenever disseminated intravascular coagulation is suspected in a critically ill patient with an appropriate triggering condition and thrombocytopenia, providing a standardized, reproducible framework that reduces the diagnostic variability that unstructured clinical impression alone would otherwise produce in this complex, multi-parameter diagnostic scenario.

Serial scoring, repeated as the clinical picture evolves rather than performed as a single point-in-time assessment, provides substantially more diagnostic and prognostic value than an isolated score, since disseminated intravascular coagulation is fundamentally a dynamic, evolving process, and a worsening trend across sequential scores, even before meeting formal diagnostic threshold criteria, should prompt the same clinical vigilance and management consideration discussed later in this chapter as a formally diagnostic score.

Distinguishing Disseminated Intravascular Coagulation From Other Consumptive Processes

Disseminated intravascular coagulation must be distinguished from the thrombotic microangiopathy syndromes developed in Chapter 12, from severe liver disease discussed later in this chapter, and from the vitamin K deficiency or anticoagulant-related coagulopathy that can independently prolong coagulation studies in a critically ill patient, each producing overlapping laboratory abnormalities that require careful, integrated interpretation to correctly distinguish. Fibrinogen level provides one of the more useful distinguishing features in this differential, since fibrinogen, an acute phase reactant, is often elevated or normal in uncomplicated sepsis or inflammation without disseminated intravascular coagulation and in the thrombotic microangiopathy syndromes discussed in Chapter 12, while a low or rapidly declining fibrinogen level more specifically supports disseminated intravascular coagulation given its consumption in the widespread fibrin formation this condition produces.

This distinguishing framework, combining the platelet count and coagulation study pattern with the specific clinical context and triggering condition, exemplifies the multi-source diagnostic integration principle that has recurred throughout this book, applied here to one of the most laboratory-complex diagnostic distinctions this book addresses, where no single test or finding definitively establishes or excludes the diagnosis in isolation.

THE PLATELET CRISIS DECISION COMPASS — Recognizing Evolving Disseminated Intravascular Coagulation Before Overt Criteria Are Met

The Presentation: A patient with severe sepsis shows a platelet count declining from 180 to 95 x10^9/L over 24 hours, prothrombin time mildly prolonged, and fibrinogen declining from 480 to 220 mg/dL, though not yet meeting formal overt disseminated intravascular coagulation scoring criteria.

Mimic Signature: Early, evolving (non-overt) disseminated intravascular coagulation; uncomplicated sepsis-associated thrombocytopenia and acute phase fibrinogen normalization without true consumptive coagulopathy; and dilutional effect from ongoing fluid resuscitation.

The Decision: Apply serial, rather than single-timepoint, disseminated intravascular coagulation scoring, recognizing the declining trend across platelet count and fibrinogen as clinically significant even before formal overt criteria are met; intensify monitoring frequency and treat the underlying sepsis aggressively rather than waiting for the score to cross the formal diagnostic threshold before escalating clinical attention.

Trap Logic: Waiting for a formal overt disseminated intravascular coagulation score before recognizing the clinical significance of a consistently worsening trend across multiple coagulation parameters ignores the dynamic, evolving nature of this condition and delays the heightened monitoring and source-control urgency this trajectory warrants.

Crisis Anchor: A consistent worsening trend across platelet count, coagulation studies, and fibrinogen in a patient with a disseminated intravascular coagulation-predisposing condition warrants intensified monitoring and aggressive treatment of the underlying trigger, regardless of whether a formal overt scoring threshold has yet been met.

Disseminated Intravascular Coagulation: Management

Treating the Underlying Trigger

The primary and most effective management intervention for disseminated intravascular coagulation is prompt, aggressive treatment of the underlying triggering condition, whether source control and antimicrobial therapy for sepsis, delivery for the obstetric triggers discussed in Chapter 13, or definitive management of an underlying malignancy or trauma-related trigger, directly paralleling the discontinuation-focused management principle developed for drug-induced and heparin-induced thrombocytopenia in Chapters 10 and 11, but applied here to the underlying systemic condition rather than a specific medication. Supportive coagulation factor and platelet replacement, discussed in the following subsection, serves as an adjunct to this underlying trigger-directed treatment rather than a substitute for it, and disseminated intravascular coagulation that fails to improve despite adequate supportive replacement should prompt reassessment of whether the underlying triggering condition has been adequately addressed.

This trigger-focused management priority reflects disseminated intravascular coagulation's fundamental nature as a secondary, reactive process rather than a primary hematologic disease, and clinicians should resist the temptation to focus management attention exclusively on the coagulation laboratory abnormalities themselves without maintaining primary focus on identifying and treating the underlying condition driving this systemic coagulation activation.

Blood Product Support

Blood product replacement in disseminated intravascular coagulation, including platelet transfusion, fresh frozen plasma, and cryoprecipitate for severe hypofibrinogenemia, is generally reserved for active clinically significant bleeding or in anticipation of an invasive procedure, following the bleeding-risk-calibrated transfusion philosophy developed throughout this book and discussed further in Chapter 19, rather than administered prophylactically based on laboratory abnormality severity alone in a patient without active bleeding, given that this replacement, however well-intentioned, provides additional substrate for the ongoing consumptive process without addressing its underlying cause. This selective, bleeding-risk-calibrated approach to blood product support represents an important management principle specific to disseminated intravascular coagulation, distinguishing it from the more liberal, prophylactic transfusion approach that might be appropriate for some of the primary marrow failure or production-limited conditions discussed elsewhere in this book, where the underlying process is not actively consuming the transfused product.

Anticoagulation, using heparin or other agents, has a more limited and controversial role in disseminated intravascular coagulation management, generally reserved for specific clinical scenarios where the thrombotic manifestations of this condition predominate over the hemorrhagic manifestations, and this nuanced, situation-specific application of anticoagulation should involve hematology consultation given the complexity of balancing thrombotic and hemorrhagic risk this specific management decision requires.

Monitoring Response to Treatment

Serial monitoring of platelet count, coagulation studies, and fibrinogen, applying the same trend-based interpretation principle developed throughout this chapter, provides the primary means of assessing treatment response, with improvement across these parameters generally following successful treatment of the underlying triggering condition, while persistent or worsening abnormalities despite apparently adequate trigger-directed treatment should prompt reconsideration of whether the underlying condition has been fully addressed or whether a superimposed additional process, applying the layered diagnostic approach discussed earlier in this chapter, requires specific additional evaluation and management. This monitoring should continue at a frequency appropriate to clinical severity and trajectory, following the individualized monitoring philosophy developed throughout Chapters 6 through 13, until sustained improvement confirms adequate resolution of the underlying disseminated intravascular coagulation process.

This monitoring-based management approach, integrating trend interpretation with treatment response assessment, exemplifies the dynamic, iterative clinical reasoning this chapter has emphasized throughout its discussion of disseminated intravascular coagulation, reflecting the condition's own dynamic, evolving nature rather than treating it as a single, static diagnostic and management event.

Thrombocytopenia in Advanced Liver Disease

Mechanisms of Liver Disease-Associated Thrombocytopenia

Advanced liver disease produces thrombocytopenia through multiple converging mechanisms, including impaired hepatic thrombopoietin production, directly extending the thrombopoietin physiology developed in Chapter 1, splenic sequestration from portal hypertension-associated splenomegaly, applying the distributional mechanism developed in Chapter 8, and, in some patients, an additional immune-mediated component, particularly in liver disease of autoimmune or viral hepatitis etiology, discussed in the secondary immune thrombocytopenia associations developed in Chapter 9. This multifactorial mechanism means that liver disease-associated thrombocytopenia, like the critical illness thrombocytopenia discussed earlier in this chapter, often does not localize cleanly to a single mechanistic category, requiring the same multi-mechanism assessment approach this chapter has emphasized throughout.

The degree of thrombocytopenia in chronic liver disease generally correlates with disease severity and the degree of portal hypertension, and platelet count has been incorporated into several validated liver disease severity and prognostic scoring systems, reflecting its value as a marker of overall hepatic synthetic function and portal hypertension severity beyond its direct hemostatic implications, a prognostic role discussed further in the final section of this chapter.

The Complex Relationship Between Platelet Count and Bleeding Risk in Liver Disease

The relationship between platelet count and bleeding risk in liver disease is more complex than in most other conditions addressed throughout this book, since advanced liver disease simultaneously produces both procoagulant and anticoagulant deficits, including reduced synthesis of both procoagulant factors and the natural anticoagulant proteins C and S, producing a rebalanced, rather than simply deficient, hemostatic system that does not necessarily carry the bleeding risk a similarly low platelet count would suggest in a patient without this compensatory rebalancing. This rebalanced hemostasis concept, an important evolution in understanding liver disease coagulopathy over recent decades, has directly influenced contemporary management practice, discussed further in this section, moving away from the historical practice of aggressive prophylactic platelet and plasma transfusion based on laboratory values alone toward a more selective, bleeding-risk and procedure-specific transfusion approach.

This rebalanced hemostasis concept should directly inform how a clinician interprets and responds to thrombocytopenia in a patient with chronic, stable liver disease, recognizing that the platelet count number alone, without consideration of this broader rebalanced hemostatic context, may substantially overestimate the true bleeding risk this specific patient population experiences relative to a similar platelet count arising from one of the other mechanisms discussed throughout this book.

Thrombopoietin Receptor Agonists in Liver Disease

Thrombopoietin receptor agonists, discussed as second-line immune thrombocytopenia therapy in Chapter 9, have an established, specific role in liver disease-associated thrombocytopenia for the distinct indication of periprocedural platelet count optimization before a planned invasive procedure, directly addressing the impaired thrombopoietin production mechanism discussed earlier in this section, and this specific, procedure-anticipatory use differs from the more chronic, ongoing management approach these agents typically serve in immune thrombocytopenia, reflecting their targeted application to the specific procedural bleeding risk window rather than indefinite chronic therapy in most liver disease patients. Careful patient selection and timing, generally initiating therapy approximately two weeks before a planned procedure to allow adequate time for platelet count response, are essential to this specific application, and portal vein thrombosis risk, a specific consideration in the cirrhotic population given the altered portal hemodynamics this condition produces, should be assessed and discussed as part of the risk-benefit evaluation for this therapy in this specific population.

This liver disease-specific application of thrombopoietin receptor agonist therapy exemplifies how a therapeutic approach developed and validated for one condition, immune thrombocytopenia, can be thoughtfully adapted and validated for a distinct clinical application, directly paralleling this book's broader theme of applying core mechanistic understanding across the full breadth of clinical contexts a given pathophysiologic principle can inform.

A Systematic Approach to New Thrombocytopenia in the ICU

Integrating This Book's Diagnostic Framework Into the Critical Care Setting

Applying the mechanistic and algorithmic framework developed in Chapter 8 to the critically ill patient requires the specific modifications this chapter has developed throughout: an explicit expectation of multifactorial contribution rather than a single unifying diagnosis, systematic screening for the specific, discretely treatable conditions including heparin-induced thrombocytopenia, drug-induced thrombocytopenia, and thrombotic microangiopathy alongside the broader critical illness and disseminated intravascular coagulation assessment this chapter has developed, and careful attention to the specific exposure timeline, applying the timeline construction principle developed in Chapter 8, given the density of potential contributing exposures characteristic of the intensive care unit environment. This integrated approach should proceed systematically rather than reactively, ideally supported by a structured institutional protocol or checklist specifically addressing critical illness thrombocytopenia evaluation, extending the structured tool and institutional reflex principles developed throughout Chapters 6 through 11 into this specific, high-complexity clinical setting.

This systematic approach should be applied consistently to every new or significantly worsening thrombocytopenia identified in the intensive care unit, rather than reserved only for the most severe or diagnostically puzzling presentations, given both the frequency with which specific, treatable causes are identified through this systematic screening and the prognostic significance thrombocytopenia carries in this population, discussed in the final section of this chapter.

Multidisciplinary Coordination in the Critically Ill Patient

Given the complexity this chapter has developed throughout, hematology consultation should be considered relatively early in the evaluation of significant or diagnostically unclear critical illness thrombocytopenia, extending the multidisciplinary coordination principle developed throughout Chapters 8 through 13 into this specific high-acuity setting, with hematology providing specific expertise in disentangling the multiple potentially contributing mechanisms this chapter has emphasized, while the primary intensive care team maintains overall coordination of the patient's broader critical illness management. This coordination should incorporate clear, structured communication regarding the working differential diagnosis, the specific tests pending, and the anticipated timeline for results, directly extending the multidisciplinary communication principles developed for the hospitalized and critically ill patient throughout Chapters 8, 11, and 12.

Given the acuity and rapid evolution characteristic of critical illness, this multidisciplinary communication should occur more frequently than the periodic reassessment appropriate to less acute settings discussed elsewhere in this book, with daily or even more frequent reassessment of the working differential diagnosis and management plan appropriate during the most acute phase of a critically ill patient's thrombocytopenia evaluation.

Avoiding Diagnostic Anchoring in the Complex Critically Ill Patient

The multifactorial nature of critical illness thrombocytopenia this chapter has emphasized throughout creates a specific risk of diagnostic anchoring, in which an initially identified plausible contributing factor, such as sepsis or recent surgery, is accepted as the complete explanation without systematic screening for the additional, potentially more specifically treatable conditions this chapter and this book's broader framework have developed, a risk that directly parallels but is amplified relative to the anchoring bias discussed for incidental thrombocytopenia in Chapter 5. Deliberately structured, checklist-based screening for the specific treatable conditions discussed throughout this chapter, applied consistently rather than only when the initial, more obvious explanation fails to adequately account for the clinical picture, provides a systematic safeguard against this diagnostic anchoring risk.

This anti-anchoring discipline exemplifies a theme that has recurred throughout this book: the availability of an initially plausible explanation should never substitute for systematic evaluation of the full relevant differential diagnosis, a principle that carries particular weight in the critically ill patient given both the density of plausible initial explanations this population presents and the potentially severe consequences of missing a specific, treatable superimposed condition.

THE PLATELET CRISIS DECISION COMPASS — Distinguishing Chronic Liver Disease Thrombocytopenia from a Superimposed Acute Process

The Presentation: A patient with known, stable cirrhosis and a chronically low platelet count around 70 x10^9/L presents with a new decline to 35 x10^9/L over the preceding week, without an obvious precipitant identified on initial review.

Mimic Signature: Worsening portal hypertension and splenic sequestration from progressive liver disease; a superimposed acute process, including infection-associated consumption, a new medication effect, or evolving disseminated intravascular coagulation from an unrecognized precipitant such as spontaneous bacterial peritonitis; and a laboratory or preanalytic artifact requiring the confirmatory approach from Chapter 6.

The Decision: Confirm the count via smear review; systematically screen for a new precipitant, including infection (with a low threshold for diagnostic paracentesis given the cirrhotic population's spontaneous bacterial peritonitis risk), new medications, and coagulation studies to assess for evolving disseminated intravascular coagulation, rather than attributing the decline reflexively to 'worsening cirrhosis' without this evaluation.

Trap Logic: Attributing a new, more rapid decline in a chronically thrombocytopenic cirrhotic patient to simple progression of known liver disease, without systematically screening for a new superimposed precipitant, risks missing a specifically treatable acute process such as infection or evolving disseminated intravascular coagulation that a stable chronic baseline would not itself explain.

Crisis Anchor: A new, more rapid platelet count decline in a patient with known chronic liver disease thrombocytopenia is evaluated for a superimposed acute precipitant (infection, new medication, evolving coagulopathy) rather than attributed reflexively to progression of the known chronic baseline.

Prognostic Significance and Long-Term Considerations

Thrombocytopenia as an Independent Prognostic Marker

Thrombocytopenia in critically ill and septic patients carries independent prognostic significance beyond its direct hemostatic implications, with multiple studies demonstrating association between thrombocytopenia, and particularly a declining platelet count trajectory, and increased mortality risk across diverse critically ill populations, reflecting thrombocytopenia's role as a marker of overall illness severity and the degree of underlying endothelial injury and systemic inflammatory activation rather than merely a laboratory abnormality requiring its own isolated management attention. This prognostic significance should inform the overall clinical assessment and communication with patients and families regarding illness severity and trajectory, incorporating platelet count trend as one component of the broader clinical picture rather than treating it as an isolated data point disconnected from overall prognosis.

This prognostic role directly parallels, while extending in severity, the trend-based prognostic reasoning developed throughout this book, including the platelet count trajectory discussion in Chapter 8 and the chronic thrombocytopenia monitoring discussion in that same chapter, reinforcing that platelet count trend carries meaningful prognostic information across the full spectrum of clinical acuity this book addresses, from the most routine ambulatory presentation through the most severely critically ill patient.

Recovery Trajectory and Post-ICU Follow-Up

Platelet count recovery following resolution of the acute critical illness generally parallels overall clinical recovery, and persistent thrombocytopenia despite apparent resolution of the acute critical illness precipitant should prompt the same systematic reevaluation this chapter and this book's broader framework have developed throughout, considering whether an underlying chronic condition, including liver disease discussed earlier in this chapter or an inherited disorder discussed in Chapter 8, might explain a platelet count that has not fully normalized despite resolution of the acute critical illness. This post-acute monitoring should be incorporated into post-intensive care unit follow-up planning, extending the longitudinal documentation and follow-up planning principles developed throughout this book into this specific post-critical-illness recovery context, ensuring that persistent hematologic abnormalities receive appropriate ongoing attention beyond the acute hospitalization itself.

This post-acute follow-up consideration reflects the broader post-intensive care syndrome awareness that has developed in contemporary critical care practice, recognizing that recovery from critical illness extends well beyond hospital discharge, and hematologic recovery, including platelet count normalization, represents one component of this broader post-critical-illness recovery trajectory that deserves continued clinical attention.

Integrating This Chapter's Framework Into Broader Practice

This chapter has developed the critically ill and liver disease patient populations as settings of maximal diagnostic complexity within this book's broader thrombocytopenia framework, requiring explicit acknowledgment of multifactorial mechanism, systematic screening for specifically treatable superimposed conditions, and integration of prognostic considerations beyond the direct hemostatic implications addressed throughout most of this book. The chapters that follow shift focus from these acquired, acute, and multifactorial presentations toward the inherited conditions addressed in Chapters 15 and 16, representing a return to the more classically single-mechanism, chronic presentations that contrast with the complexity this chapter has emphasized throughout.

The systematic, multi-mechanism diagnostic discipline this chapter has developed, while introduced specifically for the critically ill and liver disease context, exemplifies a broader analytical approach applicable whenever a patient's presentation resists the cleaner, single-mechanism categorization this book's earlier chapters have primarily emphasized, and clinicians should feel equipped to apply this same multi-mechanism, systematic screening discipline whenever a complex clinical presentation similarly resists straightforward categorization.

Extracorporeal Circuits and Mechanical Circulatory Support

Mechanical Platelet Destruction in Extracorporeal Circuits

Extracorporeal membrane oxygenation, ventricular assist devices, and other mechanical circulatory support systems produce thrombocytopenia through direct mechanical platelet destruction from shear stress as blood passes through the pump and oxygenator circuit, directly extending the shear-dependent platelet biology developed in Chapter 3, in addition to the circuit-surface-induced platelet activation and consumption that occurs as platelets contact the large synthetic surface area these circuits present. This mechanical destruction mechanism operates independently of, though often in addition to, the sepsis, disseminated intravascular coagulation, and other mechanisms discussed earlier in this chapter, meaning a patient on mechanical circulatory support frequently experiences thrombocytopenia from multiple simultaneously operating mechanisms even more densely layered than the general critical illness population this chapter has primarily addressed.

Acquired von Willebrand syndrome, discussed mechanistically in Chapter 3 in the context of shear-related loss of high molecular weight von Willebrand factor multimers, frequently accompanies mechanical circulatory support and contributes an additional platelet-adhesion-related bleeding risk component beyond the thrombocytopenia itself, and clinicians managing a patient on mechanical circulatory support with bleeding symptoms disproportionate to the platelet count alone should specifically consider this acquired von Willebrand syndrome contribution, applying the platelet function testing framework developed in Chapter 7 when this diagnosis is suspected.

Anticoagulation Management in the Extracorporeal Circuit Setting

Patients on extracorporeal circuits require ongoing anticoagulation to prevent circuit thrombosis, and this anticoagulation requirement, layered onto the already thrombocytopenic and frequently coagulopathic state this population experiences, creates a particularly narrow and challenging therapeutic window balancing circuit patency against bleeding risk, requiring the specialized, frequently reassessed anticoagulation management approach discussed in the renal replacement therapy context of Chapter 11 but applied here to the more complex extracorporeal membrane oxygenation and ventricular assist device setting. Heparin-induced thrombocytopenia, discussed in full in Chapter 11, carries particular relevance in this population given the near-universal heparin-based anticoagulation these circuits typically require, and the 4Ts scoring and alternative anticoagulation principles developed in that chapter apply directly, though with additional complexity given the circuit thrombosis risk that heparin discontinuation itself introduces in this specific setting.

This anticoagulation complexity underscores why mechanical circulatory support patients require specialized, dedicated hematology and critical care coordination, extending the multidisciplinary coordination principle developed throughout this chapter, with structured, frequently reassessed anticoagulation protocols specific to the individual circuit type and clinical scenario rather than a generic anticoagulation approach applied uniformly across this heterogeneous patient population.

Platelet Count Trends as a Circuit Function Indicator

A progressively declining platelet count in a patient on extracorporeal circulatory support can additionally serve as an early indicator of circuit thrombosis or impending circuit failure, reflecting increased platelet consumption at a developing thrombus within the circuit itself, and this specific diagnostic application of platelet count trending, distinct from its more general prognostic role discussed in the final section of this chapter, should prompt circuit inspection and, where indicated, circuit exchange consideration alongside the broader thrombocytopenia evaluation this chapter has developed throughout. This circuit-specific application of platelet count trend monitoring exemplifies how the trend-based interpretation principle developed throughout this book can carry setting-specific diagnostic value beyond its more general application to the underlying hematologic condition, extending this book's core interpretive philosophy into a highly specialized, technology-dependent clinical context.

This mechanical circulatory support discussion illustrates the outer edge of complexity this chapter has developed throughout: a patient on extracorporeal support may simultaneously experience mechanical platelet destruction, acquired von Willebrand syndrome, anticoagulation-related bleeding risk, heparin-induced thrombocytopenia risk, and the sepsis and disseminated intravascular coagulation mechanisms discussed earlier in this chapter, requiring the full breadth of this book's diagnostic framework applied simultaneously and systematically to a single, exceptionally complex clinical presentation.

Massive Transfusion and Dilutional Thrombocytopenia

The Mechanism of Dilutional Thrombocytopenia

Massive transfusion, generally defined as replacement of a patient's total blood volume within twenty-four hours or a specified high-volume transfusion rate within a shorter interval, produces dilutional thrombocytopenia because red cell and plasma products, while replacing lost blood volume, do not adequately replace the platelet mass lost through hemorrhage and consumed during the ongoing bleeding process, directly extending the distributional and dilutional mechanism introduced in Chapter 8 to this specific, high-acuity transfusion context. This dilutional mechanism compounds, rather than replaces, any consumptive or destructive thrombocytopenia mechanism already present from the underlying hemorrhage or its precipitating trauma or surgical process, meaning the massively transfused patient frequently experiences multiple simultaneously operating thrombocytopenia mechanisms directly paralleling the multifactorial theme this chapter has developed throughout.

Recognizing dilutional thrombocytopenia as an expected, mechanistically predictable consequence of massive transfusion, rather than an unexpected or diagnostically puzzling finding, allows the clinical team to anticipate and proactively address this specific contributing factor through the balanced transfusion ratio strategies discussed in the following subsection, rather than reactively identifying and addressing a declining platelet count only after it has already become clinically significant.

Balanced Massive Transfusion Protocols

Contemporary massive transfusion protocols incorporate platelet transfusion in a balanced ratio alongside red cell and plasma products, generally targeting a ratio approximating whole blood composition, specifically to prevent or minimize the dilutional thrombocytopenia and coagulopathy that historical, red-cell-predominant transfusion practice characteristically produced, and adherence to a structured, balanced massive transfusion protocol, extending the structured protocol principle developed throughout this book, represents current standard of care for the actively hemorrhaging patient requiring large-volume transfusion support. This balanced approach directly reflects the blood product support principles discussed further in Chapter 19, applied here specifically to the acute, high-volume hemorrhage resuscitation context rather than the more measured, laboratory-value-guided transfusion approach appropriate to the non-hemorrhaging thrombocytopenic patient discussed throughout most of this book.

Point-of-care viscoelastic testing, discussed in the platelet function testing context of Chapter 7, increasingly supplements or guides massive transfusion protocol administration in many trauma and surgical centers, providing real-time assessment of the evolving coagulopathy this acute hemorrhage and transfusion process produces and allowing more individualized, rather than purely ratio-based, blood product administration as the clinical and laboratory picture evolves throughout the resuscitation.

Monitoring and Transitioning From Massive Transfusion

Once hemorrhage control has been achieved and massive transfusion protocol activation is no longer required, platelet count and broader coagulation monitoring should continue at a frequency appropriate to the patient's ongoing clinical trajectory, applying the individualized, trend-based monitoring principle developed throughout this chapter and this book more broadly, transitioning from the ratio-based resuscitation approach discussed above toward the laboratory-value-guided, selective transfusion approach appropriate to the post-resuscitation, non-actively-hemorrhaging patient. This transition should be explicitly recognized and communicated across the care team, avoiding either premature discontinuation of needed ongoing blood product support or unnecessary continuation of massive transfusion protocol-level resource utilization once the acute hemorrhagic emergency has been adequately controlled.

This massive transfusion discussion further illustrates the multifactorial complexity theme this chapter has developed throughout, demonstrating how an acute, mechanistically well-understood and largely preventable contributor to critical illness thrombocytopenia can be proactively addressed through structured protocol-based practice, directly complementing the more reactive, diagnostic screening-based approach this chapter has emphasized for the less predictable contributing factors discussed in earlier sections.

Nutritional and Metabolic Contributors in Critical Illness

Vitamin and Micronutrient Deficiency in Prolonged Critical Illness

Prolonged critical illness, particularly when accompanied by inadequate nutritional intake, malabsorption, or specific gastrointestinal losses, can produce or unmask vitamin B12 and folate deficiency, contributing an additional production-limited component to the multifactorial thrombocytopenia picture this chapter has developed throughout, and this nutritional contribution is frequently overlooked in the acute critical care setting where more immediately pressing concerns dominate clinical attention, despite its straightforward identification through the routine laboratory testing discussed in the broader thrombocytopenia evaluation framework of Chapter 8. Copper deficiency, a less commonly recognized but increasingly appreciated contributor particularly in patients receiving prolonged parenteral nutrition or with significant gastrointestinal surgical history, can similarly produce cytopenias including thrombocytopenia through impaired marrow function, and this specific nutritional deficiency should be considered in a critically ill patient with prolonged, unexplained cytopenia and an appropriate nutritional or surgical history.

Identifying and correcting these nutritional contributors, while rarely the sole explanation for critical illness thrombocytopenia given the multifactorial mechanisms this chapter has emphasized throughout, represents a readily actionable component of the comprehensive evaluation this chapter has developed, and systematic nutritional assessment should be incorporated into the evaluation of any critically ill patient with prolonged, incompletely explained thrombocytopenia, particularly when the more acute mechanisms discussed earlier in this chapter have been reasonably addressed without full platelet count normalization.

Electrolyte and Acid-Base Considerations

Severe metabolic derangements, including significant acidosis and specific electrolyte abnormalities, can transiently affect platelet count assessment and, in some circumstances, genuine platelet function and survival through mechanisms that remain incompletely characterized but are increasingly recognized in the critical care literature, and correction of these underlying metabolic derangements, pursued as part of the broader critical illness management this chapter has addressed throughout, may contribute to platelet count and function improvement alongside the more specific mechanisms discussed in earlier sections of this chapter. This consideration reinforces the multifactorial, whole-patient assessment philosophy this chapter has emphasized throughout, extending beyond the hematologically specific mechanisms discussed in earlier sections to encompass the broader metabolic and physiologic derangements characteristic of severe critical illness.

While these metabolic contributors rarely represent the primary driver of clinically significant thrombocytopenia in isolation, their identification and correction as part of comprehensive critical care management exemplifies the holistic, whole-patient approach this chapter has developed throughout, reinforcing that thrombocytopenia evaluation in the critically ill patient cannot be fully separated from the broader physiologic management this population requires.

Coordinating Nutritional and Hematologic Assessment

Given the frequency with which nutritional and metabolic factors contribute to critical illness thrombocytopenia, coordination between the primary critical care team, clinical nutrition or dietetics specialists, and hematology, when involved, ensures these contributing factors receive appropriate systematic attention alongside the more acute mechanisms this chapter has primarily emphasized, extending the multidisciplinary coordination theme that has recurred throughout this chapter into this specific, often underappreciated dimension of comprehensive critical illness thrombocytopenia evaluation. This coordination should include structured nutritional assessment as part of the systematic screening checklist discussed earlier in this chapter, ensuring that this readily correctable contributing factor category receives the same systematic attention as the more immediately dramatic mechanisms, including disseminated intravascular coagulation and heparin-induced thrombocytopenia, that have appropriately received primary emphasis throughout most of this chapter.

This nutritional and metabolic dimension closes this chapter's comprehensive development of critical illness thrombocytopenia, reinforcing that a truly systematic evaluation, consistent with the multifactorial expectation this chapter has emphasized from its opening section, extends beyond the most acute and dramatic potential contributors to encompass the full range of factors, however seemingly modest individually, that together shape a critically ill patient's overall thrombocytopenia presentation and recovery trajectory.

CLINICAL CASE: A 54-year-old man with septic shock secondary to necrotizing fasciitis, receiving broad-spectrum antibiotics, vasopressor support, and prophylactic-dose heparin, develops a platelet count decline from 165 to 52 x10^9/L over three days in the intensive care unit. Applying the systematic approach developed in this chapter, the team obtains serial disseminated intravascular coagulation scoring, which reveals a rising score approaching but not yet meeting overt criteria, with fibrinogen declining from 520 to 240 mg/dL and prothrombin time mildly prolonged, consistent with evolving, non-overt disseminated intravascular coagulation in the setting of severe sepsis. Simultaneously, the team calculates a 4Ts score given the heparin exposure, which returns low given the timing pattern not matching the classic heparin-induced thrombocytopenia interval and the strong alternative explanation the sepsis and disseminated intravascular coagulation picture provides, reasonably deprioritizing that specific alternative diagnosis. Peripheral smear review excludes schistocytes, arguing against a superimposed thrombotic microangiopathy, and a thorough medication timeline review identifies no other clear drug-induced thrombocytopenia candidate beyond the already-considered heparin exposure. Management proceeds with aggressive source control, including additional surgical debridement and continued broad-spectrum antimicrobial therapy directed at the underlying necrotizing infection, following the trigger-focused management principle developed in this chapter, while platelet and coagulation factor support is reserved for the active surgical bleeding anticipated during the debridement procedure rather than administered prophylactically beforehand. Over the following five days, as source control is achieved and the septic process improves, the platelet count and coagulation parameters progressively normalize, confirming the working diagnosis of sepsis-associated evolving disseminated intravascular coagulation retrospectively through this expected treatment response trajectory. This case illustrates the complete systematic approach developed in this chapter: explicit multifactorial assessment, structured serial scoring rather than a single-timepoint evaluation, systematic screening for the specific alternative diagnoses this book has developed throughout, and trigger-focused management with selective, bleeding-risk-calibrated blood product support.

THE PLATELET CRISIS DECISION COMPASS — Critical Illness Thrombocytopenia Recognition and Management

Compass Recap: Evolving DIC: A consistent worsening trend across platelet count, coagulation studies, and fibrinogen in a patient with a disseminated intravascular coagulation-predisposing condition warrants intensified monitoring and aggressive treatment of the underlying trigger, regardless of whether a formal overt scoring threshold has yet been met.

Compass Recap: Superimposed Acute Process in Liver Disease: A new, more rapid platelet count decline in a patient with known chronic liver disease thrombocytopenia is evaluated for a superimposed acute precipitant (infection, new medication, evolving coagulopathy) rather than attributed reflexively to progression of the known chronic baseline.

Chapter Anchor: Critical illness thrombocytopenia is approached with explicit expectation of multifactorial mechanism, systematic screening for specifically treatable superimposed conditions (heparin-induced thrombocytopenia, drug-induced thrombocytopenia, thrombotic microangiopathy, evolving disseminated intravascular coagulation) alongside the general sepsis/critical illness picture, and trigger-focused management with selective, bleeding-risk-calibrated blood product support rather than reflexive prophylactic transfusion.

Summary and Key Concepts

Critical illness thrombocytopenia arises from multiple simultaneous mechanisms (marrow suppression, consumption, dilution, drug effects) rather than a single cause, requiring explicit multi-mechanism assessment rather than the cleaner single-mechanism localization appropriate to ambulatory presentations.

Disseminated intravascular coagulation combines thrombotic and hemorrhagic pathophysiology, diagnosed via structured serial scoring (platelet count, prothrombin time, fibrinogen, fibrin degradation products) and managed primarily by treating the underlying trigger, with blood product support reserved for active bleeding.

Advanced liver disease produces thrombocytopenia through impaired thrombopoietin production and splenic sequestration, but 'rebalanced hemostasis' means platelet count alone often overestimates true bleeding risk in stable chronic liver disease.

Thrombopoietin receptor agonists have a specific, procedure-anticipatory role in liver disease thrombocytopenia, distinct from their chronic use in immune thrombocytopenia.

A systematic ICU thrombocytopenia approach requires deliberate screening for specifically treatable superimposed conditions (heparin-induced thrombocytopenia, drug-induced thrombocytopenia, thrombotic microangiopathy) to avoid diagnostic anchoring on the most obvious initial explanation.

Thrombocytopenia carries independent prognostic significance in critical illness, and persistent thrombocytopenia after acute illness resolution warrants reevaluation for an underlying chronic condition.

CHAPTER 15: INHERITED THROMBOCYTOPENIA SYNDROMES

Learning Objectives

1. Classify inherited thrombocytopenia syndromes using the platelet size-based framework and apply it to direct genetic testing.
2. Describe the clinical features and diagnostic approach for MYH9-related disorders, Wiskott-Aldrich syndrome, and thrombocytopenia-absent radius syndrome.
3. Recognize the inherited thrombocytopenia syndromes carrying an increased risk of hematologic malignancy and apply appropriate surveillance.
4. Select an appropriate genetic testing strategy for a patient with suspected inherited thrombocytopenia.
5. Construct a management and family counseling plan for a confirmed inherited thrombocytopenia syndrome.
6. Coordinate the transition of care from pediatric to adult hematology for a patient with a chronic inherited platelet disorder.

Chapter Outline

This chapter develops the inherited thrombocytopenia syndromes as a distinct diagnostic category requiring the specific recognition and genetic testing approach introduced throughout Chapters 5 through 8, extending the brief inherited-pattern discussions in those chapters into comprehensive, syndrome-specific detail. It addresses the platelet size-based classification framework, the major specific syndromes including MYH9-related disorders, Wiskott-Aldrich syndrome, thrombocytopenia-absent radius syndrome, and the malignancy-predisposing syndromes, genetic testing strategy, malignancy surveillance, and long-term management including the pediatric-to-adult care transition. Two Platelet Crisis Decision Compass instances address the recognition of a macrothrombocytopenia pattern warranting genetic evaluation and the malignancy surveillance imperative in a confirmed predisposition syndrome.

Inherited thrombocytopenia syndromes, though individually uncommon, collectively represent an important and underrecognized category within the broader thrombocytopenia differential this book has developed throughout Part III, and their correct identification carries implications extending well beyond the thrombocytopenia itself, including malignancy surveillance, family counseling, and avoidance of unnecessary immune-directed therapy for a condition these therapies cannot address.

Classification by Platelet Size

The Diagnostic Value of Platelet Volume

Inherited thrombocytopenia syndromes are clinically organized into macrothrombocytopenia, microthrombocytopenia, and normal platelet volume categories based on mean platelet volume and smear-based size assessment, applying and extending the platelet indices framework developed in Chapter 6, and this size-based classification provides substantial diagnostic efficiency by directing genetic testing toward the specific gene panel most likely to identify the causative variant, since each size category is associated with a largely distinct set of causative genes. Macrothrombocytopenia, in which platelets approach or exceed red cell size, is associated with MYH9-related disorders and Bernard-Soulier syndrome among other conditions discussed throughout this chapter, while microthrombocytopenia, with characteristically small platelets, is most classically associated with Wiskott-Aldrich syndrome and X-linked thrombocytopenia, and normal platelet volume with thrombocytopenia is associated with a further set of distinct genetic causes including several of the malignancy-predisposing syndromes discussed later in this chapter.

This classification framework should be applied as the first analytical step whenever an inherited thrombocytopenia syndrome is suspected, following the smear-based morphologic assessment developed in Chapter 6, before proceeding to the syndrome-specific clinical and genetic evaluation this chapter develops throughout the remainder of the chapter, directly paralleling the mechanistic localization-before-specific-diagnosis principle developed throughout this book's diagnostic chapters.

Integrating Size Classification With Clinical Features

While platelet size classification substantially narrows the differential diagnosis, it should be integrated with the specific clinical features, including the syndromic examination findings developed in Chapter 5, family history and inheritance pattern, and any associated organ system involvement, to further refine the diagnostic hypothesis before genetic testing is pursued, since several conditions within each size category present with distinguishing clinical features that meaningfully inform testing prioritization even within a shared size classification. This integrated approach, combining laboratory classification with clinical pattern recognition, exemplifies the multi-source diagnostic synthesis principle that has recurred throughout this book, applied here to the specific challenge of navigating an expanding genetic testing landscape efficiently rather than pursuing an unfocused, exhaustive panel-based approach for every suspected inherited thrombocytopenia presentation.

This integrated classification and clinical correlation approach directly informs the genetic testing strategy developed later in this chapter, allowing the clinician to select a more targeted testing approach when specific clinical features point toward a particular syndrome, while reserving the broader panel-based approach for presentations that do not clearly localize to a single, specific suspected diagnosis based on this initial classification and clinical correlation.

Distinguishing Inherited From Acquired Macrothrombocytopenia and Microthrombocytopenia

Both macrothrombocytopenia and microthrombocytopenia can arise from acquired as well as inherited causes, discussed throughout Chapters 8 through 14, and distinguishing an inherited from an acquired explanation for an abnormal platelet size pattern requires the same longitudinal, family history, and tempo-based reasoning developed throughout this book, particularly the adult recognition pathway for inherited thrombocytopenia discussed in Chapter 8, applied here with the specific syndrome-level detail this chapter provides. A platelet count and size pattern that has remained stable across every available prior measurement, accompanied by a compatible family history or syndromic features, favors the inherited syndromes this chapter develops, while an acute or subacute change favors the acquired processes discussed throughout Chapters 8 through 14, a distinction carrying direct implications for the appropriate diagnostic pathway and, ultimately, management approach.

This distinguishing framework reinforces why the inherited thrombocytopenia possibility should remain part of the differential diagnosis at every stage of the thrombocytopenia evaluation this book has developed throughout Part III, rather than considered only after every acquired cause has been exhaustively excluded, particularly when the specific clinical clues this chapter and Chapter 5 have developed are present from the outset of evaluation.

MYH9-Related Disorders

Pathophysiology and Clinical Spectrum

MYH9-related disorders arise from pathogenic variants in the gene encoding non-muscle myosin heavy chain IIA, a component of the platelet cytoskeleton developed mechanistically in Chapter 2, producing macrothrombocytopenia through impaired proplatelet formation and platelet release from megakaryocytes, directly extending the cytoskeletal platelet formation mechanisms developed in Chapter 1. This genetically unified but clinically heterogeneous group, historically described under several separate eponymous syndrome names before their shared genetic basis was recognized, spans a spectrum from isolated macrothrombocytopenia without other organ involvement to syndromic presentations including sensorineural hearing loss, cataracts, and, most clinically significant among the associated findings, progressive nephropathy that can advance to end-stage renal disease if not identified and monitored.

This clinical heterogeneity, ranging from an isolated hematologic finding to a multi-organ syndromic presentation, means that MYH9-related disorder should be considered in the differential diagnosis of macrothrombocytopenia even in the absence of the more classically syndromic features, since a substantial proportion of affected individuals present with isolated or predominantly hematologic findings at initial evaluation, with the extrarenal and renal manifestations discussed above sometimes emerging only later in the disease course.

The Critical Importance of Nephropathy Surveillance

Given the potentially severe, progressive nature of MYH9-related nephropathy and the availability of interventions that can slow its progression when identified early, periodic renal function monitoring, including urinalysis for proteinuria and serum creatinine assessment, represents an essential component of long-term management for any patient with confirmed MYH9-related disorder, extending the syndrome-specific surveillance principle this chapter develops throughout its coverage of the major inherited thrombocytopenia syndromes. This surveillance imperative should be clearly communicated to the patient and incorporated into their long-term monitoring plan at the time of diagnosis, extending the documentation and communication principles developed throughout this book into this specific, potentially severe long-term complication.

Nephrology co-management, once proteinuria or renal function decline is identified, follows standard chronic kidney disease management principles with attention to the specific MYH9-related nephropathy natural history, and early nephrology involvement, before advanced renal impairment develops, offers the greatest opportunity to slow disease progression through the interventions this specialized co-management can provide.

Diagnostic Confirmation and Family Implications

Diagnosis of MYH9-related disorder is confirmed through genetic testing identifying a pathogenic MYH9 variant, and peripheral smear review often reveals a distinctive additional finding, Döhle body-like neutrophil cytoplasmic inclusions, that provides a valuable, readily available diagnostic clue supporting this specific diagnosis even before genetic confirmation returns, directly extending the smear-based diagnostic clue principle developed throughout Chapters 6 and 8. Given the autosomal dominant inheritance pattern characteristic of MYH9-related disorders, family testing and counseling, following the cascade testing principle discussed in Chapter 8, should be offered to first-degree relatives once an index case is confirmed, allowing affected family members to benefit from the same nephropathy surveillance this section has emphasized before symptomatic renal involvement potentially develops.

This combination of a distinctive smear finding and confirmatory genetic testing exemplifies the multi-modal diagnostic confirmation approach this book has developed throughout, and clinicians evaluating macrothrombocytopenia should specifically request attention to neutrophil inclusions during smear review whenever this diagnosis is under consideration, potentially accelerating diagnostic confidence before genetic testing results become available.

Wiskott-Aldrich Syndrome and X-Linked Thrombocytopenia

Pathophysiology and the WAS Gene Spectrum

Wiskott-Aldrich syndrome and the milder X-linked thrombocytopenia represent a phenotypic spectrum arising from pathogenic variants in the WAS gene, encoding a cytoskeletal regulatory protein essential to normal platelet formation and immune cell function, with the specific variant and its functional consequence determining where along this spectrum an affected individual's presentation falls, from the severe, classic Wiskott-Aldrich syndrome triad discussed below to the milder, predominantly hematologic X-linked thrombocytopenia phenotype. This genotype-phenotype correlation, while not absolute, provides useful prognostic information once a specific variant is identified through the genetic testing discussed later in this chapter, informing the intensity of surveillance and the anticipated clinical course a specific affected individual is likely to experience.

Given the X-linked inheritance pattern this condition follows, affected individuals are predominantly male, with carrier females generally unaffected or showing a substantially milder phenotype through skewed X-inactivation in a minority of cases, a pattern directly paralleling the X-linked inheritance discussion introduced in Chapter 5 and informing the family counseling approach discussed later in this chapter.

The Classic Triad and Associated Immunodeficiency

Classic Wiskott-Aldrich syndrome presents with the triad of microthrombocytopenia, eczema, and recurrent infections reflecting an associated combined immunodeficiency, with the immunodeficiency component distinguishing this condition from the purely hematologic inherited thrombocytopenia syndromes discussed elsewhere in this chapter and carrying its own independent management implications, including infection prophylaxis and, in severe cases, consideration of hematopoietic stem cell transplantation, which can address both the immunodeficiency and the thrombocytopenia given the underlying hematopoietic stem cell origin of the WAS gene defect. This immunodeficiency component means that management of classic Wiskott-Aldrich syndrome requires immunology or allergy-immunology co-management alongside the hematologic management this chapter primarily addresses, extending the multidisciplinary coordination principle developed throughout this book into this specific, combined hematologic-immunologic syndrome.

X-linked thrombocytopenia, the milder phenotypic variant discussed earlier in this section, typically presents with microthrombocytopenia and bleeding symptoms without the significant eczema or recurrent infection burden characteristic of classic Wiskott-Aldrich syndrome, and this milder presentation, while carrying a more favorable overall prognosis, still requires the malignancy surveillance discussed in the following subsection and periodic reassessment given the possibility of clinical evolution over time.

Malignancy Risk and Long-Term Surveillance

Wiskott-Aldrich syndrome carries an increased risk of lymphoma and, less commonly, other malignancies, reflecting both the underlying immunodeficiency-associated malignancy risk and additional factors related to the specific gene defect this condition reflects, and long-term surveillance for lymphoproliferative disease should be incorporated into the ongoing management plan for an affected individual, extending the malignancy surveillance theme developed further in the dedicated section later in this chapter. This malignancy risk consideration should be explicitly discussed with the patient and family as part of the comprehensive counseling this chapter emphasizes throughout, providing appropriate context for the ongoing surveillance recommendations without creating disproportionate anxiety about a risk that, while elevated relative to the general population, remains a minority outcome for most affected individuals with appropriate ongoing management.

This malignancy risk discussion for Wiskott-Aldrich syndrome exemplifies the broader theme this chapter develops throughout regarding inherited thrombocytopenia syndromes with additional, non-hematologic clinical implications, reinforcing why accurate syndrome-specific diagnosis, rather than a generic 'inherited thrombocytopenia' label, carries substantial clinical value for guiding the comprehensive, syndrome-appropriate long-term management this chapter has emphasized throughout.

THE PLATELET CRISIS DECISION COMPASS — Recognizing a Macrothrombocytopenia Pattern Warranting Genetic Evaluation

The Presentation: A 26-year-old man is found to have a platelet count of 95 x10^9/L on routine testing, with smear review showing giant platelets and mean platelet volume markedly elevated; he reports a lifelong history of a similarly low platelet count with only mild bruising.

Mimic Signature: An inherited macrothrombocytopenia syndrome (MYH9-related disorder or Bernard-Soulier syndrome) explaining the lifelong, stable pattern; acquired immune thrombocytopenia with compensatory giant platelet formation, distinguished by the lifelong rather than recent history; and a laboratory artifact from automated undercounting of giant platelets, requiring the confirmatory approach from Chapter 6.

The Decision: Confirm the count via smear review, specifically assessing for neutrophil inclusions suggestive of MYH9-related disorder and correlating with the ristocetin-based aggregometry pattern from Chapter 7 if Bernard-Soulier syndrome is suspected; given the lifelong, stable history, proceed to genetic testing rather than assuming an acquired immune thrombocytopenia diagnosis, and obtain baseline renal function given the MYH9-related nephropathy surveillance imperative.

Trap Logic: Diagnosing and treating this presentation as immune thrombocytopenia based on the platelet count and giant platelet morphology alone, without recognizing the lifelong stable history as a specific clue pointing toward an inherited macrothrombocytopenia syndrome, risks both ineffective immune-directed therapy and a missed opportunity for the renal surveillance this specific category of syndrome requires.

Crisis Anchor: Macrothrombocytopenia with a lifelong, stable history prompts genetic evaluation for an inherited syndrome and baseline renal function assessment, rather than default classification as acquired immune thrombocytopenia.

Thrombocytopenia-Absent Radius Syndrome and Congenital Amegakaryocytic Thrombocytopenia

Thrombocytopenia-Absent Radius Syndrome

Thrombocytopenia-absent radius syndrome, characterized by the combination of thrombocytopenia and bilateral radial aplasia with, characteristically, preserved thumbs, distinguishing it from other radial ray anomaly syndromes in which thumb involvement is typical, presents in the neonatal period with both the hematologic and skeletal findings apparent at birth, and the thrombocytopenia in this condition characteristically improves over the first years of life, in contrast to the persistent, lifelong thrombocytopenia characteristic of most other inherited thrombocytopenia syndromes discussed throughout this chapter, an important prognostic distinction to communicate to affected families. Additional associated findings can include cow's milk protein intolerance and, less commonly, cardiac and renal anomalies, and comprehensive evaluation for these associated findings should be pursued once the diagnosis is suspected or confirmed, extending the syndromic evaluation principle developed throughout this chapter.

The severe thrombocytopenia characteristic of the neonatal and early infant period in thrombocytopenia-absent radius syndrome carries substantial bleeding risk during this specific developmental window, requiring close hematologic monitoring and, at times, platelet transfusion support during infancy, following the transfusion principles discussed further in Chapter 19, before the characteristic improvement discussed above typically allows this intensive monitoring to be relaxed.

Congenital Amegakaryocytic Thrombocytopenia

Congenital amegakaryocytic thrombocytopenia, arising from pathogenic variants in the thrombopoietin receptor gene developed mechanistically in Chapter 1, produces severe thrombocytopenia from birth due to failure of normal megakaryocyte development, and, in contrast to the improving trajectory characteristic of thrombocytopenia-absent radius syndrome discussed above, this condition characteristically progresses to more generalized bone marrow failure, including aplastic anemia, over the following years if not treated with definitive therapy, reflecting the thrombopoietin receptor's broader role in hematopoietic stem cell maintenance beyond megakaryopoiesis alone. This progressive natural history distinguishes congenital amegakaryocytic thrombocytopenia as one of the more severe inherited thrombocytopenia syndromes this chapter addresses, and hematopoietic stem cell transplantation represents the only curative treatment approach, generally pursued once the diagnosis is confirmed rather than delayed until progression to overt marrow failure has already occurred.

Given this progressive, potentially life-threatening natural history, prompt genetic confirmation and early hematopoietic stem cell transplantation referral represent essential components of management for any infant with a clinical presentation and bone marrow examination findings, showing absent or markedly reduced megakaryocytes, consistent with this diagnosis, reflecting the time-sensitive treatment imperative this specific inherited thrombocytopenia syndrome carries relative to the more indolent natural history characteristic of most other conditions discussed throughout this chapter.

Distinguishing These Congenital Presentations From Other Neonatal Causes

Both thrombocytopenia-absent radius syndrome and congenital amegakaryocytic thrombocytopenia present in the neonatal period and must be distinguished from the broader neonatal thrombocytopenia differential developed in Chapter 13, including neonatal alloimmune thrombocytopenia and the placental insufficiency and sepsis-related causes discussed in that chapter, with the characteristic physical examination findings, particularly the radial ray anomaly of thrombocytopenia-absent radius syndrome, and bone marrow megakaryocyte assessment for congenital amegakaryocytic thrombocytopenia providing the key distinguishing features. This distinguishing evaluation directly extends the neonatal thrombocytopenia evaluation framework developed in Chapter 13, adding the specific syndromic and marrow-based distinguishing features this chapter provides for these particular inherited congenital presentations.

Recognizing these specific congenital thrombocytopenia syndromes promptly in the neonatal period, rather than attributing severe neonatal thrombocytopenia reflexively to the more common acquired causes discussed in Chapter 13, carries direct management implications given the transplant urgency discussed above for congenital amegakaryocytic thrombocytopenia and the distinct expected trajectory and associated findings evaluation appropriate to thrombocytopenia-absent radius syndrome.

Malignancy Predisposition Syndromes: ANKRD26 and RUNX1

ANKRD26-Related Thrombocytopenia

ANKRD26-related thrombocytopenia, arising from specific pathogenic variants in the 5' untranslated region of the ANKRD26 gene, produces mild to moderate thrombocytopenia with normal platelet size and an associated, well-documented increased lifetime risk of myeloid malignancy, including acute myeloid leukemia and myelodysplastic syndrome, discussed in the surveillance section later in this chapter. This condition follows autosomal dominant inheritance and frequently presents with a family history spanning multiple generations, and the normal platelet size characteristic of this condition means it is not captured by the size-based classification framework's macrothrombocytopenia or microthrombocytopenia categories discussed earlier in this chapter, requiring specific clinical suspicion based on the mild, stable, familial thrombocytopenia pattern this condition characteristically presents.

Given the mild hematologic severity but significant malignancy risk this condition carries, ANKRD26-related thrombocytopenia exemplifies why accurate syndrome-specific genetic diagnosis matters even for a condition whose hematologic manifestations alone might otherwise seem to warrant limited clinical attention, reinforcing the malignancy surveillance imperative this chapter develops throughout its discussion of the predisposition syndromes.

Familial Platelet Disorder With Predisposition to Myeloid Malignancy

Familial platelet disorder with predisposition to myeloid malignancy, arising from pathogenic variants in the RUNX1 gene, a critical transcription factor in normal hematopoiesis, produces mild thrombocytopenia often accompanied by platelet function abnormalities detectable through the aggregometry testing developed in Chapter 7, alongside a substantially elevated lifetime risk of myeloid malignancy that represents among the highest malignancy risk of any condition discussed throughout this chapter, with published estimates suggesting a substantial minority of affected individuals eventually developing acute myeloid leukemia or myelodysplastic syndrome over their lifetime. This substantial malignancy risk, combined with the condition's autosomal dominant inheritance and consequent relevance to multiple family members once an index case is identified, makes accurate diagnosis and appropriate surveillance, discussed in the following section of this chapter, particularly consequential for this specific inherited thrombocytopenia syndrome.

Given the significant malignancy risk this condition carries, genetic counseling and testing of at-risk family members, extending the cascade testing principle developed throughout this book, is particularly important once an index case of familial platelet disorder with predisposition to myeloid malignancy is confirmed, allowing family members carrying the same pathogenic variant to benefit from the same structured surveillance discussed in the following section before malignant transformation potentially develops.

Additional Predisposition Syndromes and Emerging Genetic Discoveries

Beyond ANKRD26-related thrombocytopenia and familial platelet disorder with predisposition to myeloid malignancy, additional inherited thrombocytopenia syndromes with recognized or suspected malignancy predisposition continue to be identified as genetic testing technology and population-scale genomic research advance, including conditions related to ETV6 and other transcription factor genes with roles in normal hematopoiesis analogous to RUNX1, and clinicians should expect this predisposition syndrome category to continue expanding as ongoing research further characterizes the genetic landscape of inherited thrombocytopenia. This expanding genetic landscape reinforces the value of comprehensive, panel-based genetic testing, discussed in the following section of this chapter, over narrowly targeted single-gene testing whenever the specific causative gene is not already strongly suggested by the clinical presentation, since a broader testing approach increases the likelihood of identifying one of these less common but clinically consequential predisposition syndromes.

This evolving genetic landscape exemplifies the broader theme developed throughout this book's discussion of genetic and molecular diagnostics in Chapter 7, reinforcing that the specific gene panels and testing approaches discussed throughout this chapter represent a snapshot of current knowledge that clinicians should expect to continue evolving as the field advances, requiring ongoing engagement with updated genetic testing resources and literature.

Diagnostic Approach: Genetic Testing Strategy

Selecting Between Targeted and Panel-Based Testing

The genetic testing strategy for suspected inherited thrombocytopenia, directly extending the genetic testing framework developed in Chapter 7, should be guided by the specificity of the clinical presentation: a patient with distinctive syndromic features strongly suggestive of a specific condition, such as the radial ray anomaly of thrombocytopenia-absent radius syndrome or the classic Wiskott-Aldrich syndrome triad, may benefit from targeted single-gene or small panel testing directed at the specific suspected diagnosis, while a patient with a less specific presentation, including isolated mild thrombocytopenia with a compatible family history but without distinguishing syndromic features, generally benefits more from a comprehensive, broader inherited thrombocytopenia gene panel encompassing the full range of conditions this chapter has developed.

This targeted-versus-panel testing selection directly parallels the platelet function disorder genetic testing selection discussed in Chapter 7, reflecting the same underlying principle that testing strategy should be calibrated to the specificity of the clinical hypothesis under evaluation, with a more targeted approach appropriate when a specific diagnosis is strongly suspected and a broader approach appropriate when the presentation is compatible with multiple potential diagnoses within the inherited thrombocytopenia category.

Variant Interpretation Challenges Specific to This Category

Variant interpretation challenges, including the frequent identification of variants of uncertain significance discussed in the general genetic testing context of Chapter 7, apply with particular relevance to inherited thrombocytopenia genetic testing given the still-evolving understanding of the full genetic landscape this chapter has emphasized throughout, and a variant of uncertain significance identified in a gene associated with inherited thrombocytopenia should be interpreted in careful correlation with the platelet size classification, clinical features, and family segregation pattern this chapter has developed throughout, rather than treated as either a definitive diagnosis or dismissed entirely without this broader clinical correlation. Functional studies, when available through specialized research or reference laboratories, can sometimes help clarify the significance of an otherwise uncertain variant, particularly for a variant in a well-characterized gene such as MYH9 or WAS where functional assays have been more extensively developed and validated.

This variant interpretation nuance reinforces the value of genetic counseling, discussed in the management section of this chapter, involving a counselor with specific expertise in inherited hematologic conditions, ensuring that both definitive findings and variants of uncertain significance are communicated to the patient and family with appropriate context and nuance, directly extending the genetic counseling principles developed in Chapter 7 into this specific, syndrome-rich diagnostic category.

Integrating Genetic Results With the Broader Clinical Picture

A confirmed pathogenic variant in a gene associated with inherited thrombocytopenia should be integrated with the platelet size classification, clinical examination findings, and family history developed throughout this chapter to confirm that the genetic finding adequately explains the clinical presentation, since occasionally a patient may carry an incidentally identified variant unrelated to their actual clinical presentation, particularly as genetic testing panels expand to encompass an increasing number of genes with sometimes incompletely characterized clinical significance. This integration exemplifies the multi-source diagnostic synthesis principle that has recurred throughout this book, ensuring that genetic testing results, however definitive they may appear in isolation, are interpreted within rather than in place of the broader clinical evaluation this chapter and this book's earlier diagnostic chapters have developed.

This integrated interpretive approach positions genetic testing as the culminating, confirmatory step within a broader diagnostic process that begins with the clinical and morphologic evaluation this chapter has emphasized throughout, rather than as a standalone diagnostic tool applied in isolation from this broader clinical context, directly extending this book's consistent diagnostic philosophy into the specific, genetically rich domain of inherited thrombocytopenia.

Malignancy Surveillance in Predisposition Syndromes

Establishing a Structured Surveillance Protocol

Patients confirmed to carry a malignancy-predisposing inherited thrombocytopenia syndrome, including ANKRD26-related thrombocytopenia and familial platelet disorder with predisposition to myeloid malignancy discussed earlier in this chapter, require a structured, lifelong surveillance protocol incorporating periodic complete blood count and clinical assessment for symptoms or signs suggestive of evolving myeloid malignancy, with the specific surveillance frequency and modality informed by evolving expert consensus guidance given the still-maturing evidence base for optimal surveillance strategy in these comparatively rare conditions. This surveillance should specifically monitor for the development of new or worsening cytopenias beyond the baseline thrombocytopenia, abnormal peripheral smear findings, or clinical symptoms suggestive of marrow failure or malignant transformation, applying the trend-based and morphologic vigilance principles developed throughout Chapters 6 and 8 to this specific, elevated-risk surveillance context.

This structured surveillance protocol should be clearly documented and communicated to the patient, extending the longitudinal documentation and transparent communication principles developed throughout this book into this specific, high-stakes long-term monitoring context, ensuring that the patient understands both the rationale for ongoing surveillance and the specific findings that would warrant more urgent evaluation between scheduled surveillance encounters.

The Role of Bone Marrow Examination in Surveillance

Periodic bone marrow examination, applying the indications framework developed in Chapter 8 with the specific surveillance context this chapter adds, is generally reserved for patients demonstrating a concerning change on routine surveillance, including new or worsening cytopenia beyond the expected baseline or abnormal peripheral smear findings, rather than performed as a routine, fixed-interval surveillance procedure in every patient with a confirmed predisposition syndrome, reflecting the invasive nature of this procedure and the current evidence base supporting a symptom- and finding-triggered rather than universally scheduled approach. This triggered surveillance approach should be clearly distinguished from the fixed-interval blood count and clinical monitoring discussed earlier in this section, which does proceed on a routine, scheduled basis regardless of interim findings.

This distinction between routine blood-based surveillance and triggered marrow-based evaluation exemplifies the risk-calibrated approach to invasive procedures that has recurred throughout this book, balancing the diagnostic value of marrow examination against its procedural burden and reserving this more invasive evaluation for the specific circumstances in which its diagnostic yield is most likely to be clinically meaningful.

Coordinating Surveillance With Hematology-Oncology

Given the specialized nature of malignancy surveillance in these comparatively rare inherited thrombocytopenia syndromes, coordination with a hematologist or hematology-oncologist experienced in this specific surveillance context, extending the multidisciplinary coordination principle developed throughout this book, ensures that the surveillance protocol reflects current, evolving expert consensus rather than a generic or outdated approach, and referral to a specialized center with specific experience in inherited bone marrow failure and malignancy predisposition syndromes should be considered for patients with these confirmed diagnoses, particularly given the comparative rarity of these conditions and the correspondingly limited experience most general hematology practices have with their specific long-term management.

This specialized coordination extends throughout the patient's lifetime given the lifelong nature of the malignancy risk these syndromes carry, and clear, durable documentation of the surveillance protocol, extending the documentation principles developed throughout this book, ensures continuity of appropriate surveillance even as the patient transitions between different clinicians or care settings over their lifetime, a transition addressed specifically in the final section of this chapter.

THE PLATELET CRISIS DECISION COMPASS — Establishing Malignancy Surveillance After Confirming a Predisposition Syndrome

The Presentation: Genetic testing confirms a pathogenic RUNX1 variant in a 22-year-old woman evaluated for mild, lifelong thrombocytopenia with a family history of two relatives who developed acute myeloid leukemia in their thirties and forties.

Mimic Signature: Confirmed familial platelet disorder with predisposition to myeloid malignancy requiring structured lifelong surveillance; a coincidental family malignancy history unrelated to the confirmed genetic finding; and a variant that, despite pathogenic classification, might carry lower penetrance in this specific family than the family history alone would suggest.

The Decision: Establish a structured, lifelong surveillance protocol with periodic complete blood count and clinical assessment, applying the surveillance framework from this chapter, and refer to a specialized center experienced in inherited malignancy predisposition syndromes; offer cascade genetic testing and counseling to at-risk first-degree relatives given the confirmed autosomal dominant pathogenic variant and the significant family malignancy history.

Trap Logic: Treating this as 'just mild thrombocytopenia' and discharging the patient to routine primary care without establishing structured hematology surveillance disregards the substantial malignancy risk this specific confirmed genetic diagnosis carries, a risk the family history in this case further reinforces rather than merely coincides with.

Crisis Anchor: A confirmed pathogenic variant in a malignancy-predisposing inherited thrombocytopenia gene establishes lifelong structured surveillance and family cascade testing, regardless of how mild the patient's own current hematologic presentation appears.

Management and Genetic Counseling

Symptomatic Management of Bleeding Manifestations

Symptomatic management for bleeding manifestations in inherited thrombocytopenia syndromes follows the general principles developed throughout Chapters 5 through 7, including bleeding risk assessment using the structured tools from Chapter 5, and periprocedural planning incorporating the platelet count and, where relevant, the platelet function assessment appropriate to the specific syndrome, discussed further in the periprocedural management context of Chapter 18. Platelet transfusion, discussed further in Chapter 19, should be used judiciously in patients with inherited thrombocytopenia given the potential for alloimmunization with repeated transfusion exposure over a lifetime of chronic disease management, a consideration carrying particular weight for a condition diagnosed early in life with an anticipated lifetime of ongoing management ahead, reserving transfusion for clinically significant bleeding or specific procedural indications rather than used to normalize a chronically stable baseline platelet count without clear clinical indication.

This judicious transfusion approach exemplifies the chronic disease management perspective this chapter has emphasized throughout, recognizing that management decisions for a lifelong inherited condition carry different long-term considerations than the analogous decisions for an acute or self-limited acquired condition discussed elsewhere in this book, warranting explicit attention to the cumulative, lifetime implications of specific management choices.

Comprehensive Genetic Counseling

Genetic counseling for a confirmed inherited thrombocytopenia syndrome should address the specific inheritance pattern and recurrence risk for future offspring, the malignancy risk discussion appropriate to the specific syndrome where relevant, reproductive options including prenatal or preimplantation genetic testing for a family planning a future pregnancy, and cascade testing recommendations for at-risk family members, extending the comprehensive genetic counseling framework developed throughout Chapters 7, 8, and this chapter into a fully integrated, syndrome-specific counseling encounter. This counseling should be delivered by a genetic counselor or physician with specific expertise in inherited hematologic conditions whenever available, ensuring the nuance and nondirective counseling approach this sensitive discussion requires, particularly for the malignancy-predisposing syndromes where the counseling stakes are highest.

This counseling should be revisited periodically over the patient's lifetime rather than delivered only at the time of initial diagnosis, since reproductive planning, family circumstances, and the evolving genetic and clinical evidence base for a given syndrome may all change over time in ways that warrant updated counseling discussion, extending the longitudinal, ongoing communication principle developed throughout this book into this specific genetic counseling context.

Patient Support and Advocacy Resources

Given the rarity of many individual inherited thrombocytopenia syndromes discussed throughout this chapter, patient advocacy organizations and peer support communities specific to these conditions, though less numerous than for the more common conditions discussed elsewhere in this book, provide valuable additional support, extending the patient support resource discussion introduced in Chapter 9 into this specific, often more isolating rare disease context where affected individuals and families may otherwise have limited opportunity to connect with others sharing their specific diagnosis. Clinicians managing patients with these conditions should be aware of and able to direct patients toward available condition-specific resources, recognizing that the rarity of these conditions can compound the psychological burden of managing a chronic, sometimes malignancy-predisposing hematologic condition.

This support resource awareness closes the management discussion this chapter has developed throughout, reinforcing that comprehensive care for inherited thrombocytopenia syndromes extends beyond the hematologic and genetic management this chapter has primarily emphasized to encompass the full range of psychological and practical support these often rare, chronic, and in some cases malignancy-predisposing conditions warrant.

Additional and Emerging Inherited Thrombocytopenia Syndromes

Beyond the syndromes profiled in detail earlier in this chapter, a growing roster of less common inherited macrothrombocytopenias has been characterized as next-generation sequencing panels have expanded the practical reach of genetic diagnosis, and awareness of this broader landscape allows the clinician to recognize that a platelet size-based classification pointing away from MYH9-related disease, Wiskott-Aldrich syndrome, or the amegakaryocytic and predisposition syndromes discussed above does not exclude an inherited cause, but instead should prompt consideration of this expanding group of rarer, gene-specific diagnoses.

GATA1-Related and ACTN1-Related Macrothrombocytopenias

X-linked GATA1-related disease produces macrothrombocytopenia with a variable accompanying phenotype that may include dyserythropoietic anemia, and because GATA1 governs a shared transcriptional program across the megakaryocytic and erythroid lineages, the clinical picture in affected males can range from isolated mild thrombocytopenia to a combined thrombocytopenia-anemia phenotype with abnormal red cell morphology, a combination that should prompt genetic evaluation for this specific diagnosis rather than separate, uncoordinated workups of the two cytopenias. ACTN1-related thrombocytopenia, by contrast, produces a typically mild, non-syndromic macrothrombocytopenia without the bleeding tendency or extra-hematologic features that characterize many of the other conditions discussed in this chapter, illustrating that not every confirmed inherited thrombocytopenia syndrome carries clinically significant bleeding risk or associated organ involvement.

Distinguishing these autosomal and X-linked macrothrombocytopenias from one another, and from the more extensively characterized syndromes profiled earlier in this chapter, increasingly depends on multi-gene panel or exome-based testing rather than single-gene sequencing directed by a specific clinical suspicion, reflecting the broader diagnostic strategy shift discussed in the genetic testing section above. Recognizing a mild, non-progressive, non-syndromic macrothrombocytopenia phenotype without a bleeding history or extra-hematologic findings, such as that typical of ACTN1-related disease, appropriately lowers the intensity of subsequent surveillance relative to the malignancy predisposition and syndromic conditions discussed earlier, once the specific molecular diagnosis has excluded those more consequential possibilities.

TUBB1-Related and Cytoskeletal Variant Thrombocytopenias

TUBB1-related thrombocytopenia arises from variants affecting the beta-1 tubulin isoform that forms the marginal microtubule band responsible for maintaining the platelet's characteristic discoid shape, and affected individuals typically present with mild to moderate macrothrombocytopenia and abnormal platelet shape on smear without a clinically significant bleeding tendency, paralleling the cytoskeletal disruption mechanism discussed for MYH9-related disease earlier in this chapter but affecting a distinct structural protein with a correspondingly distinct, generally milder phenotype. Several additional cytoskeletal and membrane-trafficking genes have been implicated in isolated inherited macrothrombocytopenia phenotypes as sequencing panels have expanded, each individually rare but collectively accounting for a meaningful fraction of the inherited thrombocytopenia cases that remain unexplained after testing directed at the more extensively characterized syndromes.

This expanding catalog of rare, gene-specific macrothrombocytopenias reinforces the diagnostic approach developed earlier in this chapter: platelet size and morphology on smear guide the initial classification, syndromic features and family history narrow the differential, and increasingly comprehensive panel-based or exome-based genetic testing, rather than serial single-gene testing, provides the most efficient path to a specific molecular diagnosis when the initial evaluation does not clearly point to one of the more common, extensively characterized syndromes discussed in detail above.

Filamin A-Related Thrombocytopenia and Periventricular Nodular Heterotopia

X-linked filamin A-related thrombocytopenia presents a distinctive syndromic association between macrothrombocytopenia and periventricular nodular heterotopia, a neuronal migration disorder that may manifest clinically as seizures beginning in adolescence or adulthood, illustrating a further example of the syndromic extra-hematologic associations that recur throughout the inherited thrombocytopenia syndromes profiled in this chapter. Because the neurologic manifestation may postdate the hematologic finding by years, a patient identified with unexplained macrothrombocytopenia in whom filamin A-related disease is confirmed genetically warrants counseling regarding the neurologic association and a low threshold for neuroimaging evaluation should suggestive symptoms subsequently develop, extending the syndromic vigilance principle established for MYH9-related disease and Wiskott-Aldrich syndrome earlier in this chapter to this additional, less common syndromic diagnosis.

The connective tissue manifestations occasionally reported in filamin A-related disease, including mitral valve prolapse and other structural cardiac findings, further reinforce the need for a comprehensive, syndrome-specific evaluation once this diagnosis is confirmed genetically, rather than treating the thrombocytopenia in isolation from the broader phenotypic spectrum this and the other syndromic conditions discussed in this chapter may express.

The Expanding Role of Next-Generation Sequencing Panels

The clinical availability of multi-gene next-generation sequencing panels targeting the inherited thrombocytopenia syndromes, and of exome sequencing when panel-based testing does not yield a diagnosis, has fundamentally reshaped the diagnostic pathway described throughout this chapter, allowing simultaneous interrogation of dozens of implicated genes rather than the sequential single-gene testing strategy that historically prolonged the diagnostic odyssey for patients with atypical or non-classic presentations. This panel-based approach is particularly valuable for the rarer syndromes profiled in this section, where the low individual prevalence of any single gene-specific diagnosis makes a targeted single-gene testing strategy an inefficient use of both time and diagnostic resources relative to comprehensive panel testing pursued from the outset.

As the catalog of genes implicated in inherited thrombocytopenia continues to expand, variant interpretation, rather than variant detection, increasingly represents the rate-limiting step in the diagnostic process, and a variant of uncertain significance identified on panel testing should prompt the same structured approach discussed earlier in this chapter: correlation with the platelet size and morphology phenotype, segregation testing within the family when informative, and, where available, functional or referral to specialized laboratories or research programs with the capacity for more detailed variant characterization, rather than either dismissing or over-interpreting an uncertain result in isolation.

Transitioning Care From Pediatric to Adult Hematology

The Unique Challenges of Transition in Rare Inherited Conditions

Many inherited thrombocytopenia syndromes discussed throughout this chapter are diagnosed in childhood, and the transition from pediatric to adult hematology care represents a critical juncture carrying particular risk for care discontinuity given the rarity of these conditions and the correspondingly limited number of adult hematologists with specific experience managing them, a transition challenge shared with many other rare, chronic pediatric-onset conditions but carrying the additional specific stakes this chapter has developed, including ongoing malignancy surveillance for the predisposition syndromes discussed earlier in this chapter. This transition should be planned proactively, beginning in adolescence rather than deferred until the abrupt transfer that reaching adult age might otherwise produce, extending the advance-planning principle developed throughout this book, particularly the pregnancy and perioperative planning discussions in Chapters 7, 8, and 13, into this specific, developmentally extended transition process.

This proactive transition planning should include identification of an appropriate adult hematology provider with relevant experience or willingness to develop that experience in collaboration with the pediatric team, comprehensive transfer of the patient's complete diagnostic and management history, and, ideally, a period of overlapping or joint care during the transition itself rather than an abrupt single-visit handoff.

Ensuring Continuity of Surveillance and Documentation

The structured surveillance protocols discussed earlier in this chapter, particularly the malignancy surveillance imperative for the predisposition syndromes, must transfer completely and accurately during the pediatric-to-adult transition, and a structured transition summary document, extending the longitudinal documentation principle developed throughout this book, specifically detailing the confirmed diagnosis, genetic findings, established surveillance protocol, and any relevant management history, should be prepared and reviewed with both the patient and the receiving adult hematology provider as a core component of this transition process. This structured transition documentation prevents the surveillance discontinuity that an incomplete or informal handoff might otherwise produce, ensuring that a young adult with a confirmed malignancy predisposition syndrome does not experience a gap in the surveillance this chapter has emphasized carries genuinely consequential long-term stakes.

This transition documentation should also explicitly address the family counseling and reproductive planning considerations discussed earlier in this chapter, ensuring these discussions continue appropriately as the patient enters adulthood and potentially begins considering their own family planning, a life stage transition that frequently coincides with or shortly follows the pediatric-to-adult care transition this section addresses.

Empowering the Patient as Their Own Advocate

As part of this transition, patients should be equipped with a clear, accessible understanding of their own diagnosis, its implications, and their ongoing surveillance and management plan, extending the patient self-advocacy principle developed throughout this book, particularly the documentation and self-advocacy discussion in Chapter 10, into this specific, developmentally important transition to independent adult healthcare navigation. This patient education and empowerment process should begin well before the formal transition to adult care, ideally incorporating developmentally appropriate discussion of the condition throughout adolescence rather than concentrated entirely into the transition period itself, allowing the young adult patient to gradually build the self-advocacy capacity this lifelong condition will require them to exercise throughout their subsequent adult life.

This chapter has developed the inherited thrombocytopenia syndromes as a diagnostically distinct, genetically rich, and clinically consequential category within this book's broader thrombocytopenia framework, extending from the platelet size-based classification through syndrome-specific detail, malignancy surveillance, and the full lifecycle of management from initial diagnosis through the pediatric-to-adult care transition this final section has addressed. The chapter that follows extends this inherited disease framework to the platelet function disorders, addressing both inherited and acquired causes of qualitative, rather than quantitative, platelet dysfunction.

CLINICAL CASE: A 16-year-old boy is referred to hematology after a routine complete blood count before a minor surgical procedure reveals a platelet count of 68 x10^9/L with markedly elevated mean platelet volume and giant platelets on smear, findings his primary care physician had not previously investigated despite documentation of a similarly low platelet count on two prior occasions over the preceding three years. Applying the framework developed in this chapter, careful review of the smear identifies Döhle body-like neutrophil inclusions, and urinalysis reveals trace proteinuria not previously assessed, together raising specific suspicion for an MYH9-related disorder. Genetic testing confirms a pathogenic MYH9 variant, and audiometry and ophthalmologic examination, pursued given the syndromic association discussed in this chapter, reveal mild high-frequency sensorineural hearing loss not previously recognized by the patient or family. Nephrology referral is arranged given the proteinuria finding, and a structured long-term surveillance plan is established incorporating periodic renal function assessment, with the family counseled regarding the autosomal dominant inheritance pattern and offered cascade testing, subsequently identifying the same pathogenic variant in the patient's mother, who had a similarly unrecognized lifelong mild thrombocytopenia never previously investigated. The surgical procedure proceeds with appropriate platelet count and bleeding risk assessment following the framework from Chapter 5, without the need for platelet transfusion given the procedure's low bleeding risk category. This case illustrates the complete diagnostic and management arc developed in this chapter: smear-based recognition of a distinctive morphologic clue, targeted genetic confirmation, systematic syndromic evaluation revealing previously unrecognized associated findings, structured long-term surveillance establishment, and family cascade testing identifying a previously undiagnosed affected relative.

THE PLATELET CRISIS DECISION COMPASS — Inherited Thrombocytopenia Recognition and Surveillance

Compass Recap: Genetic Evaluation Trigger: Macrothrombocytopenia with a lifelong, stable history prompts genetic evaluation for an inherited syndrome and baseline renal function assessment, rather than default classification as acquired immune thrombocytopenia.

Compass Recap: Malignancy Surveillance: A confirmed pathogenic variant in a malignancy-predisposing inherited thrombocytopenia gene establishes lifelong structured surveillance and family cascade testing, regardless of how mild the patient's own current hematologic presentation appears.

Chapter Anchor: Inherited thrombocytopenia syndromes are classified by platelet size to direct genetic testing, confirmed through syndrome-specific clinical correlation and genetic testing, and managed through syndrome-specific surveillance (renal for MYH9-related disorders, malignancy for ANKRD26 and RUNX1-related conditions) with structured, lifelong documentation carrying through the pediatric-to-adult care transition.

Summary and Key Concepts

Inherited thrombocytopenia syndromes are classified by platelet size (macrothrombocytopenia, microthrombocytopenia, normal volume) to efficiently direct genetic testing toward the most likely causative gene panel.

MYH9-related disorders produce macrothrombocytopenia with characteristic neutrophil inclusions and require lifelong renal surveillance given progressive nephropathy risk.

Wiskott-Aldrich syndrome and X-linked thrombocytopenia (WAS gene, X-linked) span a spectrum from isolated microthrombocytopenia to the classic triad with combined immunodeficiency and lymphoma risk.

Thrombocytopenia-absent radius syndrome improves over infancy, while congenital amegakaryocytic thrombocytopenia progresses to marrow failure and requires early transplant referral — both present neonatally and require distinction from the broader neonatal thrombocytopenia differential.

ANKRD26-related thrombocytopenia and familial platelet disorder with predisposition to myeloid malignancy (RUNX1) carry substantial lifetime myeloid malignancy risk requiring structured, lifelong surveillance and family cascade testing.

Comprehensive management integrates genetic testing strategy, syndrome-specific surveillance, genetic counseling, judicious transfusion given lifetime alloimmunization risk, and proactive pediatric-to-adult care transition planning.

CHAPTER 16: INHERITED AND ACQUIRED PLATELET FUNCTION DISORDERS

Learning Objectives

1. Distinguish quantitative platelet disorders, the subject of the preceding chapters, from qualitative platelet function disorders, in which the platelet count may be normal despite a clinically significant bleeding tendency.
2. Classify inherited platelet function disorders by the specific step of platelet activation, aggregation, or secretion they disrupt, and correlate this mechanism with the characteristic laboratory findings.
3. Describe the clinical presentation, diagnosis, and management of Glanzmann thrombasthenia and Bernard-Soulier syndrome as prototypic disorders of platelet aggregation and adhesion.
4. Recognize the platelet storage pool disorders and correlate dense granule versus alpha granule deficiency with distinct laboratory and clinical patterns.
5. Apply a systematic approach to acquired platelet dysfunction, including uremic, medication-induced, and myeloproliferative-associated platelet dysfunction.
6. Formulate a bleeding management strategy for patients with platelet function disorders undergoing surgery or experiencing acute hemorrhage.

Chapter Outline

Classification of Platelet Function Disorders by Mechanism

The Platelet Activation Sequence as an Organizing Framework

Platelet function disorders are most usefully classified by the specific step of the platelet activation sequence they disrupt, mirroring the sequence of adhesion, activation, granule secretion, and aggregation introduced in Chapter 1, because this mechanistic classification directly predicts the laboratory findings that will localize a given disorder on aggregometry and other functional testing discussed in Chapter 7. Disorders of adhesion disrupt the initial platelet tethering to subendothelial collagen and von Willebrand factor, disorders of the GPIIb/IIIa aggregation receptor disrupt the final fibrinogen-mediated cross-linking step that converts individually activated platelets into a cohesive plug, and disorders of granule content or release disrupt the amplification signals that recruit and activate additional platelets at the site of injury.

This framework, applied systematically, allows the clinician to move from a bleeding phenotype and an aggregometry pattern to a specific mechanistic diagnosis in most cases without requiring genetic testing, reserving molecular confirmation for cases where the phenotype is atypical, where a specific diagnosis carries distinct management or counseling implications, or where research or clinical trial eligibility requires molecular confirmation, an approach that parallels the tiered diagnostic strategy developed for the quantitative platelet disorders in the preceding chapters.

Inherited Versus Acquired: A Critical First Branch Point

The distinction between inherited and acquired platelet function disorders represents the first and most consequential branch point in the diagnostic approach, because inherited disorders typically present with a lifelong bleeding history dating to early childhood, a family history in autosomal or X-linked patterns depending on the specific disorder, and a stable, reproducible functional defect on repeated testing, whereas acquired disorders present with a new or evolving bleeding tendency in a patient without a prior bleeding history, an identifiable precipitating cause such as medication exposure, uremia, or an underlying hematologic malignancy, and a functional defect that may fluctuate with the underlying cause and characteristically improves or resolves when that cause is addressed.

A structured bleeding history following the standardized bleeding assessment tool framework introduced in Chapter 5, applied specifically with attention to lifelong onset versus recent onset, remains the single most valuable diagnostic instrument for establishing this inherited-versus-acquired distinction before any laboratory testing is undertaken, and this history should be revisited explicitly whenever aggregometry findings are being interpreted, since the same aggregometry pattern may arise from either an inherited or an acquired mechanism and the clinical context, not the laboratory pattern alone, ultimately establishes which is operative in a given patient.

Glanzmann Thrombasthenia and Disorders of the GPIIb/IIIa Complex

Molecular Basis and Inheritance

Glanzmann thrombasthenia arises from biallelic pathogenic variants in ITGA2B or ITGB3, the genes encoding the two subunits of the platelet fibrinogen receptor GPIIb/IIIa, and this autosomal recessive inheritance pattern means the disorder occurs with increased frequency in populations with elevated rates of consanguinity, a demographic pattern the clinician should recognize when evaluating an unexplained severe mucocutaneous bleeding phenotype in a patient from a consanguineous family. The absent or dysfunctional GPIIb/IIIa receptor prevents the fibrinogen and von Willebrand factor cross-linking between adjacent activated platelets that normally converts a loose platelet aggregate into a stable hemostatic plug, so that platelets adhere normally to the site of vascular injury but fail to aggregate with one another, producing a severe bleeding phenotype despite an entirely normal platelet count.

This mechanism explains the characteristic aggregometry pattern in Glanzmann thrombasthenia: absent or markedly reduced aggregation in response to essentially all physiologic agonists except ristocetin, which, because it triggers GPIb-mediated agglutination rather than GPIIb/IIIa-mediated aggregation, remains preserved, a pattern that immediately localizes the defect to the aggregation receptor itself rather than to a signaling or granule secretion abnormality and distinguishes Glanzmann thrombasthenia from the broad panel-agonist reduction pattern that characterizes several other platelet function disorders discussed later in this chapter.

Clinical Presentation and Bleeding Phenotype

Glanzmann thrombasthenia typically presents in infancy or early childhood with mucocutaneous bleeding of a severity disproportionate to any identifiable trauma, including easy bruising, prolonged bleeding from minor oral trauma or tooth eruption, epistaxis, and, in affected girls, potentially severe menorrhagia from menarche onward, a presentation pattern that closely parallels the severe end of the von Willebrand disease bleeding spectrum discussed in Chapter 5 and underscores why aggregometry, rather than von Willebrand factor testing alone, must be pursued when a severe mucocutaneous bleeding phenotype does not have an identified von Willebrand disease explanation. Gastrointestinal bleeding and, less commonly, intracranial or other severe internal hemorrhage may occur, particularly around the time of surgery or trauma without adequate hemostatic support, reflecting the severity of the underlying aggregation defect.

Bleeding severity in Glanzmann thrombasthenia does not correlate closely with the specific underlying genetic variant, and even within a single family sharing an identical causative variant, bleeding severity may vary considerably between affected individuals, a pattern that should temper counseling regarding expected bleeding severity based on genotype alone and instead emphasize the individual patient's own documented bleeding history as the primary guide to management intensity, paralleling the genotype-phenotype variability discussed for several inherited thrombocytopenia syndromes in Chapter 15.

Management Principles

Management of Glanzmann thrombasthenia centers on local hemostatic measures and antifibrinolytic therapy for minor mucocutaneous bleeding, with platelet transfusion reserved for more significant bleeding episodes or surgical procedures given the recognized risk of alloimmunization against the GPIIb/IIIa complex with repeated transfusion exposure, a risk that, once alloimmunization has occurred, can render subsequent platelet transfusions ineffective and substantially complicate future bleeding management, extending the judicious transfusion principle emphasized throughout this book to a condition where the alloimmunization stakes are particularly high given the specific receptor being targeted. Recombinant activated factor VII provides an important platelet transfusion-independent hemostatic option for patients with Glanzmann thrombasthenia, particularly those who have developed GPIIb/IIIa alloantibodies, working through a mechanism that generates thrombin independent of the platelet aggregation step this disorder specifically disrupts.

Hematopoietic stem cell transplantation has been pursued in selected patients with severe, transfusion-refractory Glanzmann thrombasthenia and represents the only currently available curative approach, though the decision to pursue transplantation must weigh the procedure-related risks against the specific bleeding severity and alloimmunization status of the individual patient, a risk-benefit calculation requiring the specialized input of centers with specific experience managing this rare disorder.

THE PLATELET CRISIS DECISION COMPASS — Aggregometry Pattern Recognition Arc

The Presentation: A neonate develops severe bleeding from the umbilical stump and circumcision site, prompting hematology referral. Platelet count is normal, but bleeding time and closure times are markedly prolonged.

Mimic Signature: Von Willebrand disease type 3 can produce a similarly severe mucocutaneous bleeding phenotype with normal platelet count, but von Willebrand factor antigen and activity are severely reduced or absent in that disorder, whereas both are normal in Glanzmann thrombasthenia; factor VIII deficiency produces a distinct bleeding pattern favoring deep tissue and joint hemorrhage rather than the mucocutaneous predominance seen here.

The Decision: Aggregometry is obtained, revealing absent aggregation to ADP, collagen, epinephrine, and arachidonic acid, with preserved ristocetin-induced agglutination, a pattern that localizes the defect to the GPIIb/IIIa receptor itself.

Trap Logic: The preserved ristocetin response is the critical discriminator: because ristocetin agglutination depends on GPIb-von Willebrand factor interaction rather than GPIIb/IIIa-mediated aggregation, its preservation distinguishes Glanzmann thrombasthenia from Bernard-Soulier syndrome, in which ristocetin-induced agglutination is characteristically absent or markedly reduced alongside giant platelets and a low-normal platelet count.

Crisis Anchor: Absent aggregation to all agonists except ristocetin, in a patient with a normal platelet count and normal platelet size, is the aggregometry signature of Glanzmann thrombasthenia and should prompt GPIIb/IIIa flow cytometric confirmation and genetic counseling for this autosomal recessive disorder.

Bernard-Soulier Syndrome and Disorders of Platelet Adhesion

The GPIb-IX-V Complex and Its Role in Platelet Adhesion

Bernard-Soulier syndrome arises from biallelic pathogenic variants affecting the genes encoding the GPIb-IX-V complex, the platelet surface receptor responsible for the initial tethering interaction with von Willebrand factor bound to exposed subendothelial collagen at the site of vascular injury, an interaction that, as discussed in Chapter 1, is particularly critical under the high shear stress conditions of arteriolar and capillary flow where this initial tethering step must occur before platelets can engage in the firmer, integrin-mediated adhesion and subsequent aggregation. Loss of this receptor prevents the initial platelet adhesion step entirely, producing a bleeding phenotype that, like Glanzmann thrombasthenia, is severe and predominantly mucocutaneous despite occurring through a mechanistically distinct disruption of an earlier step in the platelet activation sequence.

Bernard-Soulier syndrome is distinguished from most other inherited platelet disorders by its characteristic association with macrothrombocytopenia, in which giant platelets are visible on peripheral smear alongside a mildly to moderately reduced platelet count, a combined quantitative and qualitative phenotype that places Bernard-Soulier syndrome at the intersection of the platelet size-based classification framework introduced in Chapter 15 and the mechanistic, aggregometry-based classification developed in this chapter, and that should prompt the clinician encountering unexplained macrothrombocytopenia to consider Bernard-Soulier syndrome alongside the MYH9-related and other macrothrombocytopenia syndromes discussed in the preceding chapter.

Laboratory Diagnosis and Distinguishing Features

The aggregometry pattern in Bernard-Soulier syndrome shows absent or markedly reduced ristocetin-induced platelet agglutination, in direct contrast to the preserved ristocetin response that characterizes Glanzmann thrombasthenia, while aggregation responses to ADP, collagen, and other agonists that act through the GPIIb/IIIa-dependent aggregation pathway remain relatively preserved, producing a mirror-image aggregometry pattern relative to Glanzmann thrombasthenia that, together with the giant platelets and reduced platelet count on smear, should reliably distinguish the two disorders. Flow cytometric confirmation of absent or markedly reduced GPIb expression on the platelet surface provides definitive diagnostic confirmation and should be pursued whenever the clinical and aggregometry findings suggest this diagnosis.

Because Bernard-Soulier syndrome combines mild to moderate thrombocytopenia with severely impaired platelet function, the bleeding phenotype is frequently more severe than the platelet count alone would predict, a discordance the clinician should specifically anticipate and communicate to other treating clinicians, since a bleeding risk assessment based on platelet count alone, following the general quantitative framework discussed in Chapter 5, will substantially underestimate the true hemorrhagic risk in a patient with this specific combined disorder.

Management Considerations

Management parallels that of Glanzmann thrombasthenia, with local measures and antifibrinolytic therapy for minor bleeding, judicious platelet transfusion reserved for significant hemorrhage or surgical procedures given the alloimmunization risk this population shares with Glanzmann thrombasthenia patients, and recombinant activated factor VII as a transfusion-independent option for patients who have developed platelet alloantibodies, extending the shared management framework for the severe inherited platelet disorders discussed throughout this section of the chapter. Desmopressin has been used with variable and generally limited efficacy in Bernard-Soulier syndrome, in contrast to its more established role in certain other bleeding disorders discussed in Chapter 5, reflecting the fundamentally structural, rather than releasable-pool, nature of the underlying receptor defect.

Platelet Storage Pool Disorders and Secretion Defects

Dense Granule Deficiency

Dense granule deficiency, sometimes termed delta storage pool disease, impairs the release of ADP, ATP, serotonin, and calcium normally secreted from platelet dense granules during activation, and because this secreted ADP amplifies the initial platelet activation signal and recruits additional platelets to the growing hemostatic plug, its absence produces a mild to moderate bleeding phenotype characterized by a distinctive aggregometry pattern showing normal primary aggregation in response to most agonists followed by absent or markedly reduced secondary aggregation, reflecting preserved initial receptor-mediated activation but impaired amplification through the missing secreted granule contents. Dense granule deficiency occurs both in isolation and as a component of several recognizable syndromes, most notably Hermansky-Pudlak syndrome and Chediak-Higashi syndrome, in which the platelet defect accompanies oculocutaneous albinism and, in Hermansky-Pudlak syndrome specifically, a risk of progressive pulmonary fibrosis and granulomatous colitis that carries independent and substantial prognostic significance beyond the bleeding tendency itself.

Recognition of the syndromic features accompanying dense granule deficiency, particularly the characteristic hypopigmentation of Hermansky-Pudlak and Chediak-Higashi syndromes, should prompt referral for the syndrome-specific evaluation and surveillance these conditions warrant beyond the hematologic management this chapter addresses, extending the syndromic vigilance principle established for the inherited thrombocytopenia syndromes discussed in Chapter 15 to this related category of inherited platelet function disorders.

Alpha Granule Deficiency and Gray Platelet Syndrome

Alpha granule deficiency, characteristic of gray platelet syndrome, impairs the release of a broad array of proteins normally secreted from platelet alpha granules, including platelet factor 4, von Willebrand factor, fibrinogen, and numerous growth factors, and the resulting depletion of alpha granule content produces the pathognomonic gray or pale appearance of platelets on Wright-stained peripheral smear from which the syndrome derives its name, a distinctive morphologic finding that, once recognized, should prompt specific consideration of this diagnosis in a patient with an otherwise unexplained mild bleeding tendency. Gray platelet syndrome frequently presents with progressive marrow fibrosis and splenomegaly over time, thought to reflect the chronic release of growth factors from megakaryocytes within the marrow microenvironment in the absence of normal alpha granule packaging, a long-term complication that warrants periodic surveillance distinct from the acute bleeding management this and the preceding subsection primarily address.

Aggregometry in alpha granule deficiency shows a variable pattern that may include reduced aggregation to collagen and thrombin, reflecting the loss of granule-derived amplification signals analogous to, though mechanistically distinct from, the pattern seen in dense granule deficiency, and definitive diagnosis increasingly relies on electron microscopy demonstrating absent or markedly reduced alpha granules, given the relatively nonspecific nature of the peripheral smear and aggregometry findings in isolation.

Combined and Other Secretion Defects

Combined alpha-delta granule deficiency, affecting both granule populations simultaneously, produces a bleeding phenotype and aggregometry pattern reflecting the additive impairment of both amplification pathways, and several additional, less common defects affecting platelet signal transduction pathways upstream of granule release, including defects in thromboxane synthesis and specific receptor signaling defects, produce clinically and aggregometrically similar secondary aggregation abnormalities that require specialized testing beyond standard aggregometry, including thromboxane B2 measurement or specific signaling pathway assays, to fully characterize when a definitive molecular diagnosis is pursued. In practice, many patients with a mild, lifelong mucocutaneous bleeding tendency and a nonspecific secondary aggregation defect on aggregometry will not receive a fully specific molecular diagnosis even after extensive evaluation, and management in this circumstance appropriately focuses on the bleeding phenotype itself, following the general principles discussed later in this chapter, rather than on achieving diagnostic certainty regarding the precise underlying molecular defect.

Additional Rare Inherited Platelet Function Disorders

Beyond the prototypic disorders of aggregation, adhesion, and secretion profiled above, several additional rare inherited platelet function disorders illustrate further mechanistic steps in the platelet activation sequence whose disruption produces a distinct, recognizable clinical and laboratory phenotype, and awareness of this broader landscape prevents premature closure of the diagnostic process when a patient's aggregometry and clinical findings do not fit neatly into the more commonly encountered categories discussed earlier in this chapter.

Scott Syndrome and Impaired Procoagulant Activity

Scott syndrome arises from impaired platelet membrane phospholipid scramblase activity, disrupting the normal activation-dependent externalization of phosphatidylserine to the outer platelet membrane leaflet that provides the catalytic surface for coagulation factor complex assembly, so that affected platelets adhere and aggregate entirely normally but fail to support the subsequent thrombin generation step, producing a bleeding phenotype despite a normal aggregometry pattern, a mechanistic and diagnostic distinction from every other disorder profiled in this chapter. This normal-aggregometry, abnormal-procoagulant-activity pattern means Scott syndrome will be missed by standard aggregometry alone and requires specific flow cytometric assessment of activation-dependent phosphatidylserine exposure, typically using annexin V binding, to establish the diagnosis in a patient with an unexplained bleeding phenotype and otherwise unremarkable platelet testing.

This distinctive mechanism illustrates a broader diagnostic principle this chapter has developed throughout: a normal aggregometry result does not fully exclude a platelet-based bleeding disorder, and a sufficiently convincing bleeding history in a patient with normal standard testing warrants consideration of these rarer, mechanistically distinct disorders and, where clinically indicated, referral to a specialized coagulation laboratory capable of the additional functional assays these diagnoses require.

Quebec Platelet Disorder

Quebec platelet disorder, an autosomal dominant condition first described in a French-Canadian kindred, arises from increased platelet content of urokinase-type plasminogen activator, producing intraplatelet proteolytic degradation of several alpha granule proteins, most notably factor V, and a distinctive delayed-onset bleeding phenotype in which initial hemostasis appears adequate but bleeding recurs hours after the initial injury or procedure as the abnormally fibrinolytic local clot degrades prematurely. This delayed-bleeding pattern, together with the disorder's characteristic favorable response to antifibrinolytic therapy rather than platelet transfusion, which may paradoxically provide additional abnormal platelets without correcting the underlying fibrinolytic mechanism, distinguishes Quebec platelet disorder from every other condition discussed in this chapter and underscores why establishing a specific mechanistic diagnosis directly informs management rather than serving only an academic diagnostic purpose.

P2Y12 Receptor Deficiency and Other ADP Receptor Defects

Inherited P2Y12 receptor deficiency impairs the platelet response to secreted ADP, producing a mild to moderate bleeding phenotype with an aggregometry pattern showing markedly reduced or absent aggregation specifically to ADP while responses to other agonists remain relatively preserved, a pattern that should be distinguished from the pharmacologic P2Y12 blockade produced by clopidogrel and other P2Y12 inhibitor medications discussed in the acquired platelet dysfunction section below through careful medication history, since the laboratory pattern alone cannot reliably distinguish an inherited receptor defect from its pharmacologic mimic. Several additional rare inherited defects affecting other specific signaling receptors or downstream pathway components have been described, each individually rare but collectively reinforcing that the aggregometry-based mechanistic classification framework developed throughout this chapter extends well beyond the handful of prototypic disorders discussed in greatest detail.

Acquired Platelet Dysfunction

Uremic Platelet Dysfunction

Uremic platelet dysfunction, arising in the setting of advanced chronic kidney disease, reflects a multifactorial mechanism including accumulation of uremic toxins that impair platelet-vessel wall interaction, abnormal von Willebrand factor multimer function in the uremic milieu, and the frequently coexisting anemia of chronic kidney disease, which itself impairs platelet margination toward the vessel wall through the same rheologic mechanism discussed for severe anemia in Chapter 5, together producing a clinically significant bleeding tendency in advanced renal failure despite a typically normal platelet count. This multifactorial mechanism explains why uremic platelet dysfunction improves with dialysis, erythropoietin-stimulating agent correction of the accompanying anemia, and desmopressin, each of which addresses a distinct component of the overall pathophysiology, and why the bleeding tendency of uremia does not respond reliably to platelet transfusion alone, since transfused platelets entering the same uremic milieu remain subject to the same functional impairment affecting the patient's endogenous platelets.

Desmopressin provides a rapid, though transient, improvement in uremic platelet dysfunction through its effect on von Willebrand factor release, making it a useful bridging measure before urgent procedures in patients with advanced renal failure, while dialysis intensification and correction of anemia provide the more durable, though slower-onset, improvement appropriate for elective procedure preparation, illustrating the same acute-bridging-versus-durable-correction distinction that recurs throughout the platelet disorder management framework developed across this book.

Medication-Induced Platelet Dysfunction

Antiplatelet medications, discussed in detail in their periprocedural management context in Chapter 18, represent the most common cause of acquired platelet dysfunction encountered in clinical practice, with aspirin producing irreversible cyclooxygenase-1 inhibition lasting the roughly ten-day lifespan of the affected platelet, and the P2Y12 inhibitors producing variable-duration ADP receptor blockade depending on the specific agent, together accounting for the large majority of medication-induced platelet dysfunction cases evaluated in clinical hematology. Numerous additional medications, including selective serotonin reuptake inhibitors, which impair platelet dense granule serotonin content through a mechanism distinct from cyclooxygenase or ADP receptor inhibition, certain beta-lactam antibiotics at high doses, and several herbal supplements including fish oil and ginkgo, have been associated with mild acquired platelet dysfunction and should be specifically elicited on medication reconciliation when evaluating an otherwise unexplained mild bleeding tendency or unexpected perioperative bleeding.

A systematic medication history, extending the comprehensive medication reconciliation principle emphasized in the drug-induced thrombocytopenia discussion in Chapter 10 to the qualitative platelet disorders addressed in this chapter, remains the single most important step in evaluating suspected acquired platelet dysfunction, since identifying and, where clinically appropriate, discontinuing or substituting the causative agent typically resolves the functional abnormality without requiring further specific intervention.

Myeloproliferative Neoplasm-Associated Platelet Dysfunction

Platelet dysfunction complicating the myeloproliferative neoplasms, discussed in their quantitative aspect in Chapter 17, reflects an intrinsically abnormal platelet population produced by the clonal megakaryocytic proliferation characteristic of these disorders, producing a paradoxical clinical picture in which the same patient may experience both thrombotic complications from the elevated platelet count and, particularly at very high platelet counts, bleeding complications from acquired von Willebrand syndrome and intrinsic platelet dysfunction, a combination requiring the same nuanced, individualized management discussed in the periprocedural pharmacology context of Chapter 18 rather than a uniform approach based on platelet count alone. Acquired von Willebrand syndrome in this setting arises from shear-mediated cleavage of high-molecular-weight von Willebrand factor multimers at markedly elevated platelet counts, a mechanism that improves with cytoreductive therapy lowering the platelet count toward the normal range, illustrating the count-dependent nature of this specific acquired bleeding mechanism.

THE PLATELET CRISIS DECISION COMPASS — Acquired Dysfunction Recognition Arc

The Presentation: A 68-year-old man with essential thrombocythemia and a platelet count of 1,450 x10^9/L presents with epistaxis and easy bruising despite having no prior bleeding history.

Mimic Signature: New-onset thrombocytopenia from marrow fibrotic transformation would present with a falling, not elevated, platelet count; an inherited platelet function disorder would typically have presented earlier in life rather than as a new finding in a 68-year-old without prior bleeding history.

The Decision: Acquired von Willebrand syndrome secondary to shear-mediated high-molecular-weight multimer cleavage at the markedly elevated platelet count is suspected, and von Willebrand factor multimer analysis confirms loss of the highest-molecular-weight multimers.

Trap Logic: The temptation to attribute new bleeding in essential thrombocythemia solely to antiplatelet therapy, if the patient is taking aspirin, would miss the count-dependent acquired von Willebrand syndrome mechanism, which requires cytoreductive therapy targeting the platelet count itself rather than antiplatelet therapy adjustment alone.

Crisis Anchor: New bleeding at a markedly elevated platelet count in a myeloproliferative neoplasm should prompt von Willebrand factor multimer analysis for acquired von Willebrand syndrome, and cytoreductive therapy lowering the platelet count, rather than platelet transfusion, is the mechanistically appropriate corrective measure.

Diagnostic Approach to Suspected Platelet Function Disorders

When to Suspect a Platelet Function Disorder

A platelet function disorder should be suspected in any patient with a mucocutaneous bleeding phenotype, whether lifelong or newly acquired, in whom the platelet count is normal or does not fully explain the observed bleeding severity, following the same structured bleeding assessment framework introduced in Chapter 5 and applied throughout the diagnostic approach to quantitative platelet disorders in the preceding chapters. The distinction between a lifelong and a newly acquired bleeding pattern, established through careful history, directs the subsequent evaluation toward either the inherited disorders profiled earlier in this chapter or the acquired causes discussed in the preceding section, and this distinction should be made explicitly before proceeding to specialized functional testing rather than pursuing an undirected battery of tests.

Screening coagulation studies, including prothrombin time and activated partial thromboplastin time, are typically normal in isolated platelet function disorders, since these assays interrogate the coagulation cascade rather than the platelet phase of hemostasis, and a normal platelet count with normal screening coagulation studies in a patient with a convincing mucocutaneous bleeding history should specifically prompt platelet function testing rather than being interpreted as excluding a bleeding disorder.

Sequential Testing Strategy

Light transmission aggregometry, discussed in its technical aspects in Chapter 7, remains the diagnostic cornerstone for platelet function disorders, and the resulting agonist-specific pattern, interpreted alongside platelet size and count on peripheral smear, localizes most disorders to a specific category among those discussed in this chapter without requiring further specialized testing in the majority of cases. Von Willebrand factor testing should be performed alongside aggregometry in any patient being evaluated for a mucocutaneous bleeding phenotype, given the substantial phenotypic overlap between von Willebrand disease and the inherited platelet function disorders discussed in this chapter, and a diagnosis of one does not exclude the coexistence of the other in an individual patient.

Electron microscopy, flow cytometric receptor quantification, and targeted or panel-based genetic testing provide progressively more specific diagnostic confirmation for cases where aggregometry and clinical findings suggest a specific inherited disorder, following the same tiered diagnostic escalation strategy developed for the inherited thrombocytopenia syndromes in Chapter 15, with the specific choice of confirmatory testing directed by the aggregometry pattern and clinical phenotype rather than pursued as an undirected panel in every patient.

Interpreting Nonspecific or Borderline Results

Aggregometry results in mild platelet function disorders may be borderline or difficult to interpret with confidence, particularly given the assay's sensitivity to preanalytic variables including recent medication exposure, specimen handling, and patient hydration status, and a borderline or equivocal initial result should prompt repeat testing under carefully controlled preanalytic conditions, including a medication washout period where clinically feasible, rather than either dismissing a potentially real abnormality or over-diagnosing a disorder based on a technically compromised specimen. This diagnostic uncertainty is particularly relevant for the mild secondary aggregation defects discussed earlier in this chapter, where the clinical and laboratory findings may never converge on a fully specific molecular diagnosis despite a genuine and clinically significant underlying bleeding tendency.

Laboratory Considerations: Preanalytic Variables and Emerging Assays

Preanalytic Variables Affecting Aggregometry

Light transmission aggregometry is highly sensitive to preanalytic variables including recent medication or supplement exposure, specimen age and handling, ambient temperature during transport, and patient factors such as recent exercise or caffeine intake, and failure to control for these variables represents a common and under-recognized cause of spurious or nonreproducible aggregometry results, extending the preanalytic vigilance principle emphasized for platelet count and morphology assessment in Chapter 6 to this technically demanding functional assay. A structured preanalytic checklist, confirming an adequate medication washout period where clinically feasible, specimen processing within the assay's validated time window, and avoidance of specimen agitation or temperature extremes during transport, should precede interpretation of any aggregometry result, particularly one that will inform a significant management decision such as preoperative planning or genetic counseling.

Point-of-Care and Viscoelastic Platelet Function Assessment

Point-of-care platelet function analyzers, most notably the PFA-100 and PFA-200 systems, provide a rapid global assessment of platelet-mediated primary hemostasis under high shear conditions and offer a useful, though nonspecific, screening tool that can raise suspicion for a platelet function disorder or acquired von Willebrand syndrome before more definitive aggregometry and specialized testing are pursued, though a normal result does not fully exclude a mild platelet function disorder and an abnormal result requires confirmatory testing rather than standing alone as a definitive diagnosis. Viscoelastic testing, including thromboelastography and rotational thromboelastometry, assesses global clot formation and stability incorporating platelet, coagulation factor, and fibrinolytic contributions simultaneously, providing particular value in the acute perioperative or trauma setting where rapid, integrated hemostatic assessment guides real-time blood product and antifibrinolytic therapy decisions rather than the more granular, mechanism-specific characterization aggregometry provides.

These point-of-care and viscoelastic modalities complement rather than replace standard aggregometry and specialized testing in the definitive diagnostic evaluation of a suspected platelet function disorder, and the clinician should recognize their appropriate role as rapid screening or acute perioperative management tools distinct from the mechanistic, diagnosis-establishing role aggregometry and the specialized confirmatory assays discussed earlier in this chapter serve.

Perioperative and Acute Bleeding Management

Preoperative Risk Assessment

Preoperative bleeding risk assessment in a patient with a known or suspected platelet function disorder follows the structured framework introduced in Chapter 5, incorporating the specific bleeding history, the underlying disorder's typical severity, and the planned procedure's bleeding risk category, with this integrated assessment directing the specific hemostatic support plan rather than a uniform approach applied regardless of the individual patient's documented bleeding phenotype. Patients with a known severe disorder, such as Glanzmann thrombasthenia or Bernard-Soulier syndrome, warrant preoperative hematology consultation and a specific, individualized hemostatic support plan established well in advance of elective surgery, extending the advance-planning principle emphasized throughout this book's perioperative discussions to this population.

Desmopressin trial, where the underlying disorder is one known to respond, should be assessed in advance of elective surgery rather than for the first time on the day of the procedure, since establishing whether an individual patient demonstrates the expected functional and clinical response allows this information to directly inform the perioperative hemostatic plan rather than requiring a reactive adjustment during the procedure itself.

Acute Bleeding Management

Acute significant bleeding in a patient with a known platelet function disorder should be managed with local hemostatic measures, antifibrinolytic therapy, and, for the severe inherited disorders discussed earlier in this chapter, platelet transfusion or recombinant activated factor VII as clinically indicated, following the same disorder-specific management principles discussed in the corresponding sections above rather than a generic bleeding management protocol undifferentiated by the specific underlying mechanism. For acquired platelet dysfunction, addressing the underlying cause, whether through medication discontinuation, dialysis intensification, or cytoreductive therapy as discussed earlier in this chapter, provides the most durable resolution, with desmopressin and platelet transfusion serving as bridging measures for acute bleeding while the underlying cause-directed therapy takes effect.

Coordination between hematology, the surgical or procedural team, and, where relevant, anesthesiology should be established well in advance for patients with known severe platelet function disorders undergoing planned procedures, extending the multidisciplinary coordination principle emphasized throughout the perioperative discussions in this book to this population, in which the combination of a structural platelet defect and the hemostatic demands of surgery creates a particularly narrow margin for error without careful advance planning.

CLINICAL CASE: A 22-year-old woman with a lifelong history of easy bruising, prolonged bleeding after dental extractions, and heavy menstrual bleeding since menarche is referred for evaluation before a planned tonsillectomy. Platelet count, prothrombin time, and activated partial thromboplastin time are all normal. Applying the diagnostic framework developed in this chapter, a structured bleeding assessment tool score confirms a clinically significant bleeding phenotype, and von Willebrand factor testing is normal, prompting light transmission aggregometry. Aggregometry reveals normal primary aggregation to ADP and collagen with absent secondary aggregation and absent aggregation to epinephrine, a pattern consistent with a platelet secretion defect. Peripheral smear shows normal platelet size and number without the gray platelet appearance of alpha granule deficiency, and mepacrine uptake and release studies confirm reduced dense granule content, establishing a diagnosis of dense granule deficiency. Preoperative planning for the tonsillectomy incorporates desmopressin, to which the patient demonstrates a favorable trial response, along with tranexamic acid, and the procedure proceeds without excess bleeding. The patient is counseled regarding the diagnosis, its implications for future procedures and pregnancy, and the absence of an associated syndrome given the isolated nature of her dense granule deficiency without the hypopigmentation or other features of Hermansky-Pudlak or Chediak-Higashi syndrome. This case illustrates the complete diagnostic arc developed in this chapter: structured bleeding history establishing a lifelong mucocutaneous phenotype, exclusion of von Willebrand disease, aggregometry localizing the defect to the secretion phase, and desmopressin trial informing a successful perioperative management plan.

Pediatric Presentation and the Diagnostic Odyssey

Recognizing Platelet Function Disorders in Childhood

Inherited platelet function disorders frequently first come to clinical attention in early childhood through bleeding events that, in isolation, might otherwise be attributed to normal childhood trauma, including prolonged bleeding after minor lacerations, unusually severe bruising from routine falls and play, and, for the more severe disorders discussed earlier in this chapter, bleeding from the umbilical stump or circumcision site in the neonatal period, and a pattern of bleeding events disproportionate to the inciting trauma across multiple, temporally separate episodes should prompt structured bleeding assessment following the framework introduced in Chapter 5 rather than being individually dismissed as isolated, unremarkable childhood injuries. Oral cavity bleeding surrounding tooth eruption and, later, tooth extraction provides a particularly informative early diagnostic window, since the oral mucosa's rich vascularity and the essentially universal nature of tooth eruption and loss in childhood create a natural, recurring hemostatic challenge whose outcome offers the clinician meaningful diagnostic information.

Because normal childhood bruising and minor bleeding are themselves common, distinguishing a genuine underlying platelet function disorder from normal childhood variation requires the same structured, standardized bleeding assessment tool approach emphasized throughout this book rather than reliance on parental impression alone, which, while valuable and worth eliciting in detail, benefits from the additional structure and standardized comparison population a validated bleeding assessment tool provides.

The Diagnostic Odyssey in Mild Platelet Function Disorders

Patients with mild platelet function disorders, particularly the secondary aggregation defects and mild storage pool disorders discussed earlier in this chapter, frequently experience a prolonged diagnostic odyssey spanning years and multiple clinical encounters before a specific diagnosis is established, reflecting both the nonspecific nature of mild mucocutaneous bleeding symptoms and the technical complexity and limited availability of specialized platelet function testing outside major academic centers, a diagnostic delay pattern that parallels the extended diagnostic timelines discussed for several inherited thrombocytopenia syndromes in Chapter 15. This prolonged diagnostic odyssey carries genuine clinical consequences beyond diagnostic frustration alone, including unnecessary or inadequately hemostatically supported procedures performed before the underlying disorder is recognized, and underscores the clinical value of a low threshold for referral to a hematologist with specific platelet function disorder expertise once a structured bleeding assessment tool has identified a clinically significant bleeding phenotype.

Establishing a specific diagnosis, even when it does not immediately change day-to-day management for a mild disorder, provides substantial value through informed perioperative planning for future procedures, appropriate genetic counseling regarding inheritance and family implications, and validation of the patient's bleeding history, which not infrequently has been previously dismissed or minimized before a specific diagnosis is established, extending the diagnostic validation and patient-centered communication principle emphasized throughout this book to this population.

Multidisciplinary Care Coordination for Severe Inherited Disorders

Children with severe inherited platelet function disorders, most notably Glanzmann thrombasthenia and Bernard-Soulier syndrome, benefit from coordinated, longitudinal care involving pediatric hematology, dentistry with specific attention to atraumatic dental care techniques, and, as the patient approaches adolescence, the same structured pediatric-to-adult care transition planning discussed for the inherited thrombocytopenia syndromes in Chapter 15, extending that transition framework to this related category of severe inherited bleeding disorders. School and childcare personnel should receive age-appropriate guidance regarding the child's specific bleeding risk and an individualized action plan for managing bleeding events at school or during childcare, developed collaboratively with the family and treating hematology team, ensuring consistent, informed response across the settings in which the child spends significant time outside direct parental supervision.

This multidisciplinary coordination extends to sports and activity counseling, in which the family and treating team collaboratively weigh the developmental and psychosocial benefits of activity participation against the specific bleeding risk the child's diagnosis and severity confer, generally favoring a individualized, activity-specific risk discussion over a uniform activity restriction applied without regard to the specific disorder and its severity, consistent with the person-centered, shared decision-making approach this book emphasizes throughout.

Special Populations and Long-Term Considerations

Pregnancy in Inherited Platelet Function Disorders

Pregnancy in a woman with a known inherited platelet function disorder, most critically Glanzmann thrombasthenia or Bernard-Soulier syndrome, requires multidisciplinary planning extending the framework developed for thrombocytopenia in pregnancy in Chapter 13 to this distinct but analogously high-stakes population, addressing peripartum hemostatic support planning, the mode of delivery, and, for Glanzmann thrombasthenia specifically, the small but described risk of neonatal alloimmune thrombocytopenia-like maternal antiplatelet antibody formation with potential fetal or neonatal platelet transfusion refractoriness in a subsequent affected pregnancy. This planning should begin early in pregnancy or, ideally, preconception, given the complexity of coordinating hematology, maternal-fetal medicine, and anesthesiology input the peripartum period for these severe inherited disorders requires.

Patient Education and Self-Management

Patients with platelet function disorders, particularly the severe inherited disorders discussed earlier in this chapter, benefit from structured education regarding their specific diagnosis, expected bleeding triggers, appropriate first-line self-management measures for minor bleeding, and clear guidance regarding when to seek urgent medical evaluation, extending the patient education and self-advocacy framework developed throughout this book, particularly in Chapters 10 and 15, to this population. Medical alert identification specifically noting the diagnosis and any established management protocol should be recommended for patients with severe inherited platelet function disorders, ensuring that treating clinicians unfamiliar with the patient's history have immediate access to the diagnosis-specific management guidance an acute bleeding presentation or urgent procedure might require.

This chapter has developed the qualitative platelet function disorders as a mechanistically distinct but clinically parallel counterpart to the quantitative disorders addressed throughout the preceding chapters, extending the aggregometry-based classification framework from the prototypic inherited disorders of aggregation and adhesion through the storage pool disorders and the diverse acquired causes of platelet dysfunction encountered in general clinical practice. The chapter that follows shifts attention to the thrombocytoses, addressing both reactive and clonal causes of an elevated platelet count and the distinct diagnostic and management considerations this quantitative abnormality presents.

THE PLATELET CRISIS DECISION COMPASS — Platelet Function Disorder Pattern Recognition

Compass Synthesis: This chapter's Decision Compass instances established the mirror-image aggregometry patterns distinguishing Glanzmann thrombasthenia from Bernard-Soulier syndrome, and the count-dependent mechanism of acquired von Willebrand syndrome complicating markedly elevated platelet counts in the myeloproliferative neoplasms.

Crisis Anchor: Applied together, these patterns direct the clinician from a mucocutaneous bleeding phenotype and an aggregometry tracing to a specific mechanistic diagnosis, whether inherited or acquired, and toward the disorder-specific management strategy this chapter has developed throughout.

Summary and Key Concepts

Platelet function disorders present with mucocutaneous bleeding despite a normal or near-normal platelet count and are classified by the specific step of platelet adhesion, aggregation, or secretion they disrupt.

Glanzmann thrombasthenia, from GPIIb/IIIa deficiency, shows absent aggregation to all agonists except ristocetin; Bernard-Soulier syndrome, from GPIb-IX-V deficiency, shows the mirror-image pattern with absent ristocetin agglutination and coexisting macrothrombocytopenia.

Dense granule and alpha granule storage pool disorders impair secondary aggregation through loss of amplification signals normally released during platelet activation, and may occur in isolation or as components of syndromes including Hermansky-Pudlak and gray platelet syndrome.

Acquired platelet dysfunction arises from uremia, medications including aspirin and P2Y12 inhibitors, and myeloproliferative neoplasm-associated acquired von Willebrand syndrome at markedly elevated platelet counts.

A structured bleeding history distinguishing lifelong from newly acquired bleeding, combined with aggregometry and von Willebrand factor testing, localizes most platelet function disorders without requiring genetic testing in every case.

Perioperative management is disorder-specific, combining local measures, antifibrinolytic therapy, desmopressin where responsive, and judicious platelet transfusion or recombinant activated factor VII for the severe inherited disorders, with careful advance multidisciplinary planning for known cases.

CHAPTER 17: THE THROMBOCYTOSES: REACTIVE AND CLONAL DISEASE

Learning Objectives

1. Define thrombocytosis and distinguish reactive from clonal causes using clinical context, laboratory findings, and molecular testing.
2. Identify the common causes of reactive thrombocytosis and recognize when an elevated platelet count requires no further hematologic evaluation.
3. Apply the diagnostic criteria for essential thrombocythemia and distinguish it from other myeloproliferative neoplasms presenting with thrombocytosis.
4. Formulate a risk-stratified management approach to essential thrombocythemia incorporating thrombotic risk assessment and cytoreductive therapy selection.
5. Recognize the distinctive management considerations for essential thrombocythemia in pregnancy and in young patients.
6. Describe the approach to extreme thrombocytosis and its associated bleeding and thrombotic risks.

Chapter Outline

Definition and Classification of Thrombocytosis

Defining the Threshold and Degree of Elevation

Thrombocytosis is conventionally defined as a platelet count exceeding 450 x10^9/L, though the clinical significance of an elevated platelet count varies considerably depending on the specific degree of elevation, the clinical context in which it arises, and whether the elevation is an isolated finding or accompanies other hematologic abnormalities, a threshold-plus-context framework that parallels the approach to thrombocytopenia developed throughout the preceding chapters of this book. Mild to moderate thrombocytosis, generally in the range of 450 to 700 x10^9/L, is common in general clinical practice and overwhelmingly reflects a reactive process rather than a primary hematologic disorder, whereas more marked elevations, particularly those exceeding 1,000 x10^9/L, carry a substantially higher likelihood of an underlying clonal myeloproliferative process and warrant more focused hematologic evaluation.

This degree-dependent likelihood is a probabilistic guide rather than a rigid diagnostic rule, since reactive thrombocytosis occasionally reaches marked elevations, particularly in the setting of severe or prolonged inflammatory states, and clonal thrombocytosis occasionally presents with only mild platelet count elevation, so the overall clinical context, including the presence or absence of an identifiable reactive trigger, must always be integrated with the platelet count itself rather than relying on the count in isolation to establish the reactive-versus-clonal distinction.

The Fundamental Reactive-Clonal Distinction

The distinction between reactive, or secondary, thrombocytosis and clonal, or primary, thrombocytosis represents the central organizing framework for this chapter, mirroring the fundamental distinction the preceding chapters have applied to thrombocytopenia, in which an identifiable secondary cause is systematically sought before a primary clonal hematologic disorder is diagnosed. Reactive thrombocytosis arises as a physiologic or pathophysiologic response to an identifiable underlying process, mediated substantially through increased thrombopoietin production and the megakaryopoiesis-stimulating cytokine cascade discussed in Chapter 1, and resolves as the underlying trigger is treated or resolves, whereas clonal thrombocytosis arises from an acquired somatic mutation conferring a proliferative or survival advantage to the megakaryocytic lineage independent of physiologic regulatory signals, producing a platelet count elevation that persists independent of any external trigger and requires a fundamentally different management framework.

Establishing this reactive-versus-clonal distinction correctly at the outset of the evaluation directly determines the subsequent management pathway: reactive thrombocytosis requires investigation and management of the underlying trigger rather than platelet-directed therapy, while clonal thrombocytosis requires the specific myeloproliferative neoplasm evaluation and, where indicated, cytoreductive management framework developed later in this chapter, making accurate initial classification the single most consequential decision point in the evaluation of an elevated platelet count.

Reactive Thrombocytosis

Common Causes and Mechanisms

Reactive thrombocytosis arises from a diverse array of underlying processes sharing the common mechanistic thread of increased thrombopoietin availability or direct inflammatory cytokine stimulation of megakaryopoiesis, including acute and chronic infection, active inflammatory conditions such as inflammatory bowel disease and rheumatoid arthritis, iron deficiency, discussed further below given its particular diagnostic relevance, malignancy, tissue injury and surgery, and splenectomy or functional asplenia, which removes the spleen's normal platelet sequestration reservoir discussed in Chapter 1 and thereby increases the circulating platelet count independent of any change in total body platelet production. Postoperative thrombocytosis follows a characteristic time course, typically becoming apparent within the first one to two weeks after surgery and resolving over the subsequent several weeks as the acute-phase inflammatory response resolves, a predictable pattern that, when recognized, allows the clinician to reassure the patient and avoid unnecessary hematologic evaluation of an expected postoperative laboratory finding.

Iron deficiency deserves particular diagnostic attention as a cause of reactive thrombocytosis because it is common, readily identified through the same iron studies discussed in the context of thrombocytopenia evaluation in earlier chapters, and because the platelet count elevation resolves predictably with iron repletion, providing both a diagnostic and therapeutic confirmation of the underlying mechanism. The mechanistic basis for iron deficiency-associated thrombocytosis remains incompletely understood but is thought to relate to shared regulatory pathways between iron metabolism and megakaryopoiesis, and recognizing this association allows the clinician to avoid unnecessary myeloproliferative neoplasm evaluation in a patient whose thrombocytosis fully resolves with iron repletion.

Clinical Approach to Suspected Reactive Thrombocytosis

The evaluation of thrombocytosis should begin with a careful clinical history and examination directed at identifying a reactive trigger among the causes discussed above, including a review of recent surgery, active or recent infection, symptoms suggesting an underlying inflammatory or malignant process, and screening iron studies, following an approach that parallels the systematic secondary-cause evaluation applied to thrombocytopenia in Chapter 8 before more specialized clonal disorder testing is pursued. In a patient with a clear, identifiable reactive trigger and a platelet count in the mild to moderate range, repeat platelet count after the trigger has resolved, rather than immediate myeloproliferative neoplasm evaluation, is the appropriate initial approach, reserving molecular testing for cases where thrombocytosis persists despite resolution of the apparent trigger or where no reactive cause is identified.

Persistent thrombocytosis without an identifiable reactive cause, thrombocytosis markedly out of proportion to an identified reactive trigger, or thrombocytosis accompanying other findings suggestive of a myeloproliferative neoplasm, including splenomegaly, thrombotic or unusual bleeding events, or accompanying abnormalities in other blood counts, should prompt the clonal disorder evaluation discussed in the following section rather than continued attribution to an incompletely explanatory reactive cause.

Essential Thrombocythemia: Diagnosis

Diagnostic Criteria and Molecular Landscape

Essential thrombocythemia is diagnosed according to World Health Organization criteria requiring a sustained platelet count exceeding 450 x10^9/L, bone marrow biopsy showing proliferation mainly of the megakaryocytic lineage with increased numbers of enlarged, mature megakaryocytes without significant increase or left shift of neutrophil granulopoiesis or erythropoiesis, exclusion of other myeloid neoplasms including chronic myeloid leukemia, polycythemia vera, primary myelofibrosis, and myelodysplastic syndromes, and demonstration of a JAK2, CALR, or MPL mutation or, in the absence of these mutations, exclusion of a reactive cause of thrombocytosis and evidence supporting a clonal rather than reactive process. This molecular testing requirement reflects the substantial diagnostic advance the discovery of these driver mutations has provided, allowing confident distinction of clonal from reactive thrombocytosis in the large majority of cases through molecular testing that has become standard practice since these mutations were characterized.

JAK2 V617F, present in approximately 50 to 60 percent of essential thrombocythemia cases, activates constitutive JAK-STAT signaling downstream of the thrombopoietin receptor discussed in Chapter 1, producing thrombopoietin-independent megakaryocytic proliferation, while CALR mutations, present in roughly 20 to 25 percent of cases, and the less common MPL mutations, present in approximately 3 to 5 percent, converge on activation of the same downstream signaling pathway through distinct upstream mechanisms, and the residual 10 to 15 percent of cases lacking any of these three driver mutations, termed triple-negative essential thrombocythemia, require particularly careful exclusion of a reactive cause given the absence of the molecular confirmation that streamlines diagnosis in the majority of cases.

Distinguishing Essential Thrombocythemia From Related Myeloproliferative Neoplasms

Essential thrombocythemia must be distinguished from prefibrotic primary myelofibrosis, which can present with a similar degree of thrombocytosis but shows distinct bone marrow morphology on careful histologic review, including megakaryocyte morphologic atypia and, even in the prefibrotic stage, subtle reticulin fibrosis increase, a distinction carrying substantial prognostic significance given prefibrotic myelofibrosis's less favorable natural history relative to essential thrombocythemia, making expert hematopathology review of the bone marrow biopsy an essential, rather than optional, component of the diagnostic evaluation. Polycythemia vera presenting with thrombocytosis as a prominent feature alongside erythrocytosis, and chronic myeloid leukemia, which must be excluded through BCR-ABL1 testing given its distinct management implications despite a shared myeloproliferative lineage origin, round out the differential diagnosis this systematic evaluation must address before an essential thrombocythemia diagnosis is confirmed.

This careful differential diagnostic process, integrating molecular testing, bone marrow morphology, and exclusion of the related myeloproliferative neoplasms discussed above, reflects the broader diagnostic principle this book has emphasized throughout: an elevated platelet count, like an abnormal platelet count in either direction, requires systematic evaluation proportionate to its clinical context rather than either reflexive extensive workup of every mild, reactively explained elevation or premature acceptance of an unexplained, potentially clonal elevation without appropriate evaluation.

THE PLATELET CRISIS DECISION COMPASS — Reactive Versus Clonal Recognition Arc

The Presentation: A 45-year-old woman has a platelet count of 620 x10^9/L identified incidentally on routine bloodwork, with no symptoms and an unremarkable examination.

Mimic Signature: Recent surgery, active infection, and iron deficiency can each produce a similar degree of thrombocytosis; the absence of any of these identifiable triggers, combined with persistence on repeat testing, shifts the differential toward a clonal process.

The Decision: Iron studies are normal, there is no history of recent surgery or active infection, and repeat platelet count six weeks later remains elevated at 640 x10^9/L, prompting JAK2 V617F testing, which returns positive.

Trap Logic: Attributing persistent, unexplained thrombocytosis to a presumed but unidentified reactive cause without pursuing molecular testing risks delaying the essential thrombocythemia diagnosis and the thrombotic risk assessment this chapter's management framework depends upon.

Crisis Anchor: Persistent thrombocytosis without an identifiable reactive trigger, confirmed on repeat testing, warrants JAK2, CALR, and MPL mutation testing before further reactive causes are pursued, since a positive result establishes essential thrombocythemia and directs the risk-stratified management pathway.

Essential Thrombocythemia: Risk Stratification and Management

Thrombotic Risk Stratification

Management of essential thrombocythemia is guided by risk stratification for the thrombotic and hemorrhagic complications that represent its principal clinical concern, with the International Prognostic Score for Thrombosis in Essential Thrombocythemia incorporating age greater than 60 years, prior thrombosis, presence of the JAK2 V617F mutation, and cardiovascular risk factors to stratify patients into very low, low, intermediate, and high thrombotic risk categories, an approach that mirrors the risk-stratified management philosophy this book has applied to bleeding and thrombotic risk assessment throughout its clinical chapters. This risk stratification directly determines the intensity of antithrombotic and cytoreductive therapy recommended for an individual patient, moving essential thrombocythemia management away from a uniform approach based on platelet count alone toward an individualized strategy incorporating the full constellation of thrombotic risk factors this scoring system captures.

Very low and low-risk patients, typically younger patients without prior thrombosis and without the JAK2 mutation, may require only low-dose aspirin, or in the very lowest risk category with additional favorable features, observation alone without specific antithrombotic therapy, reflecting the recognition that the absolute thrombotic risk in this population, while somewhat elevated relative to the general population, does not clearly justify the bleeding risk that antiplatelet or cytoreductive therapy would introduce.

Cytoreductive Therapy Selection

High-risk patients, defined by age greater than 60 years, prior thrombosis, or, in some risk models, extreme thrombocytosis, warrant cytoreductive therapy in addition to antiplatelet therapy, with hydroxyurea representing the standard first-line cytoreductive agent for most patients given its established efficacy in reducing thrombotic events and its generally favorable tolerability profile, while anagrelide, which selectively reduces platelet production through a distinct mechanism from hydroxyurea's broader myelosuppressive effect, and interferon-based therapy, particularly favored in younger patients and during pregnancy given the absence of the teratogenic and, in prolonged use, leukemogenic concerns associated with hydroxyurea, provide important alternative or second-line options. Cytoreductive therapy selection should be individualized based on patient age, pregnancy status or reproductive planning, comorbidities, and treatment tolerability, following the general principle that no single agent is universally preferred and the specific choice requires integration of the individual patient's circumstances with the comparative efficacy and toxicity profile of each available option.

Response to cytoreductive therapy is monitored through serial platelet counts with a general target of reducing the platelet count below 400 to 450 x10^9/L, alongside assessment of symptom control and, particularly for hydroxyurea, monitoring for cytopenias and other treatment-related toxicity that would prompt dose adjustment, following a treat-to-target monitoring framework analogous to the therapeutic monitoring approaches discussed for other chronic hematologic conditions throughout this book.

Special Management Considerations

Aspirin use in essential thrombocythemia requires specific attention to extreme thrombocytosis, discussed in greater detail later in this chapter, given the association between very high platelet counts and acquired von Willebrand syndrome introduced in Chapter 16, in which aspirin may paradoxically increase bleeding risk rather than providing the intended thrombotic risk reduction if the platelet count is not first addressed through cytoreductive therapy, making platelet count-informed sequencing of aspirin and cytoreductive therapy initiation an important management nuance rather than a uniform simultaneous initiation of both interventions. Cardiovascular risk factor modification, including blood pressure control, lipid management, and smoking cessation, should be pursued alongside disease-directed therapy in all essential thrombocythemia patients, recognizing that traditional cardiovascular risk factors contribute meaningfully to the overall thrombotic risk this disease confers and represent a modifiable component of the comprehensive risk stratification framework discussed above.

Essential Thrombocythemia in Pregnancy and Young Patients

Pregnancy Management Considerations

Essential thrombocythemia in pregnancy requires specialized multidisciplinary management given the disease's association with increased risk of pregnancy loss, particularly in the first trimester, placental insufficiency, and preeclampsia, alongside the maternal thrombotic risk this chapter has discussed throughout, extending the high-risk pregnancy management framework developed for thrombocytopenic conditions in Chapter 13 to this distinct but analogously complex hematologic condition complicating pregnancy. Low-dose aspirin is generally recommended throughout pregnancy for essential thrombocythemia given its favorable safety profile and evidence supporting improved pregnancy outcomes, while interferon-based therapy, given its lack of teratogenic risk in contrast to hydroxyurea, represents the preferred cytoreductive agent when cytoreductive therapy is indicated during pregnancy, a preference that should be established and, where a transition from another cytoreductive agent is needed, implemented preconception whenever possible given the importance of avoiding hydroxyurea exposure during the critical early first-trimester organogenesis period.

Postpartum thrombotic risk is particularly elevated in essential thrombocythemia, mirroring the general postpartum thrombotic risk elevation discussed in other contexts throughout this book, and extended postpartum thromboprophylaxis, typically continuing for at least six weeks after delivery, should be considered for essential thrombocythemia patients, particularly those with additional thrombotic risk factors, as part of the comprehensive peripartum management plan this population requires.

Considerations Specific to Young Patients

Young patients diagnosed with essential thrombocythemia, often identified incidentally on routine bloodwork performed for unrelated reasons, present specific long-term management considerations given the anticipated decades of subsequent disease management, including the cumulative leukemogenic risk associated with prolonged hydroxyurea exposure, which, while individually modest, accrues over a lifetime of use in a way that has prompted increasing consideration of interferon-based therapy as a preferred first-line agent in younger patients specifically to avoid this cumulative exposure concern. Reproductive planning discussions should be initiated proactively in young patients of reproductive age at the time of diagnosis, extending the advance-planning principle emphasized throughout this book to essential thrombocythemia, ensuring that cytoreductive therapy selection and pregnancy planning are coordinated well before pregnancy occurs rather than requiring reactive adjustment after a pregnancy is already underway.

Long-term surveillance for disease progression, including transformation to myelofibrosis or, less commonly, acute leukemia, should be incorporated into the longitudinal management plan for young essential thrombocythemia patients, following periodic assessment of blood counts, symptoms, and, where clinically indicated, repeat bone marrow evaluation, extending the long-term surveillance framework developed for the malignancy predisposition syndromes discussed in Chapter 15 to this related category of clonal hematologic conditions carrying a distinct but analogous long-term progression risk.

THE PLATELET CRISIS DECISION COMPASS — Extreme Count Dual-Risk Arc

The Presentation: A 52-year-old man with known essential thrombocythemia on hydroxyurea presents with new epistaxis and bruising, and his platelet count is found to be 1,420 x10^9/L, up from 780 x10^9/L at his last visit three months ago.

Mimic Signature: Hydroxyurea nonadherence or dose inadequacy could explain the rising count, but the new bleeding, rather than a thrombotic event, is the key feature distinguishing this presentation from the more commonly anticipated thrombotic complication of undertreated essential thrombocythemia.

The Decision: Von Willebrand factor multimer analysis is obtained given the marked platelet count elevation and bleeding phenotype, confirming loss of high-molecular-weight multimers consistent with acquired von Willebrand syndrome.

Trap Logic: Increasing aspirin or adding an additional antiplatelet agent in response to the marked platelet count elevation, without first recognizing the bleeding phenotype as a signal for acquired von Willebrand syndrome, would worsen rather than improve this patient's hemostatic status.

Crisis Anchor: New bleeding accompanying a rising platelet count at extreme levels should prompt von Willebrand factor multimer testing before any antiplatelet therapy escalation, since cytoreductive therapy intensification to lower the platelet count, not additional antiplatelet therapy, is the mechanistically appropriate correction.

Extreme Thrombocytosis and Its Complications

Defining Extreme Thrombocytosis

Extreme thrombocytosis, generally defined as a platelet count exceeding 1,000 to 1,500 x10^9/L, though thresholds vary somewhat across the literature, carries a distinctive and clinically important paradox in which the markedly elevated platelet count is associated with both increased thrombotic risk, reflecting the same mechanism underlying the broader thrombotic risk elevation in essential thrombocythemia, and, at the same time, increased bleeding risk through the acquired von Willebrand syndrome mechanism introduced in Chapter 16, in which shear-mediated cleavage of high-molecular-weight von Willebrand factor multimers becomes increasingly prominent as the platelet count rises. This dual thrombotic-and-hemorrhagic risk profile at extreme platelet count elevations requires the clinician to actively assess for both complications simultaneously, rather than assuming that a very high platelet count uniformly favors a thrombotic rather than bleeding risk profile.

Extreme thrombocytosis may arise from either reactive or clonal causes, though the reactive causes capable of producing this degree of elevation, most notably severe or prolonged inflammatory states, splenectomy, particularly in the immediate postoperative period, and, less commonly, severe iron deficiency, are less common than the moderate reactive elevations discussed earlier in this chapter, making a clonal myeloproliferative process proportionately more likely, though not certain, at this degree of platelet count elevation.

Acquired Von Willebrand Syndrome at Extreme Platelet Counts

Acquired von Willebrand syndrome secondary to extreme thrombocytosis, discussed in its clinical recognition context in Chapter 16, should be specifically screened for through von Willebrand factor multimer analysis in any patient with extreme thrombocytosis and a bleeding history or before a planned procedure, given the distinctive management implication this diagnosis carries: cytoreductive therapy lowering the platelet count, rather than antifibrinolytic therapy or desmopressin alone, addresses the underlying count-dependent mechanism and represents the most effective corrective approach for this specific bleeding phenotype. Aspirin therapy should be withheld or used with particular caution in patients with extreme thrombocytosis and confirmed or suspected acquired von Willebrand syndrome, extending the platelet count-informed aspirin sequencing principle discussed earlier in this chapter to this population where the bleeding risk from acquired von Willebrand syndrome may specifically outweigh the intended antithrombotic benefit until the platelet count has been reduced through cytoreductive therapy.

Urgent Management of Extreme Thrombocytosis

Extreme thrombocytosis presenting with acute thrombotic or significant hemorrhagic complications may warrant urgent cytoreductive intervention, including hydroxyurea initiation with close monitoring or, in selected cases of severe, life-threatening complications, plateletpheresis to achieve rapid platelet count reduction while definitive cytoreductive therapy takes effect, a management approach reserved for genuinely urgent presentations given plateletpheresis's invasive nature and the general preference for pharmacologic cytoreduction in less acute circumstances. Coordination with a hematologist experienced in myeloproliferative neoplasm management should be established promptly whenever extreme thrombocytosis is identified, particularly in the setting of an acute thrombotic or hemorrhagic complication, given the specialized, individualized decision-making this presentation requires beyond the general management framework this chapter provides.

CLINICAL CASE: A 58-year-old man presents to the emergency department with sudden-onset left-sided weakness and is found to have an acute ischemic stroke on imaging. Complete blood count reveals a platelet count of 1,380 x10^9/L, previously undocumented, alongside a normal hemoglobin and white blood cell count. Applying the diagnostic framework developed in this chapter, the markedly elevated platelet count in the setting of an acute thrombotic event prompts urgent hematology consultation. Bone marrow biopsy shows increased, enlarged, mature megakaryocytes without significant fibrosis or granulocytic or erythroid proliferation, and JAK2 V617F mutation testing returns positive, establishing a diagnosis of essential thrombocythemia presenting with a thrombotic complication, placing the patient in the high-risk category by virtue of the thrombotic event itself. Hydroxyurea is initiated promptly alongside standard acute stroke management and secondary prevention measures, with a treatment target of reducing the platelet count below 400 x10^9/L. Von Willebrand factor multimer analysis, obtained given the markedly elevated platelet count, shows preserved high-molecular-weight multimers, and aspirin is added once the platelet count begins trending downward. The patient is counseled regarding the new diagnosis, the high-risk classification based on this presenting thrombotic event, and the long-term cytoreductive therapy and monitoring plan this diagnosis requires. This case illustrates the complete diagnostic and management arc developed in this chapter: an incidentally discovered marked thrombocytosis presenting acutely through its most serious complication, bone marrow and molecular confirmation of essential thrombocythemia, and immediate high-risk category cytoreductive management integrating both the thrombotic presentation and the extreme platelet count.

Laboratory and Diagnostic Pitfalls in Thrombocytosis Evaluation

Accurate interpretation of an elevated platelet count requires attention to several laboratory and diagnostic pitfalls that can mislead the evaluation process, extending the general vigilance for spurious or artifactual laboratory findings this book has emphasized throughout its discussion of both thrombocytopenia and, now, thrombocytosis.

Spurious and Artifactual Elevations

Automated hematology analyzers occasionally overestimate the platelet count through misclassification of red or white blood cell fragments, microcytes, or cryoglobulin precipitates as platelets, an artifactual elevation that, unlike the pseudothrombocytopenia discussed in Chapter 6, produces a spuriously high rather than spuriously low count, and this possibility should be considered whenever an unexpectedly elevated platelet count does not fit the overall clinical picture, particularly in a patient with a coexisting condition, such as severe hemolysis or a paraproteinemia, known to produce this specific analyzer artifact. Peripheral smear review, following the same principle emphasized for suspected pseudothrombocytopenia in Chapter 6, resolves this ambiguity by allowing direct visual confirmation of true platelet morphology and number rather than reliance on the automated count alone when an artifactual elevation is suspected.

Extreme leukocytosis, particularly in the setting of chronic myeloid leukemia or other myeloproliferative processes with markedly elevated white blood cell counts, can similarly produce automated platelet count artifacts in either direction, reinforcing that peripheral smear correlation remains an essential, rather than optional, component of the diagnostic evaluation whenever the automated platelet count is unexpectedly discordant with the overall clinical and hematologic picture.

Distinguishing Essential Thrombocythemia From Reactive Thrombocytosis in Ambiguous Cases

A subset of patients presents with genuinely ambiguous features, including moderate thrombocytosis without a clearly identifiable reactive trigger but also without a driver mutation on standard JAK2, CALR, and MPL testing, a triple-negative scenario in which the reactive-versus-clonal distinction cannot be resolved through molecular testing alone and instead requires the fuller diagnostic evaluation discussed earlier in this chapter, including bone marrow biopsy with expert hematopathology review and careful, sometimes prolonged, clinical observation to determine whether the thrombocytosis persists, progresses, or eventually resolves as an occult reactive trigger becomes apparent or is successfully treated. Serial platelet count monitoring over an extended interval, rather than a single time-point assessment, often provides the most informative diagnostic information in these ambiguous cases, since a genuinely reactive process typically shows some fluctuation or eventual resolution over subsequent months, whereas a clonal process typically shows sustained or gradually progressive elevation.

Referral to a hematologist with specific myeloproliferative neoplasm expertise is particularly valuable in these diagnostically ambiguous triple-negative cases, given the specialized interpretation of bone marrow morphology and the individualized clinical judgment this scenario requires beyond the more straightforward molecularly confirmed cases that constitute the majority of essential thrombocythemia diagnoses.

The Role of Serum Thrombopoietin and Additional Molecular Testing

Serum thrombopoietin measurement has been explored as an additional diagnostic tool in ambiguous thrombocytosis cases, based on the principle that reactive thrombocytosis is typically driven by elevated thrombopoietin levels while clonal thrombocytosis in essential thrombocythemia often shows relatively normal or only mildly elevated thrombopoietin despite the markedly elevated platelet count, reflecting the thrombopoietin-independent proliferative signal the driver mutations discussed earlier in this chapter provide, though this test has not achieved the diagnostic centrality that JAK2, CALR, and MPL molecular testing now occupy and is generally reserved for select ambiguous cases at specialized centers. Additional molecular testing beyond the three canonical driver mutations, including next-generation sequencing panels assessing for additional somatic mutations associated with clonal hematopoiesis and myeloid neoplasm progression, may be pursued in triple-negative cases or when there is specific concern for disease progression, extending the expanding role of comprehensive molecular testing discussed in the context of the inherited thrombocytopenia syndromes in Chapter 15 to this related diagnostic context within acquired clonal hematologic disease.

Essential Thrombocythemia: Natural History and Disease Transformation

Understanding the long-term natural history of essential thrombocythemia, including its generally favorable prognosis alongside the specific, if uncommon, risks of disease transformation, provides essential context for the long-term monitoring and patient communication framework this chapter addresses in its closing section.

Long-Term Prognosis and Life Expectancy

Essential thrombocythemia carries a generally favorable long-term prognosis for most patients, with life expectancy in appropriately risk-stratified and managed patients approaching that of the age-matched general population, particularly for lower-risk patients without significant thrombotic complications, a reassuring natural history that should form a central component of the patient communication approach discussed later in this chapter, tempering the understandable anxiety a new diagnosis of a clonal hematologic disorder often provokes. This generally favorable prognosis nonetheless coexists with the small but clinically meaningful long-term risks of thrombotic complications, bleeding complications particularly at extreme platelet counts as discussed earlier in this chapter, and, less commonly, disease transformation, each of which the risk-stratified management framework developed in this chapter is specifically designed to mitigate.

Transformation to Myelofibrosis

A minority of essential thrombocythemia patients experience transformation to secondary myelofibrosis over an extended disease course, typically manifesting as progressive anemia, increasing splenomegaly, constitutional symptoms, and, on repeat bone marrow biopsy, progression of reticulin or collagen fibrosis beyond the findings present at initial diagnosis, a transformation risk that increases with longer disease duration and underscores the value of the long-term surveillance framework discussed later in this chapter rather than assuming a stable disease course indefinitely following initial diagnosis. Recognizing early signs of myelofibrotic transformation, including a new or worsening anemia, new or increasing splenomegaly on examination, or new constitutional symptoms, should prompt repeat bone marrow evaluation and reassessment of the management plan, since myelofibrotic transformation carries distinct management implications and a less favorable prognosis than uncomplicated essential thrombocythemia.

Transformation to Acute Leukemia and Associated Risk Factors

Transformation to acute myeloid leukemia represents the most serious, though least common, long-term complication of essential thrombocythemia, occurring in a small percentage of patients over an extended disease course and associated with risk factors including longer disease duration, prior exposure to certain cytoreductive agents, particularly with prolonged use, and specific additional molecular abnormalities beyond the primary driver mutation, a risk profile that has specifically informed the increasing preference for interferon-based therapy over prolonged hydroxyurea exposure in younger patients discussed earlier in this chapter. This leukemic transformation risk, while important to acknowledge in the overall risk-benefit discussion surrounding long-term cytoreductive therapy, should be communicated with appropriate proportion, since the absolute risk remains low for most patients and should not overshadow the substantial benefit cytoreductive therapy provides in reducing the more common thrombotic and hemorrhagic complications this chapter has emphasized throughout.

Perioperative and Procedural Management of Essential Thrombocythemia

Patients with essential thrombocythemia undergoing surgery or other invasive procedures require specific perioperative planning that integrates the thrombotic risk this disease confers with the bleeding risk of the planned procedure, extending the structured perioperative risk assessment framework developed throughout this book's clinical chapters to this population.

Preoperative Risk Assessment and Platelet Count Optimization

Preoperative evaluation should assess current platelet count control, with particular attention to whether the count is adequately controlled below the treat-to-target range discussed earlier in this chapter, since a poorly controlled or extreme platelet count elevation at the time of a planned procedure carries the combined thrombotic and, at extreme levels, hemorrhagic risk this chapter has emphasized throughout, warranting cytoreductive therapy optimization in the weeks preceding an elective procedure whenever the clinical timeline allows this advance planning. Von Willebrand factor multimer analysis should be considered preoperatively in patients with extreme thrombocytosis, following the same acquired von Willebrand syndrome screening principle discussed earlier in this chapter, given its direct implication for perioperative antiplatelet and hemostatic management planning.

Antiplatelet and Cytoreductive Therapy Perioperative Management

Perioperative management of antiplatelet therapy in essential thrombocythemia follows the general periprocedural antiplatelet management principles discussed in detail in Chapter 18, balancing the procedure-specific bleeding risk against the disease-specific thrombotic risk this chapter has developed throughout, with the specific decision to continue, hold, or bridge antiplatelet therapy individualized to the patient's risk stratification category and the planned procedure's bleeding risk. Cytoreductive therapy is generally continued through the perioperative period given its role in maintaining platelet count control rather than providing an acute antithrombotic effect analogous to antiplatelet therapy, though the specific perioperative management plan should be established collaboratively between the treating hematologist and the surgical or procedural team well in advance of the planned procedure.

Special Procedural Considerations

Emergency or urgent procedures in patients with poorly controlled or newly diagnosed essential thrombocythemia present particular management challenges given the limited opportunity for the advance platelet count optimization available for elective procedures, and in this circumstance, close coordination with hematology for expedited assessment and, where clinically appropriate, urgent cytoreductive intervention or plateletpheresis as discussed earlier in this chapter, alongside intraoperative and postoperative vigilance for both thrombotic and hemorrhagic complications, becomes the primary management strategy rather than the more deliberate advance-planning approach preferred for elective procedures.

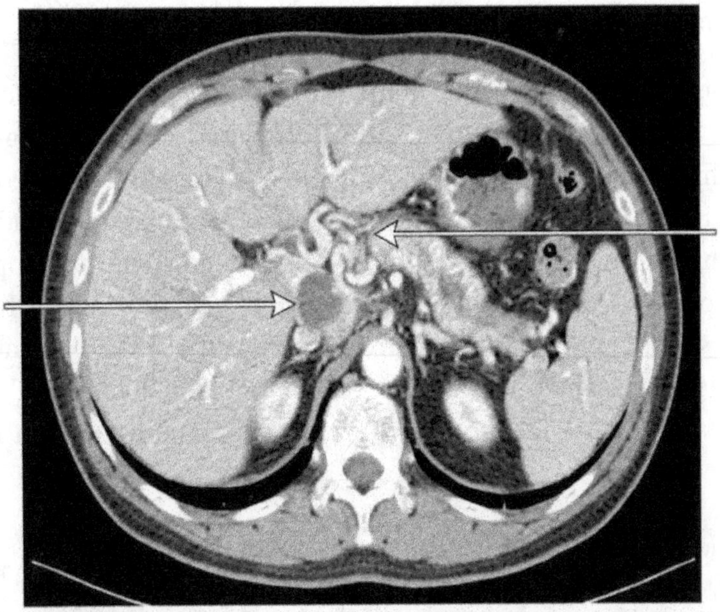

Figure 17.2 — Diagnostic Imaging: Portal Vein Thrombosis on Contrast-Enhanced Abdominal CT — Axial CT slice at the level of the portal hilum showing a filling defect within the main portal vein with surrounding cavernous transformation collateral vessels; venous phase contrast.

Splanchnic Vein Thrombosis in Myeloproliferative Neoplasms

Splanchnic vein thrombosis, encompassing portal vein thrombosis, hepatic vein thrombosis producing Budd-Chiari syndrome, and mesenteric vein thrombosis, represents a distinctive and clinically important thrombotic manifestation of the myeloproliferative neoplasms, occurring at these unusual anatomic sites with disproportionate frequency in essential thrombocythemia and polycythemia vera relative to the general population and warranting specific discussion beyond the general thrombotic risk framework developed earlier in this chapter.

Splanchnic Thrombosis as a Presenting Feature

Splanchnic vein thrombosis not infrequently represents the initial presenting manifestation of an underlying myeloproliferative neoplasm, preceding the recognition of thrombocytosis or other blood count abnormalities in a meaningful proportion of cases, and this recognized association means that any patient presenting with unexplained splanchnic vein thrombosis, particularly a younger patient without other clear prothrombotic risk factors, warrants myeloproliferative neoplasm evaluation, including JAK2 V617F testing, which is present with particularly high frequency in myeloproliferative neoplasm-associated splanchnic thrombosis, even when the platelet count and other blood counts remain within the normal range at presentation. Budd-Chiari syndrome, arising from hepatic vein thrombosis, presents with the classic triad of abdominal pain, ascites, and hepatomegaly, while portal vein thrombosis may present more insidiously with abdominal pain or be discovered incidentally on imaging obtained for other indications, and mesenteric vein thrombosis carries the specific additional risk of bowel ischemia requiring urgent surgical evaluation when clinically suspected.

Diagnostic Evaluation of Unexplained Splanchnic Thrombosis

The diagnostic evaluation of unexplained splanchnic vein thrombosis should include JAK2 V617F testing as a routine component given the strong association discussed above, alongside evaluation for other inherited and acquired thrombophilic conditions and, where clinically indicated, imaging assessment for local anatomic contributing factors such as cirrhosis or malignancy that can independently predispose to splanchnic thrombosis through mechanisms distinct from an underlying myeloproliferative neoplasm. A finding of JAK2 V617F positivity in a patient with splanchnic vein thrombosis but a normal platelet count and other blood counts should prompt bone marrow biopsy to evaluate for an underlying, early-stage myeloproliferative neoplasm, recognizing that the classic blood count abnormalities discussed throughout this chapter may not yet be manifest at the time the thrombotic complication first brings the patient to medical attention.

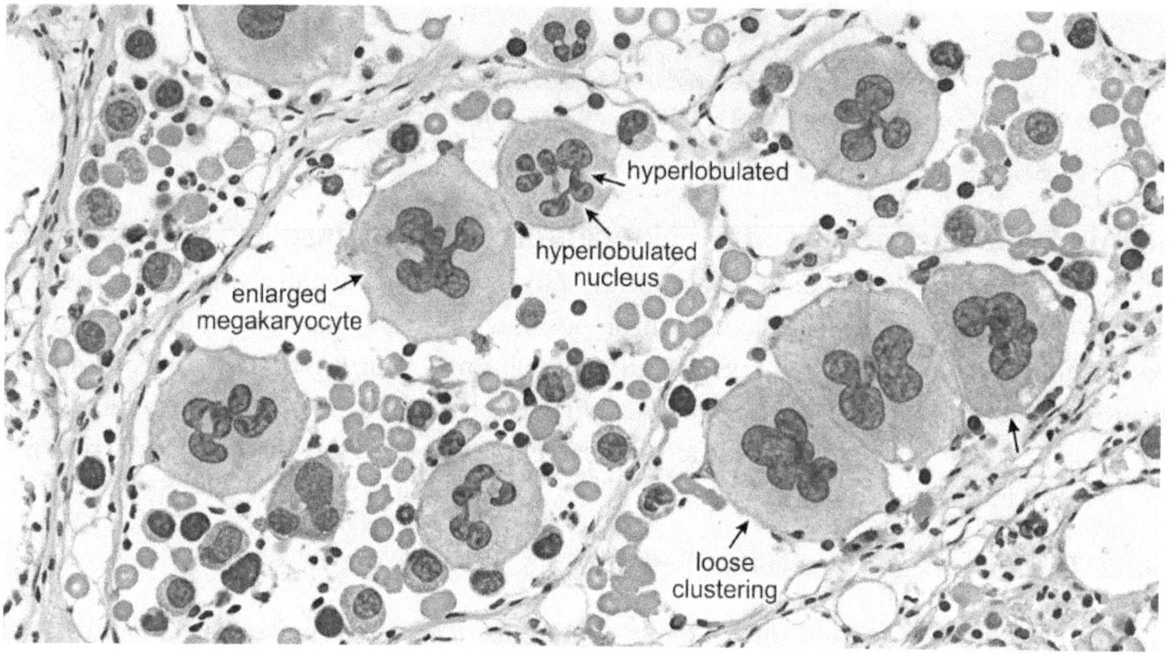

Anticoagulation and Cytoreductive Therapy in Splanchnic Vein Thrombosis

Management of myeloproliferative neoplasm-associated splanchnic vein thrombosis requires both therapeutic anticoagulation, typically continued long-term given the persistent underlying prothrombotic state the myeloproliferative neoplasm confers, and cytoreductive therapy directed at the underlying disease, reflecting the dual local-anatomic and systemic prothrombotic contributors this specific thrombotic complication involves, an approach that differs from the risk-stratified, sometimes observation-only approach applied to lower-risk essential thrombocythemia patients without a qualifying thrombotic event as discussed earlier in this chapter. The specific anticoagulant selection and duration should be individualized in collaboration with hematology and, for Budd-Chiari syndrome specifically, hepatology given the potential need for additional interventions addressing hepatic venous outflow obstruction in more severe or refractory cases, extending the multidisciplinary coordination principle this book has emphasized throughout to this specific, anatomically complex thrombotic presentation.

Long-Term Implications for Disease Classification

A myeloproliferative neoplasm diagnosis established through splanchnic vein thrombosis evaluation carries the same long-term monitoring and risk-stratified management implications discussed throughout this chapter, and the thrombotic event itself, having already occurred, automatically places the patient in the high thrombotic risk category for subsequent management purposes regardless of the specific platelet count or other risk factors present at diagnosis, directly informing the cytoreductive therapy decision discussed earlier in this chapter without requiring further risk stratification calculation for this particular management decision.

Risk Category	Defining Criteria	Recommended Therapy
Very Low Risk	Age under 60, no prior thrombosis, JAK2 wild-type	Observation, or low-dose aspirin if additional cardiovascular risk factors present
Low Risk	Age under 60, no prior thrombosis, JAK2-mutated	Low-dose aspirin
Intermediate Risk	Age over 60, no prior thrombosis, JAK2 wild-type	Low-dose aspirin, individualized cytoreductive consideration
High Risk	Age over 60 with JAK2 mutation, or any prior thrombosis, or extreme thrombocytosis	Low-dose aspirin plus cytoreductive therapy (hydroxyurea, anagrelide, or interferon)

Quality of Life and Psychosocial Considerations

Living with essential thrombocythemia as a chronic clonal hematologic condition carries psychosocial dimensions beyond the thrombotic and hemorrhagic risk management this chapter has emphasized throughout, and attending to these dimensions represents an integral, rather than peripheral, component of comprehensive care for this population.

Symptom Burden Beyond Thrombosis and Bleeding

A subset of essential thrombocythemia patients experiences meaningful symptom burden beyond the thrombotic and hemorrhagic complications this chapter has primarily addressed, including fatigue, difficulty concentrating, pruritus, and vasomotor symptoms such as erythromelalgia, a painful erythematous burning sensation typically affecting the extremities that reflects microvascular platelet aggregation and responds characteristically well to aspirin therapy, providing both diagnostic recognition value and a specific therapeutic target distinct from the systemic thrombotic risk reduction aspirin otherwise provides. Systematic symptom assessment using validated myeloproliferative neoplasm symptom burden instruments, rather than reliance on spontaneous patient reporting alone, allows the clinician to identify and address this symptom burden, which may substantially affect quality of life even in patients whose thrombotic risk is otherwise well controlled through the risk-stratified management framework developed earlier in this chapter.

Psychological Adjustment to a Chronic Clonal Diagnosis

The diagnosis of a clonal hematologic condition, even one carrying the generally favorable prognosis essential thrombocythemia typically confers, can provoke significant anxiety related to its cancer-adjacent classification, uncertainty regarding long-term disease course, and the small but real risk of transformation discussed earlier in this chapter, and clinicians should proactively address this psychological dimension rather than assuming it is adequately managed simply by delivering accurate prognostic information, extending the mental health awareness and support principle this book has emphasized throughout its discussion of chronic and life-altering hematologic diagnoses. Peer support communities and myeloproliferative neoplasm-specific patient advocacy organizations provide valuable additional support for many patients navigating this psychological adjustment, complementing rather than replacing the clinical relationship and offering connection with others managing the same specific diagnosis and its associated uncertainties.

Sustaining Long-Term Treatment Adherence

Long-term adherence to cytoreductive and antiplatelet therapy, essential given the chronic, indefinite nature of essential thrombocythemia management, benefits from explicit clinician attention to treatment burden, side effect management, and the patient's own understanding of and engagement with the rationale for ongoing therapy, extending the shared decision-making and treatment adherence principles emphasized throughout this book's chronic disease management discussions to this specific, lifelong therapeutic relationship. Regular reassessment of treatment tolerability and quality of life impact, rather than a narrow focus on platelet count and thrombotic risk markers alone, supports sustained long-term adherence and allows earlier identification of a treatment regimen that may warrant adjustment given accumulating side effects or declining quality of life, even when the platelet count target itself remains adequately controlled.

Long-Term Monitoring and Patient Communication

Longitudinal Disease Monitoring

Long-term monitoring of essential thrombocythemia incorporates periodic complete blood count assessment to confirm cytoreductive therapy is achieving and maintaining the target platelet count range, symptom assessment for constitutional symptoms and disease-related complications, and periodic reassessment of thrombotic risk factors that may evolve over time, including the development of new cardiovascular risk factors or, less commonly, a first thrombotic event that would reclassify a previously low-risk patient into the high-risk category requiring treatment intensification. This ongoing risk reassessment reflects the same principle of individualized, evolving management this book has emphasized throughout its chronic disease management discussions, in which the initial risk stratification and treatment plan established at diagnosis is not fixed but rather revisited and adjusted as the patient's clinical circumstances change over time.

Communicating the Diagnosis and Long-Term Outlook

Patient education regarding essential thrombocythemia should address the generally favorable long-term prognosis for most patients, the chronic nature of the condition requiring ongoing monitoring and management rather than a single definitive treatment, the specific rationale for the individualized risk-stratified treatment approach the patient has been placed on, and the small but clinically important long-term risk of disease transformation to myelofibrosis or acute leukemia, delivered with the same balanced, honest, and hope-preserving communication approach this book has emphasized throughout its discussion of chronic and potentially serious hematologic diagnoses. Patients should be specifically counseled regarding symptoms that would warrant prompt medical attention, including new neurologic symptoms suggesting stroke or transient ischemic attack, symptoms of venous thromboembolism, and unusual bleeding, extending the patient self-advocacy and symptom-recognition education framework developed throughout this book to this population living with a chronic condition carrying ongoing thrombotic and hemorrhagic risk.

This chapter has developed the thrombocytoses as a quantitative platelet disorder category requiring, in parallel with the thrombocytopenia framework developed across Chapters 8 through 14, careful distinction between reactive and clonal causes before the risk-stratified essential thrombocythemia management framework is applied, and has addressed the distinctive dual thrombotic-and-hemorrhagic risk profile that emerges at extreme degrees of platelet count elevation. The chapter that follows shifts from disease-directed management to pharmacology, addressing the antithrombotic medications whose periprocedural management this and the preceding chapters have repeatedly referenced.

Figure 17.3 Therapeutic Plateletpheresis Circuit

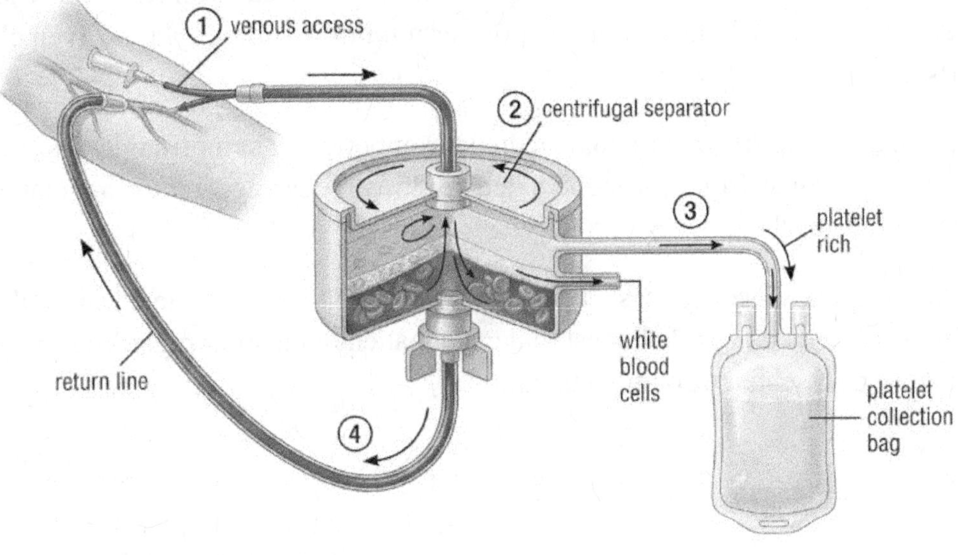

Figure 17.3 Therapeutic Plateletpheresis Circuit

THE PLATELET CRISIS DECISION COMPASS — Thrombocytosis Recognition and Risk Stratification

Compass Synthesis: This chapter's Decision Compass instance established the systematic approach to distinguishing persistent, unexplained thrombocytosis from a resolving reactive elevation, directing molecular testing at the appropriate diagnostic juncture rather than either premature testing of every mild reactive elevation or delayed testing of a genuinely clonal, persistent process.

Crisis Anchor: An elevated platelet count without an identifiable or resolving reactive trigger warrants JAK2, CALR, and MPL testing, and once essential thrombocythemia is confirmed, thrombotic risk stratification, rather than platelet count alone, should direct the intensity of antiplatelet and cytoreductive therapy.

Summary and Key Concepts

Thrombocytosis is classified as reactive or clonal; reactive causes, including infection, inflammation, iron deficiency, and postoperative states, are common and resolve as the underlying trigger is addressed.

Essential thrombocythemia is diagnosed by WHO criteria integrating bone marrow morphology, exclusion of other myeloproliferative neoplasms, and JAK2, CALR, or MPL mutation testing, which distinguishes clonal from reactive thrombocytosis in the majority of cases.

Management of essential thrombocythemia is risk-stratified using the IPSET-thrombosis score, with low-risk patients managed conservatively and high-risk patients receiving cytoreductive therapy, typically hydroxyurea, anagrelide, or interferon, alongside antiplatelet therapy.

Essential thrombocythemia in pregnancy requires interferon-based cytoreduction when indicated, given hydroxyurea's teratogenic risk, and extended postpartum thromboprophylaxis given elevated postpartum thrombotic risk.

Extreme thrombocytosis carries a paradoxical dual thrombotic and hemorrhagic risk profile, with acquired von Willebrand syndrome from shear-mediated multimer cleavage requiring platelet count-lowering cytoreductive therapy as the primary corrective measure.

Long-term monitoring incorporates periodic risk reassessment and surveillance for disease transformation, delivered alongside honest, balanced patient education regarding the generally favorable but chronic nature of essential thrombocythemia.

CHAPTER 18: ANTITHROMBOTIC PHARMACOLOGY, REVERSAL, AND PERIPROCEDURAL MANAGEMENT

Learning Objectives

1. Describe the mechanism of action of aspirin, P2Y12 inhibitors, and other antiplatelet agents and correlate mechanism with periprocedural management implications.
2. Formulate a periprocedural antiplatelet management plan integrating procedural bleeding risk, thrombotic risk, and specific antiplatelet agent pharmacokinetics.
3. Describe the available strategies for reversing or mitigating antiplatelet effect in the setting of urgent surgery or life-threatening bleeding.
4. Distinguish the periprocedural management principles for antiplatelet therapy from those for anticoagulant therapy, and recognize situations requiring management of both simultaneously.
5. Apply bridging therapy principles appropriately, recognizing situations in which bridging is and is not indicated.
6. Formulate a management approach for antiplatelet-associated intracranial and gastrointestinal hemorrhage.

Chapter Outline

Pharmacology of Aspirin and Cyclooxygenase Inhibition

Mechanism of Action

Aspirin irreversibly acetylates cyclooxygenase-1 within the platelet, permanently disabling the enzyme's capacity to generate thromboxane A2 from arachidonic acid for the remaining lifespan of that individual platelet, a mechanism that distinguishes aspirin from every other antiplatelet agent discussed in this chapter through its irreversibility, since platelets, lacking a nucleus, cannot synthesize new cyclooxygenase-1 protein to replace the permanently inactivated enzyme, meaning full recovery of thromboxane-dependent platelet function requires generation of an entirely new platelet population through the megakaryopoiesis process discussed in Chapter 1 rather than simple clearance of the drug itself from the circulation. This irreversible mechanism explains why aspirin's antiplatelet effect persists for the full approximately ten-day circulating lifespan of the platelet population present at the time of dosing, far outlasting the drug's own plasma half-life of well under one hour, a pharmacokinetic-pharmacodynamic dissociation that directly informs the periprocedural withholding intervals discussed later in this chapter.

Because aspirin's irreversible cyclooxygenase-1 inhibition affects only the fraction of the platelet population circulating at the time of each dose, and because approximately ten percent of the total platelet population is replaced daily through ongoing megakaryopoiesis, full recovery of aggregate thromboxane-dependent platelet function following aspirin discontinuation follows a predictable, gradual trajectory over the subsequent seven to ten days as progressively larger fractions of the circulating platelet population represent newly produced, unaffected platelets, a recovery curve that underlies the standard five-to-seven-day preoperative aspirin discontinuation window recommended for procedures where aspirin discontinuation is deemed appropriate.

Clinical Indications and Dosing

Low-dose aspirin, typically in the 75 to 100 mg daily range, provides near-maximal cyclooxygenase-1 inhibition and represents the standard dosing for both primary and secondary cardiovascular and cerebrovascular prevention, with higher doses providing no meaningful additional antiplatelet benefit while increasing gastrointestinal toxicity risk, reflecting the essentially complete cyclooxygenase-1 inhibition achieved even at these low doses given the enzyme's specific irreversible susceptibility to aspirin's acetylation mechanism. This low-dose, ceiling-effect pharmacology distinguishes aspirin from many other medication classes in which dose escalation produces proportionally greater therapeutic effect, and understanding this ceiling effect should inform clinical practice away from higher aspirin dosing under the mistaken assumption that more aspirin provides more antiplatelet benefit.

Aspirin resistance, a term describing incomplete laboratory or clinical response to standard aspirin therapy, remains an incompletely characterized and clinically controversial phenomenon, with true pharmacologic resistance, reflecting genuine failure to achieve adequate cyclooxygenase-1 inhibition, distinguished from pseudoresistance related to medication nonadherence or, less commonly, alternative thromboxane generation pathways not fully suppressed by cyclooxygenase-1 inhibition alone, and routine laboratory testing for aspirin resistance is not currently recommended in standard clinical practice given the limited evidence that resistance testing meaningfully changes clinical management or outcomes.

P2Y12 Inhibitors: Clopidogrel, Prasugrel, and Ticagrelor

Mechanism and Comparative Pharmacology

The P2Y12 inhibitors block the platelet ADP receptor responsible for amplifying and sustaining platelet activation following the initial activation signal, and this drug class encompasses agents with clinically important pharmacologic differences: clopidogrel and prasugrel are irreversible inhibitors requiring hepatic metabolic activation to their active metabolite, sharing aspirin's irreversible mechanism and correspondingly extended recovery timeline following discontinuation, while ticagrelor provides reversible P2Y12 inhibition through direct receptor binding without requiring metabolic activation, producing a more rapid onset and, critically for periprocedural management, a shorter recovery interval following discontinuation given its reversible rather than irreversible mechanism. Clopidogrel's dependence on hepatic CYP2C19-mediated metabolic activation introduces clinically significant interindividual variability in antiplatelet response related to CYP2C19 genetic polymorphisms, with poor metabolizers achieving substantially reduced active metabolite generation and correspondingly attenuated antiplatelet effect, a pharmacogenomic consideration that has prompted selective use of CYP2C19 genotyping or platelet function testing in specific high-risk clinical scenarios, though routine testing is not universally recommended.

Prasugrel provides more potent and consistent platelet inhibition than clopidogrel through a more efficient metabolic activation pathway less subject to the CYP2C19 variability affecting clopidogrel, but this increased potency comes with correspondingly increased bleeding risk, and prasugrel carries specific contraindications in patients with prior stroke or transient ischemic attack and is generally avoided in patients over 75 years of age or under 60 kg body weight given the disproportionate bleeding risk observed in these populations in clinical trials, illustrating the general pharmacologic principle that greater antiplatelet potency trades directly against increased bleeding risk rather than providing benefit without corresponding cost.

Recovery Timelines and Periprocedural Implications

The irreversible mechanism shared by clopidogrel and prasugrel produces a recovery timeline following discontinuation that parallels aspirin's, requiring approximately five to seven days for clopidogrel and seven to ten days for prasugrel given its more complete platelet inhibition, for adequate recovery of platelet function through the same new-platelet-generation mechanism discussed for aspirin above, whereas ticagrelor's reversible mechanism allows for a shorter recommended discontinuation interval of approximately three to five days before elective procedures, reflecting its combination of reversible receptor binding and a relatively short plasma half-life that together allow more rapid pharmacodynamic recovery than the irreversible agents provide. This mechanism-based difference in recovery timeline represents a clinically important distinction the treating clinician must specifically account for when planning periprocedural P2Y12 inhibitor management, since applying a uniform discontinuation interval across all three agents would either unnecessarily prolong the bleeding-risk-reduction benefit of earlier discontinuation for ticagrelor or inadequately allow platelet function recovery before a procedure if the shorter ticagrelor-appropriate interval were mistakenly applied to clopidogrel or prasugrel.

Indications for P2Y12 inhibitor therapy, most centrally dual antiplatelet therapy following acute coronary syndrome or coronary stent placement, carry their own specific minimum duration requirements before elective discontinuation should be considered, discussed further in the periprocedural risk stratification section below, reflecting the competing consideration that premature P2Y12 inhibitor discontinuation, particularly in the setting of a recently placed coronary stent, carries a substantial and specifically recognized risk of stent thrombosis that must be weighed against any procedural bleeding risk reduction discontinuation might provide.

THE PLATELET CRISIS DECISION COMPASS — Antiplatelet Recovery Timeline Arc

The Presentation: A 66-year-old man on clopidogrel following a coronary stent placed four months ago requires an elective inguinal hernia repair, and the surgical team asks hematology for periprocedural antiplatelet guidance.

Mimic Signature: Treating this request as a simple 'hold for five to seven days' instruction without further evaluation would overlook the critical distinction between elective discontinuation timing and whether discontinuation is safe at all given the specific stent type and time since placement.

The Decision: Cardiology consultation confirms the stent is a drug-eluting stent placed four months ago, within the minimum recommended dual antiplatelet therapy duration, making elective clopidogrel discontinuation inappropriate at this time regardless of the procedure's bleeding risk category.

Trap Logic: Focusing exclusively on the pharmacologic recovery timeline for clopidogrel discontinuation, without first establishing whether discontinuation is appropriate at all given the specific stent thrombosis risk this patient's recent drug-eluting stent placement confers, risks a catastrophic stent thrombosis and myocardial infarction that would far outweigh the bleeding risk the hernia repair itself presents.

Crisis Anchor: Before addressing how long to hold a P2Y12 inhibitor before a procedure, first establish whether holding it at all is safe given the specific indication, stent type, and time since placement — cardiology co-management is mandatory whenever a recent coronary stent is present, and elective surgery should be deferred rather than the antiplatelet therapy discontinued when the minimum dual antiplatelet therapy duration has not yet elapsed.

Periprocedural Risk Stratification

Integrating Thrombotic and Bleeding Risk

Periprocedural antiplatelet management requires systematic integration of two independent risk assessments: the thrombotic risk of temporarily discontinuing antiplatelet therapy, determined primarily by the underlying indication (recent acute coronary syndrome, recent coronary stent placement and its type, cerebrovascular disease, or peripheral arterial disease) and, where applicable, time elapsed since the qualifying event, and the procedural bleeding risk, determined by the specific procedure's inherent hemorrhagic risk and the consequences of bleeding at that particular anatomic site, following a two-axis risk integration framework that parallels the bleeding-risk-versus-thrombotic-risk balancing this book has applied throughout its discussion of periprocedural management in other bleeding and clotting disorders. Neither axis alone determines the appropriate management plan, and a systematic, explicit consideration of both, rather than reflexive discontinuation of all antiplatelet therapy before any procedure, represents the appropriate periprocedural management approach this chapter develops.

Procedures carrying minimal bleeding risk, including most minor dermatologic procedures, cataract surgery, and many routine dental procedures, generally do not require antiplatelet discontinuation regardless of the underlying thrombotic risk category, since the bleeding risk reduction discontinuation would provide is outweighed by even a modest thrombotic risk in most clinical scenarios, whereas procedures carrying substantial bleeding risk, particularly those involving closed spaces where even modest bleeding produces serious consequences such as intracranial or intraspinal procedures, require more careful individualized risk-benefit assessment incorporating the full thrombotic risk evaluation discussed above.

Figure 18.3: Epidural Space Anatomy and Neuraxial Bleeding Risk

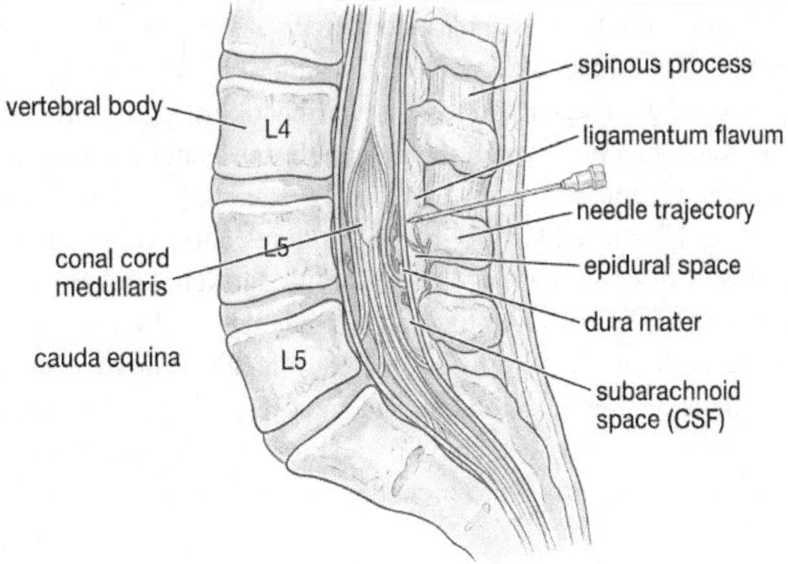

Minimum Dual Antiplatelet Therapy Durations

Current guidelines recommend minimum dual antiplatelet therapy durations following coronary stent placement that vary by stent type and clinical indication, generally ranging from one month for bare-metal stents placed for stable indications to six or twelve months for drug-eluting stents, with shorter minimum durations increasingly supported by evidence for newer-generation drug-eluting stents, and elective surgery requiring antiplatelet discontinuation should be deferred until this minimum duration has elapsed whenever clinically feasible, extending the advance-planning principle emphasized throughout this book to this specific, cardiology-coordinated periprocedural planning context. When elective surgery cannot reasonably be deferred and falls within the minimum dual antiplatelet therapy window, cardiology consultation to weigh individualized stent thrombosis risk against the specific procedural bleeding risk, rather than a unilateral surgical or hematologic decision, represents the appropriate management approach given the specialized, patient-specific risk assessment this scenario requires.

Continuing aspirin alone while discontinuing only the P2Y12 inhibitor component of dual antiplatelet therapy provides a partial risk-mitigation strategy for procedures requiring some reduction in antiplatelet intensity but not full discontinuation, reflecting the recognition that single-agent aspirin therapy provides meaningfully more thrombotic protection than complete antiplatelet discontinuation while still reducing bleeding risk relative to continued dual antiplatelet therapy, an intermediate strategy that should be specifically considered and discussed with the surgical and cardiology teams for appropriate cases rather than defaulting to the binary choice of continuing or discontinuing all antiplatelet therapy.

Anticoagulant Pharmacology and Periprocedural Management

Direct Oral Anticoagulants

The direct oral anticoagulants, including the direct thrombin inhibitor dabigatran and the direct factor Xa inhibitors apixaban, rivaroxaban, and edoxaban, have become the predominant anticoagulant class for most indications given their predictable pharmacokinetics, lack of routine laboratory monitoring requirement, and generally favorable safety profile relative to vitamin K antagonist therapy, and periprocedural management of these agents follows a pharmacokinetically-based discontinuation interval determined primarily by renal function, given their variable but generally substantial renal elimination, and the specific procedural bleeding risk category, with standard discontinuation intervals typically ranging from one to two days for low-bleeding-risk procedures and two to four days for high-bleeding-risk procedures, extended further in patients with significant renal impairment given the resulting prolongation of drug elimination half-life. Unlike the antiplatelet agents discussed earlier in this chapter, the direct oral anticoagulants do not require the extended, platelet-turnover-dependent recovery interval those irreversible agents demand, since anticoagulant effect resolves directly with drug clearance rather than requiring generation of a new, unaffected cell population, making periprocedural planning for these agents more directly tied to renal function and procedure-specific bleeding risk than to a fixed universal interval.

Bridging anticoagulation with a shorter-acting parenteral agent during the periprocedural direct oral anticoagulant discontinuation interval is generally not indicated given the direct oral anticoagulants' relatively rapid onset and offset compared to vitamin K antagonist therapy, and unnecessary bridging in this population has been associated with increased bleeding risk without a clearly demonstrated thrombotic risk reduction benefit, an important departure from the vitamin K antagonist bridging framework discussed below that reflects the fundamentally different pharmacokinetic profile of these two anticoagulant classes.

Vitamin K Antagonist Therapy and Bridging Principles

Warfarin and other vitamin K antagonists, though used less frequently than in the past given the direct oral anticoagulants' generally favorable profile, remain the anticoagulant of choice for specific indications including mechanical heart valves and, in many practice settings, antiphospholipid syndrome, and periprocedural management requires discontinuation approximately five days before an elective procedure given warfarin's longer half-life and the time required for International Normalized Ratio normalization, with bridging anticoagulation using a shorter-acting parenteral agent, typically low molecular weight heparin, considered for patients at high thrombotic risk during the resulting anticoagulation gap. Bridging therapy decisions should be individualized based on the specific thrombotic risk the underlying indication confers, since evidence has demonstrated that bridging itself carries meaningful bleeding risk without clear thrombotic risk reduction benefit for many lower-risk indications, reflecting a broader shift in periprocedural anticoagulation management away from routine bridging toward a more selective, risk-stratified approach reserved for genuinely high-risk patients such as those with mechanical mitral valves or very recent thromboembolic events.

This selective bridging approach represents an important evolution in periprocedural anticoagulation management, and clinicians should recognize that the historical default toward routine bridging for any patient on chronic anticoagulation no longer reflects current evidence-based practice, with the specific decision instead requiring individualized assessment of the underlying thrombotic risk against the bridging-associated bleeding risk for the specific clinical scenario at hand.

Reversal Strategies for Antiplatelet-Associated Bleeding

Platelet Transfusion as Reversal Strategy

Platelet transfusion provides the most direct reversal strategy for antiplatelet-associated bleeding, supplying functionally normal platelets to dilute the circulating population of drug-affected platelets, though its efficacy depends substantially on the specific antiplatelet agent and timing relative to the last dose, since transfused platelets entering a circulation still containing substantial active drug, particularly for agents with ongoing plasma presence such as ticagrelor given its reversible receptor-binding mechanism discussed earlier in this chapter, may themselves become inhibited by the still-circulating drug, limiting the effectiveness of platelet transfusion for reversal of this specific agent relative to the irreversible agents where transfused platelets, once introduced, remain functionally intact regardless of ongoing drug clearance. This mechanism-dependent variability in platelet transfusion efficacy should inform the clinician's expectations and, where feasible, the timing of platelet transfusion relative to the specific antiplatelet agent's pharmacokinetic profile when reversal is urgently needed for life-threatening bleeding.

Platelet transfusion for antiplatelet reversal is generally reserved for significant or life-threatening bleeding or urgent surgical procedures where the bleeding risk is judged to substantially outweigh the risks and resource utilization platelet transfusion entails, rather than used routinely for minor bleeding or elective procedures where the periprocedural discontinuation timelines discussed earlier in this chapter provide a more appropriate, non-transfusion-dependent management approach.

Desmopressin and Adjunctive Measures

Desmopressin, discussed in its broader hemostatic role throughout this book, provides a modest but clinically useful adjunctive measure for antiplatelet-associated bleeding through its effect on von Willebrand factor release and platelet adhesion enhancement, offering a rapid-onset, non-transfusion option particularly useful as a bridging measure while platelet transfusion or other definitive interventions are being arranged, though its effect is generally more modest for antiplatelet-associated bleeding than for the primary bleeding disorders discussed in earlier chapters where desmopressin plays a more central therapeutic role. Antifibrinolytic therapy with tranexamic acid provides an additional adjunctive measure for antiplatelet-associated mucocutaneous or surgical bleeding, working through a mechanism independent of platelet function correction and therefore providing benefit regardless of the specific antiplatelet agent or its reversibility, making it a broadly applicable adjunct across the range of antiplatelet-associated bleeding scenarios this chapter addresses.

Emerging Specific Reversal Agents

Specific reversal agents targeting individual antiplatelet mechanisms remain more limited than the specific reversal agents available for anticoagulant therapy discussed later in this chapter, reflecting the underlying biology in which platelet transfusion, rather than a pharmacologic antagonist, provides the most direct means of restoring platelet function following irreversible cyclooxygenase or P2Y12 receptor inhibition, though continued research into specific reversal strategies, including monoclonal antibody-based approaches targeting specific antiplatelet agents, may expand the available reversal armamentarium in coming years, an area of active clinical investigation the treating clinician should remain attentive to given its potential to meaningfully improve the management of urgent antiplatelet-associated bleeding.

THE PLATELET CRISIS DECISION COMPASS — Reversal Agent Selection Arc

The Presentation: A patient on rivaroxaban for atrial fibrillation presents with major gastrointestinal bleeding and hemodynamic instability, and the emergency team asks whether to give fresh frozen plasma, prothrombin complex concentrate, or a specific reversal agent.

Mimic Signature: Treating this as a generic 'major bleeding on anticoagulation' scenario and defaulting to fresh frozen plasma, the traditional reversal agent for vitamin K antagonist bleeding, would overlook that fresh frozen plasma provides minimal direct reversal benefit for a factor Xa inhibitor specifically.

The Decision: Andexanet alfa, the specific factor Xa inhibitor reversal agent, is administered given the life-threatening nature of the bleeding, with four-factor prothrombin complex concentrate as an alternative if andexanet alfa is unavailable.

Trap Logic: Reflexively reaching for fresh frozen plasma because it is the traditional 'reversal' product risks both delaying effective factor Xa inhibitor reversal and unnecessarily exposing the patient to a large-volume infusion that provides little specific benefit for this particular anticoagulant class.

Crisis Anchor: Reversal strategy must match the specific anticoagulant mechanism: andexanet alfa for factor Xa inhibitors, idarucizumab for dabigatran, and four-factor prothrombin complex concentrate with vitamin K for vitamin K antagonist therapy — fresh frozen plasma is not the default reversal agent for direct oral anticoagulants.

Reversal Strategies for Anticoagulant-Associated Bleeding

Reversal of Direct Oral Anticoagulants

Specific reversal agents are now available for both major direct oral anticoagulant classes: idarucizumab provides rapid, specific reversal of dabigatran through direct monoclonal antibody-mediated binding, and andexanet alfa provides reversal of the factor Xa inhibitors apixaban and rivaroxaban through a decoy factor Xa mechanism that sequesters the circulating anticoagulant, together representing a substantial advance in the management of life-threatening direct oral anticoagulant-associated bleeding relative to the nonspecific reversal strategies that were previously the only available option for this anticoagulant class. Four-factor prothrombin complex concentrate provides a nonspecific but clinically useful reversal strategy for direct oral anticoagulant-associated bleeding when specific reversal agents are unavailable or cost-prohibitive, working through provision of concentrated coagulation factors that overwhelm the anticoagulant effect rather than directly neutralizing the specific drug, an approach that, while less mechanistically elegant than the specific reversal agents, has demonstrated clinical utility in this setting.

Reversal of Vitamin K Antagonist Therapy

Vitamin K antagonist reversal is achieved through vitamin K administration, which corrects the underlying mechanism of anticoagulation but requires hours to days for full effect given the time required for hepatic synthesis of new, functional vitamin K-dependent coagulation factors, and four-factor prothrombin complex concentrate, which provides immediate reversal through direct replacement of the depleted vitamin K-dependent factors and represents the preferred reversal strategy for life-threatening warfarin-associated bleeding given its substantially faster onset relative to fresh frozen plasma, the historical standard reversal approach that has been largely supplanted by prothrombin complex concentrate given its more concentrated factor content, smaller volume, and correspondingly more rapid and complete reversal. Combined vitamin K and prothrombin complex concentrate administration provides both the immediate reversal prothrombin complex concentrate offers and the sustained reversal vitamin K provides as the prothrombin complex concentrate's effect wanes, representing the standard approach for significant vitamin K antagonist-associated bleeding requiring urgent reversal.

CAUTION: Andexanet alfa has been associated with a recognized risk of subsequent thrombotic events following its administration, thought to relate to a rebound procoagulant effect, and its use should be reserved for genuinely life-threatening bleeding where the reversal benefit clearly outweighs this thrombotic risk rather than used for less severe bleeding where alternative management strategies would provide an adequate margin of safety.

Special Populations and Combined Antithrombotic Therapy

Triple Therapy: Combined Antiplatelet and Anticoagulant Regimens

Patients requiring both anticoagulation, most commonly for atrial fibrillation, and dual antiplatelet therapy following coronary stent placement present a particularly high bleeding risk combined regimen, historically termed triple therapy, that has increasingly moved toward shortened dual antiplatelet therapy duration and, where clinically appropriate, single rather than dual antiplatelet therapy combined with anticoagulation for the majority of the required combined treatment period, reflecting accumulating evidence that the bleeding risk of prolonged triple therapy frequently outweighs its incremental thrombotic risk reduction benefit relative to a de-escalated regimen. This evolving management approach requires close, ongoing cardiology and, where relevant, hematology coordination given the complexity of balancing coronary stent thrombosis risk, atrial fibrillation-associated stroke risk, and the substantial bleeding risk this combined antithrombotic regimen confers, extending the multidisciplinary coordination principle this book has emphasized throughout to this particularly high-stakes combined therapy scenario.

Renal Impairment and Antithrombotic Dosing

Renal impairment substantially affects the pharmacokinetics of several antithrombotic agents, particularly the renally eliminated direct oral anticoagulants discussed earlier in this chapter, requiring dose adjustment or, in severe renal impairment, avoidance of specific agents given the risk of drug accumulation and correspondingly increased bleeding risk, and periprocedural discontinuation intervals should be extended in patients with significant renal impairment to account for the prolonged elimination half-life this population experiences, following the renal function-informed dosing framework applied throughout the antithrombotic pharmacology discussed in this chapter. Confirmation against current formulary and manufacturer dosing guidance, rather than reliance on standard dosing without regard to renal function, represents essential practice for any patient with renal impairment requiring antithrombotic therapy, given the clinically significant bleeding risk inadequate dose adjustment in this population can produce.

Neuraxial Anesthesia and Antithrombotic Therapy

Neuraxial anesthesia, including spinal and epidural techniques, carries a specific and serious risk of spinal or epidural hematoma in patients on antithrombotic therapy given the closed, non-compressible anatomic space involved, and specific, agent-dependent minimum discontinuation intervals before neuraxial procedure placement and catheter removal have been established by anesthesiology society guidelines, generally more conservative than the discontinuation intervals applied for other procedures given the severe neurologic consequences a spinal or epidural hematoma can produce. Close coordination with anesthesiology regarding these specific neuraxial timing requirements, which may differ meaningfully from the general periprocedural discontinuation framework discussed elsewhere in this chapter, represents essential practice whenever neuraxial anesthesia is planned for a patient on antithrombotic therapy.

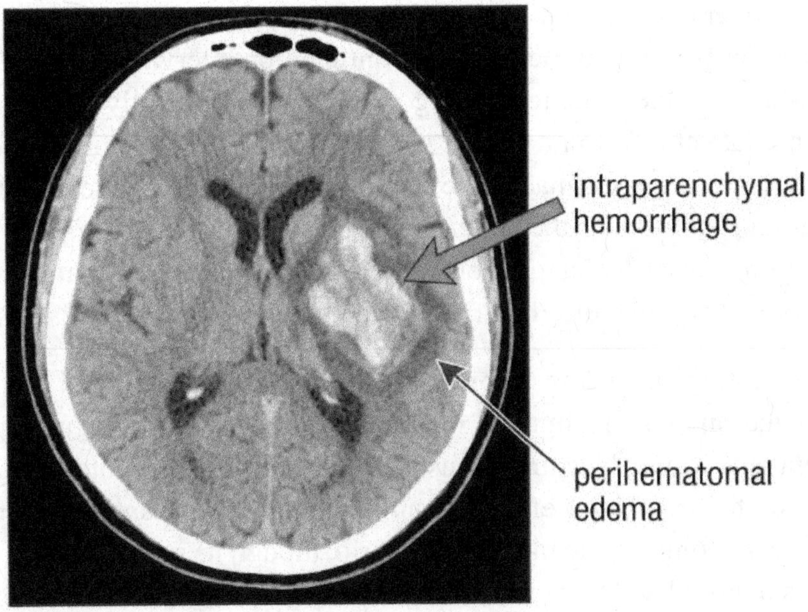

Figure 18.1: Intracranial Hemorrhage on Noncontrast CT

CLINICAL CASE: A 74-year-old woman on apixaban for atrial fibrillation and aspirin following a myocardial infarction six years ago presents with acute-onset severe headache and is found to have a large intraparenchymal hemorrhage on CT imaging. Applying the reversal framework developed in this chapter, andexanet alfa is administered promptly given the life-threatening nature of the intracranial hemorrhage, and platelet transfusion is given to address the concurrent aspirin effect, while neurosurgery is emergently consulted regarding potential surgical evacuation. Given the patient's renal function is normal, apixaban's expected elimination is confirmed to be consistent with standard pharmacokinetics rather than prolonged accumulation. Following stabilization, the multidisciplinary team, including neurology, cardiology, and hematology, discusses long-term antithrombotic management, weighing the patient's ongoing atrial fibrillation stroke risk and coronary artery disease against the substantial risk of recurrent intracranial hemorrhage this event has now established, ultimately favoring a reduced-intensity regimen with careful ongoing surveillance rather than resumption of the prior combined regimen. This case illustrates the complete reversal and long-term management arc developed in this chapter: prompt recognition of a life-threatening bleeding emergency in a patient on combined antithrombotic therapy, agent-specific reversal addressing both the anticoagulant and antiplatelet components, and a subsequent multidisciplinary discussion recalibrating the long-term antithrombotic strategy in light of the demonstrated bleeding risk.

Laboratory Monitoring of Antithrombotic Therapy

The Limited Role of Platelet Function Testing in Antiplatelet Monitoring

Platelet function testing, discussed in its technical aspects in Chapter 7, has been explored as a tool for guiding antiplatelet therapy intensity, confirming adequate response to therapy, or informing periprocedural timing decisions, but routine platelet function testing to guide antiplatelet dosing has not been consistently shown to improve clinical outcomes across large randomized trials and is not currently recommended for routine use outside specific research or highly selected clinical scenarios, a conclusion that should temper any expectation that platelet function testing offers a precise, individualized alternative to the population-based periprocedural discontinuation intervals discussed earlier in this chapter. Selected scenarios where platelet function testing may provide clinically useful information include confirming adequate antiplatelet effect in a patient with recurrent stent thrombosis despite standard dual antiplatelet therapy, where genuine pharmacologic resistance or nonadherence might be distinguished, and, in some practice settings, informing the timing of surgery in patients on P2Y12 inhibitors when the standard discontinuation interval has elapsed but confirmation of adequate platelet function recovery is specifically desired before a very high bleeding risk procedure.

Viscoelastic testing, including thromboelastography and rotational thromboelastometry introduced in Chapter 16, has an evolving but still incompletely defined role in guiding periprocedural antithrombotic management and acute bleeding resuscitation, offering the potential advantage of rapid, integrated assessment of the combined effect of antiplatelet therapy, anticoagulant therapy, and any coexisting coagulopathy in a single acute bleeding scenario, though its specific utility for guiding antiplatelet-focused decisions, as opposed to the broader trauma and massive transfusion contexts where it is more established, remains an area of ongoing clinical investigation rather than settled standard practice.

Figure 18.2: Viscoelastic Tracing Patterns

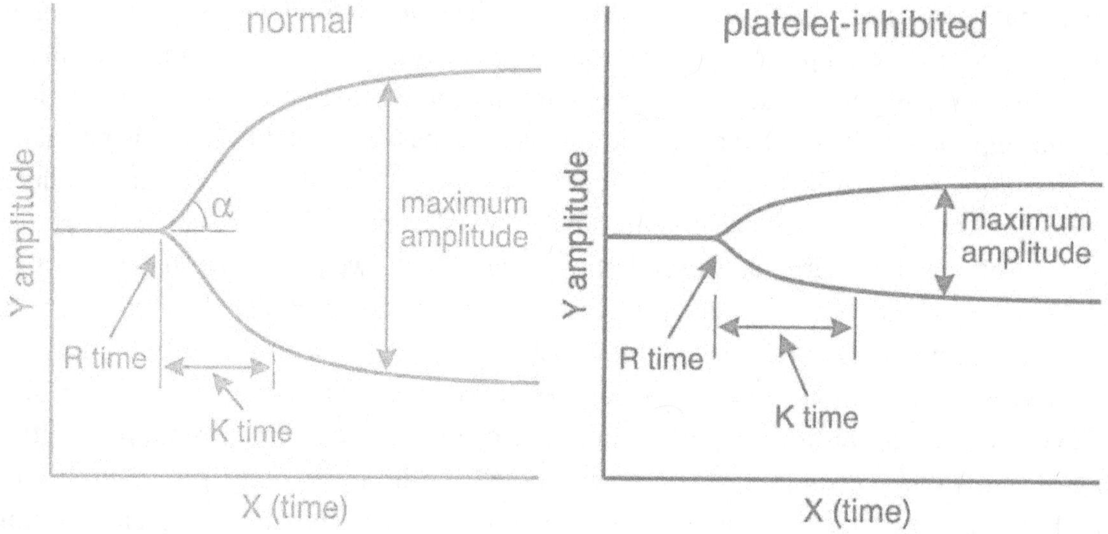

Anticoagulant Monitoring: When and How

Vitamin K antagonist therapy requires routine International Normalized Ratio monitoring given warfarin's substantial interindividual pharmacokinetic variability and numerous drug and dietary interactions, with the specific therapeutic target range determined by the underlying indication, and this routine monitoring requirement, in contrast to the direct oral anticoagulants discussed earlier in this chapter, represents one of the specific practical burdens that has driven the broader shift toward direct oral anticoagulant use for eligible indications. Direct oral anticoagulants do not require routine monitoring given their predictable pharmacokinetics, but specific clinical scenarios, including suspected drug accumulation in renal impairment, need for urgent reversal decision-making, or assessment of anticoagulant effect before urgent surgery, may warrant specific anti-Xa or dilute thrombin time assays calibrated to the specific agent, since standard coagulation assays such as prothrombin time and activated partial thromboplastin time provide only qualitative, agent-dependent information regarding direct oral anticoagulant effect and should not be relied upon for precise quantitative assessment.

Confirming the specific anti-Xa or dilute thrombin time assay ordered is properly calibrated for the specific direct oral anticoagulant in question, rather than assuming interchangeability across agents, represents an essential practical point given that a standard anti-Xa assay calibrated for heparin monitoring will not provide accurate quantitative information regarding rivaroxaban or apixaban effect without the specific drug-calibrated assay, a laboratory nuance that should be confirmed with the local laboratory whenever precise direct oral anticoagulant quantification is clinically needed.

Agent	Mechanism	Reversibility	Standard Preoperative Hold
Aspirin	Irreversible COX-1 inhibition	Irreversible	5-7 days
Clopidogrel	Irreversible P2Y12 inhibition (prodrug)	Irreversible	5-7 days
Prasugrel	Irreversible P2Y12 inhibition (prodrug)	Irreversible	7-10 days
Ticagrelor	Reversible P2Y12 inhibition	Reversible	3-5 days
Apixaban/Rivaroxaban	Direct factor Xa inhibition	Reversible (pharmacokinetic)	1-2 days (low risk); 2-4 days (high risk), renal-adjusted
Warfarin	Vitamin K-dependent factor synthesis inhibition	Reversible (pharmacokinetic)	~5 days, INR-confirmed

Newer Antithrombotic Agents and Emerging Pharmacologic Considerations

Cangrelor: A Rapid-Onset, Rapid-Offset Intravenous P2Y12 Inhibitor

Cangrelor provides intravenous, reversible P2Y12 inhibition with a plasma half-life of only several minutes and platelet function recovery within approximately one hour of infusion discontinuation, a pharmacokinetic profile that makes it particularly useful as a bridging antiplatelet strategy for patients requiring urgent surgery who cannot safely tolerate complete antiplatelet discontinuation given a recent coronary stent or acute coronary syndrome, allowing near-immediate cessation of antiplatelet effect at the time of surgery followed by rapid resumption of adequate platelet inhibition once the bleeding risk of the immediate perioperative period has passed. This bridging application addresses a genuine gap in periprocedural management for the highest-thrombotic-risk patients, for whom even the shortest available oral P2Y12 inhibitor discontinuation interval, discussed earlier in this chapter for ticagrelor, may represent an unacceptable duration of complete antiplatelet cessation, and cangrelor's rapid onset and offset allow this gap to be substantially narrowed under close monitoring.

Factor XI Inhibitors: An Emerging Anticoagulant Class

Factor XI inhibitors represent an emerging anticoagulant class in active clinical development, targeting a coagulation factor whose contribution to pathologic thrombosis appears to substantially exceed its contribution to normal hemostasis, based on the clinical observation that congenital factor XI deficiency produces a comparatively mild bleeding phenotype relative to deficiencies of other coagulation factors, and this favorable efficacy-to-bleeding-risk ratio observed in early clinical trials has generated substantial interest in factor XI inhibition as a potential anticoagulant strategy that might achieve meaningful thrombotic risk reduction with a more favorable bleeding risk profile than currently available anticoagulants, a claim that will require confirmation in larger, longer-term clinical trials before these agents, discussed further in their investigational context in Chapter 20, become part of standard clinical practice.

Individualizing Antithrombotic Selection in an Expanding Therapeutic Landscape

The expanding array of available and emerging antiplatelet and anticoagulant agents, each with a distinct mechanism, pharmacokinetic profile, and periprocedural management implication, underscores the importance of the mechanism-based, individualized approach this chapter has developed throughout rather than a memorized, agent-specific protocol applied without understanding of the underlying pharmacologic principles, since new agents will continue to enter clinical practice and the clinician equipped with a mechanistic understanding of how reversibility, half-life, and platelet turnover interact to determine periprocedural management will be able to appropriately incorporate each new agent into this same conceptual framework rather than requiring an entirely new decision paradigm for each new drug.

Antithrombotic Therapy in Special Hematologic Populations

Antithrombotic Therapy in the Setting of Thrombocytopenia

Managing antithrombotic therapy in a patient with coexisting thrombocytopenia, whether from the immune, drug-induced, or marrow-based causes discussed throughout the earlier chapters of this book, presents a distinctive dual bleeding risk in which the platelet count deficit and the antithrombotic agent's mechanism compound rather than operate independently, requiring individualized dose reduction, temporary discontinuation, or, for anticoagulation specifically, careful selection of the anticoagulant intensity appropriate to the specific platelet count threshold, an integration this book has referenced throughout its discussion of thrombocytopenic conditions but that receives its fullest pharmacologic treatment here. General practice patterns, developed largely from oncology and critical care experience, suggest full-intensity anticoagulation can often be continued down to a platelet count of approximately 50 x10^9/L, with dose reduction considered between 25 and 50 x10^9/L, and anticoagulation generally held below 25 x10^9/L absent a specifically compelling indication, though these thresholds represent general guidance rather than rigid rules and must be individualized to the specific thrombotic indication, bleeding history, and trajectory of the thrombocytopenia.

Antiplatelet therapy in thrombocytopenic patients follows an analogous individualized approach, with the specific platelet count threshold for continuing, reducing, or discontinuing therapy informed by the underlying cardiovascular or cerebrovascular indication's acuity and the thrombocytopenia's cause and expected trajectory, extending the same dual-risk integration principle to this related but mechanistically distinct antithrombotic class.

Antithrombotic Therapy in Myeloproliferative Neoplasms

Patients with essential thrombocythemia or other myeloproliferative neoplasms, discussed in Chapter 17, frequently require both disease-directed antiplatelet therapy and, for a subset with coexisting atrial fibrillation or venous thromboembolism, anticoagulation, and the periprocedural and bleeding management principles developed throughout this chapter apply directly to this population with the additional layer of extreme thrombocytosis-associated acquired von Willebrand syndrome discussed in Chapter 17 that must be specifically screened for and factored into the overall bleeding risk assessment whenever antithrombotic therapy intensity or periprocedural management decisions are being made in this population. This layered risk assessment, integrating the general antithrombotic pharmacology framework developed in this chapter with the disease-specific considerations addressed in Chapter 17, exemplifies the kind of multi-chapter clinical integration this book has aimed to develop throughout, in which no single chapter's framework operates in isolation from the broader platelet and hemostatic physiology this book has built cumulatively.

Hepatic and Renal Disease: Compounded Pharmacokinetic and Hemostatic Risk

Advanced liver disease and advanced kidney disease each independently alter antithrombotic drug pharmacokinetics, discussed for renal impairment specifically earlier in this chapter, while simultaneously conferring an intrinsic bleeding risk through the coagulopathy of liver disease and the uremic platelet dysfunction discussed in Chapter 16, together producing a population in which antithrombotic therapy decisions require unusually careful individualized risk-benefit assessment rather than application of the standard dosing and periprocedural intervals developed for patients with normal hepatic and renal function. Hepatic impairment specifically affects the direct oral anticoagulants and vitamin K antagonist therapy differently, with vitamin K antagonist dosing already complicated by impaired synthesis of the vitamin K-dependent factors this therapy targets, warranting particularly close monitoring and, in some cases, specific agent avoidance in this population given the compounded pharmacokinetic and intrinsic hemostatic risk advanced liver disease confers.

Systems-Level Safety Measures and Error Prevention

Standardized Order Sets and Electronic Decision Support

Standardized periprocedural antithrombotic order sets and electronic health record-based clinical decision support tools, incorporating the specific agent, indication, procedural bleeding risk category, and renal function into an automated discontinuation and resumption timing recommendation, reduce the risk of the manual calculation errors and communication gaps that represent a recognized and preventable source of periprocedural antithrombotic management errors, extending the systems-level safety principle this book has emphasized in other high-stakes medication contexts, including the perioperative platelet transfusion and heparin management discussions in earlier chapters, to this specific periprocedural antithrombotic context. These decision support tools work best when integrated directly into the procedural scheduling workflow, prompting the antithrombotic management plan at the time a procedure is scheduled rather than relying on a separate, manual process that may not reliably occur before every scheduled procedure, particularly for patients whose antithrombotic therapy is prescribed by a different clinician or practice than the one scheduling the procedure.

Pharmacist-led periprocedural antithrombotic management programs, in which a clinical pharmacist reviews and confirms the appropriateness of the planned discontinuation and resumption schedule before the procedure, have been associated with reduced periprocedural bleeding and thrombotic complications in health systems that have implemented them, reflecting the value of a dedicated, systematic review layer beyond the individual prescribing clinician's own assessment, particularly for the more complex combined antithrombotic regimens and special populations discussed earlier in this chapter.

Structured Handoff at Care Transitions

Transitions of care, including hospital discharge following a procedure, transfer between inpatient services, and handoff between the prescribing outpatient clinician and the proceduralist, represent recognized high-risk points for periprocedural antithrombotic management errors, particularly regarding antithrombotic therapy resumption timing, which may be inadvertently delayed or omitted entirely if responsibility for confirming resumption is not explicitly assigned and confirmed at each care transition. A structured discharge and handoff communication tool specifically addressing antithrombotic therapy status, including explicit confirmation of the planned resumption date and responsible party for ensuring resumption occurs, should be incorporated into standard discharge and transfer documentation for any patient whose antithrombotic therapy was periprocedurally interrupted, extending the structured transition communication principle developed for the pediatric-to-adult hematology transition discussed in Chapter 15 to this distinct but analogously consequential care transition context.

Learning From Periprocedural Antithrombotic Errors

Systematic review of periprocedural antithrombotic management errors and near-misses, whether through formal morbidity and mortality conferences, incident reporting systems, or dedicated antithrombotic stewardship program review, provides an essential mechanism for identifying recurring systems-level vulnerabilities, such as a specific care transition point or a particular combination of antithrombotic agents that repeatedly proves error-prone, and directing targeted process improvement efforts at these identified vulnerabilities rather than addressing each individual error in isolation without examining the broader systemic pattern it may represent. This continuous quality improvement approach to periprocedural antithrombotic safety reflects the same systematic, evidence-informed rigor this chapter has applied to the underlying pharmacology and clinical decision-making, extending it to the systems and processes through which that clinical knowledge is actually implemented in day-to-day practice.

Communicating Periprocedural Plans and Patient Education

Structured Communication Across the Care Team

Periprocedural antithrombotic management requires explicit, structured communication among the prescribing clinician, the proceduralist or surgeon, and, where relevant, cardiology or neurology, given the complexity of the risk integration this chapter has developed and the serious consequences of miscommunication in either direction, whether inadvertent bleeding from failure to appropriately discontinue therapy or thrombotic complications from inappropriate or premature discontinuation, extending the structured multidisciplinary communication principle emphasized throughout this book to this specific, time-sensitive periprocedural context. A written periprocedural antithrombotic plan, specifying the exact discontinuation date, any bridging therapy plan, and the planned resumption date and any resumption-specific considerations, should be documented and communicated to the patient and all involved clinicians well in advance of the planned procedure, reducing the risk of the communication breakdowns that represent a recognized and preventable cause of periprocedural antithrombotic management errors.

Patient Education and Self-Management

Patients should receive clear, written instructions regarding their specific periprocedural antithrombotic plan, including the exact dates for discontinuation and resumption and specific guidance regarding what to do if a dose is inadvertently missed or taken outside the planned schedule, extending the patient education and self-advocacy framework developed throughout this book to this population managing a temporary but clinically consequential medication interruption. Patients on long-term antithrombotic therapy should also receive general education regarding recognizing bleeding complications warranting urgent medical attention, applicable both in the periprocedural period specifically addressed in this chapter and during their ongoing, chronic antithrombotic therapy more broadly, ensuring the self-advocacy and symptom recognition capacity this book has emphasized throughout extends to this common and growing population of patients managed with long-term antithrombotic therapy.

This chapter has developed the pharmacology, periprocedural management, and reversal strategies for both antiplatelet and anticoagulant therapy as an integrated framework requiring systematic risk-benefit assessment rather than reflexive discontinuation or continuation, extending the individualized, mechanism-based decision-making this book has applied throughout its discussion of platelet and hemostatic disorders to this specific pharmacologic and periprocedural context. The chapter that follows shifts to platelet transfusion medicine, addressing the products, indications, and refractoriness considerations that several chapters, including this one, have referenced throughout this book.

THE PLATELET CRISIS DECISION COMPASS — Periprocedural Antithrombotic Decision Arc

Compass Synthesis: This chapter's Decision Compass instance established that periprocedural antiplatelet decisions require first confirming whether discontinuation is safe at all, given the specific indication and, for coronary stents, minimum dual antiplatelet therapy duration, before addressing the pharmacokinetically appropriate discontinuation interval.

Crisis Anchor: Cardiology or the relevant specialist co-management is mandatory whenever a recent thrombotic indication for antiplatelet or anticoagulant therapy is present, and elective procedures should be deferred rather than antithrombotic therapy prematurely discontinued when the minimum required treatment duration has not yet elapsed.

Summary and Key Concepts

Aspirin and the irreversible P2Y12 inhibitors clopidogrel and prasugrel require a five-to-ten-day recovery interval following discontinuation given their irreversible mechanism and dependence on new platelet generation, while reversible ticagrelor allows a shorter three-to-five-day interval.

Periprocedural antiplatelet management requires integrating thrombotic risk, determined by the underlying indication and, for coronary stents, minimum dual antiplatelet therapy duration, with procedural bleeding risk, rather than reflexive discontinuation before every procedure.

Direct oral anticoagulants are managed periprocedurally based on renal function and procedural bleeding risk, generally without bridging, while vitamin K antagonist therapy requires longer discontinuation and selective, risk-stratified bridging with parenteral anticoagulation.

Specific reversal agents, idarucizumab for dabigatran and andexanet alfa for factor Xa inhibitors, provide rapid direct oral anticoagulant reversal, while four-factor prothrombin complex concentrate provides nonspecific reversal and remains the preferred rapid reversal strategy for vitamin K antagonist therapy.

Platelet transfusion provides the primary reversal strategy for antiplatelet-associated bleeding, though efficacy varies by agent given ticagrelor's ongoing reversible receptor binding, with desmopressin and tranexamic acid serving as useful adjunctive measures.

Combined antiplatelet-anticoagulant regimens, renal impairment, and neuraxial anesthesia each require specific, individualized periprocedural management considerations beyond the general framework applied to single-agent antithrombotic therapy.

CHAPTER 19: PLATELET TRANSFUSION MEDICINE: PRODUCTS, INDICATIONS, AND REFRACTORINESS

Learning Objectives

1. Describe the platelet products available for transfusion, including their preparation, storage, and dosing conventions.
2. Apply evidence-based platelet transfusion thresholds for prophylactic and therapeutic indications across distinct clinical scenarios.
3. Recognize the risks and complications of platelet transfusion, including alloimmunization, transfusion reactions, and infectious risk.
4. Define platelet transfusion refractoriness and apply a systematic diagnostic approach distinguishing immune from nonimmune causes.
5. Formulate a management strategy for alloimmunized, transfusion-refractory patients requiring platelet support.
6. Describe special platelet transfusion considerations in neonatal, pediatric, and massively transfused patients.

Chapter Outline

Platelet Products: Preparation, Storage, and Dosing

Whole Blood-Derived and Apheresis Platelet Products

Platelet products for transfusion are prepared through two distinct methods that produce functionally comparable but logistically different final products: whole blood-derived platelets, prepared by centrifugation of individual whole blood donations and typically pooled from four to six donors to achieve an adult therapeutic dose, and single-donor apheresis platelets, collected directly from a single donor through an apheresis procedure that yields a full adult therapeutic dose from one donor, reducing the number of distinct donor exposures a transfused patient experiences relative to pooled whole blood-derived products. This donor-exposure reduction carries specific relevance for alloimmunization risk, discussed later in this chapter, since each additional donor exposure incrementally increases the cumulative opportunity for alloantibody development against human leukocyte antigens or platelet-specific antigens, making apheresis platelets the generally preferred product for patients anticipated to require multiple platelet transfusions over an extended period, such as those undergoing intensive chemotherapy or hematopoietic stem cell transplantation.

Figure 19.1: Apheresis Platelet Collection Circuit

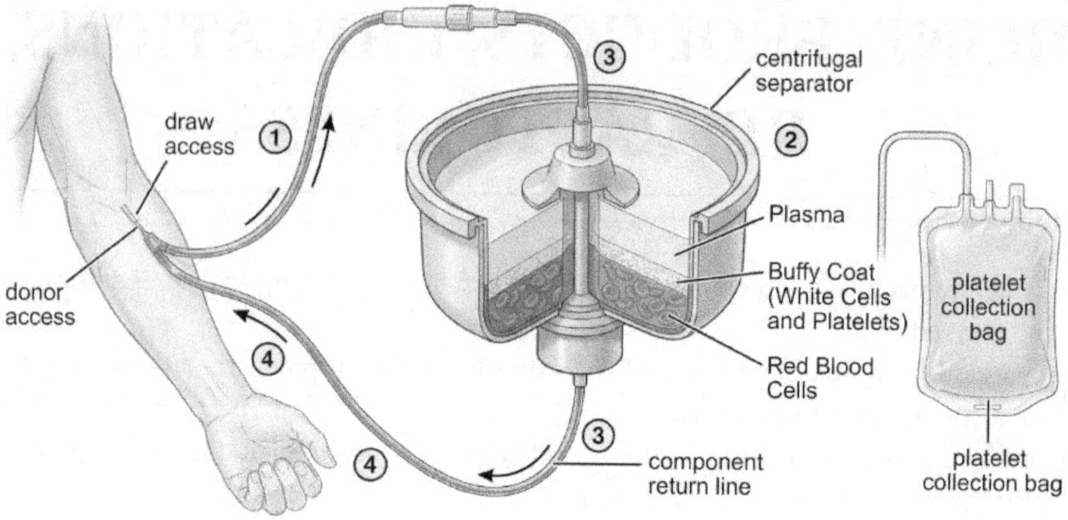

Platelet products are stored at room temperature with continuous gentle agitation to maintain platelet metabolic function and viability, a storage requirement that, unlike the refrigerated storage used for red blood cell products, creates a distinctive bacterial contamination risk given room temperature storage's permissiveness for bacterial growth should contamination occur during collection or processing, a risk this chapter addresses further in its discussion of transfusion-associated infectious complications. This room-temperature storage requirement also limits platelet product shelf life to approximately five to seven days depending on specific collection and processing methods and local regulatory standards, a substantially shorter shelf life than red blood cell products and one that creates ongoing inventory management challenges for blood banks given the balance required between maintaining adequate platelet supply and minimizing product expiration and waste.

Dosing Conventions and Expected Platelet Count Increment

A standard adult therapeutic platelet dose, whether from a pooled whole blood-derived product or a single apheresis unit, is expected to raise the platelet count by approximately 30 to 50 x10^9/L in a patient without factors predisposing to reduced increment, though this expected increment varies considerably based on patient size, splenic platelet sequestration, and the presence of consumptive or destructive processes discussed later in this chapter under refractoriness, making the corrected count increment, rather than the raw platelet count increase alone, the more precise and clinically useful metric for assessing transfusion response since it accounts for the specific platelet dose transfused and the recipient's body surface area. Pediatric platelet dosing is typically weight-based, generally in the range of 5 to 10 mL per kilogram of apheresis platelet product, reflecting the smaller total blood volume and correspondingly smaller absolute platelet dose required to achieve an equivalent proportional platelet count increase relative to the fixed adult unit dosing convention.

The timing of the post-transfusion platelet count assessment meaningfully affects interpretation, with a count obtained approximately ten minutes to one hour after transfusion completion, termed the immediate or early post-transfusion count, providing the most sensitive assessment of the transfusion's inherent effectiveness before splenic redistribution and normal platelet clearance begin to reduce the count, whereas a count obtained eighteen to twenty-four hours later reflects both the initial transfusion effectiveness and subsequent survival of the transfused platelets in the recipient's circulation, and distinguishing which timepoint is being assessed is essential when interpreting a suboptimal response in the refractoriness evaluation discussed later in this chapter.

Special Platelet Products and Modifications

Leukoreduction

Leukoreduced platelet products, in which residual white blood cells are removed through filtration during processing, are now standard practice in most transfusion services given leukoreduction's role in reducing febrile nonhemolytic transfusion reactions, reducing cytomegalovirus transmission risk to a level generally considered comparable to specifically cytomegalovirus-seronegative products, and, most importantly for the topic of this chapter, reducing human leukocyte antigen alloimmunization risk by removing the leukocyte-derived antigen-presenting cells that substantially contribute to the alloimmunization process discussed later in this chapter. This alloimmunization risk reduction benefit provided the primary evidence basis supporting the widespread adoption of universal leukoreduction, reflecting a landmark clinical trial demonstrating meaningfully reduced alloimmunization rates with leukoreduced platelet products relative to standard, non-leukoreduced products in a population of patients requiring repeated platelet transfusion.

Irradiation

Irradiated platelet products, in which gamma or x-ray irradiation inactivates residual donor lymphocytes, are indicated specifically to prevent transfusion-associated graft-versus-host disease, a rare but nearly universally fatal complication arising when viable donor lymphocytes engraft and attack the recipient's tissues, a risk specifically elevated in immunocompromised patients, patients receiving transfusion from a blood relative, and patients undergoing hematopoietic stem cell transplantation, making irradiation a standard requirement for platelet products transfused to these specific at-risk populations rather than a universal processing requirement applied to all platelet products. Irradiation does not affect platelet function or viability and specifically targets the residual lymphocyte population responsible for transfusion-associated graft-versus-host disease, distinguishing its mechanism and purpose from leukoreduction, which removes rather than inactivates leukocytes and provides distinct, complementary benefits addressed separately above.

Washed and Volume-Reduced Platelet Products

Washed platelet products, in which the plasma component is removed and replaced with a platelet additive solution, are indicated for patients with recurrent or severe allergic transfusion reactions attributed to plasma proteins, or for IgA-deficient patients with anti-IgA antibodies at risk for anaphylactic transfusion reactions, though washing reduces platelet yield and viability to some degree and should be reserved for these specific indications rather than used routinely given this trade-off. Volume-reduced platelet products, in which excess plasma volume is removed while preserving the platelet content itself, are indicated for patients at risk of volume overload from standard-volume platelet products, particularly small infants and patients with significant cardiac or renal dysfunction, extending the volume-conscious transfusion approach this chapter's neonatal and pediatric section addresses in greater detail to this broader population.

Prophylactic Platelet Transfusion Thresholds

Thresholds in Hypoproliferative Thrombocytopenia

Prophylactic platelet transfusion, given in the absence of active bleeding to reduce the risk of subsequent spontaneous hemorrhage, is most extensively studied and applied in patients with hypoproliferative thrombocytopenia from chemotherapy or hematopoietic stem cell transplantation, where randomized trial evidence supports a threshold of 10 x10^9/L for routine prophylactic transfusion in stable patients without additional bleeding risk factors, a threshold that reflects the recognition that further prophylactic transfusion at higher platelet counts does not meaningfully reduce bleeding risk while unnecessarily increasing transfusion exposure and its associated risks discussed later in this chapter. Higher prophylactic thresholds, generally in the 20 to 50 x10^9/L range depending on the specific clinical scenario, are applied for patients with additional bleeding risk factors, including fever, coagulopathy, rapidly falling platelet count, or before specific invasive procedures discussed in the following subsection, reflecting an individualized rather than uniform application of the prophylactic transfusion threshold framework.

This threshold-based prophylactic transfusion approach represents a substantial evolution from historical practice, which favored substantially higher and less evidence-based prophylactic thresholds, and the current, more restrictive evidence-based thresholds reflect the same judicious transfusion philosophy this book has emphasized throughout its discussion of platelet transfusion in specific disease contexts, recognizing that platelet transfusion, while lifesaving when appropriately indicated, carries genuine risks that argue against transfusion beyond what the evidence demonstrates provides meaningful clinical benefit.

Procedure-Specific Thresholds

Platelet count thresholds before invasive procedures vary by the specific procedure's bleeding risk, generally following a graduated framework in which low-bleeding-risk procedures such as routine central venous catheter placement may be safely performed at platelet counts as low as 20 x10^9/L, moderate-bleeding-risk procedures such as lumbar puncture or liver biopsy generally require a threshold of 50 x10^9/L, and high-bleeding-risk procedures, particularly neurosurgical procedures given the closed, non-compressible intracranial space discussed in the neuraxial anesthesia context in Chapter 18, require substantially higher thresholds, often 100 x10^9/L, reflecting the severe consequences of even modest bleeding at this anatomic site. These procedure-specific thresholds should be applied as general guidance individualized to the specific patient's bleeding history, the specific proceduralist's assessment of technical bleeding risk, and any additional coagulopathy or antithrombotic therapy discussed in Chapter 18 that might further elevate the overall bleeding risk beyond the platelet count consideration alone.

Thresholds in Specific High-Risk Scenarios

Certain clinical scenarios warrant specific threshold considerations distinct from the general framework discussed above, including active central nervous system bleeding or very high-risk neurosurgical procedures, where thresholds up to 100 x10^9/L are often applied, and extracorporeal membrane oxygenation, discussed in its critical illness context in Chapter 14, where the extracorporeal circuit's platelet-consumptive effect combined with the anticoagulation typically required during circuit operation creates a distinctive bleeding risk warranting individualized, often higher, prophylactic thresholds than would be applied to a comparably thrombocytopenic patient without extracorporeal circuit support. These high-risk scenario thresholds should be established collaboratively with the relevant specialists, extending the multidisciplinary coordination principle this book has emphasized throughout to the specific platelet transfusion threshold decisions these complex clinical scenarios require.

Figure 19.2: Splenomegaly on Abdominal CT

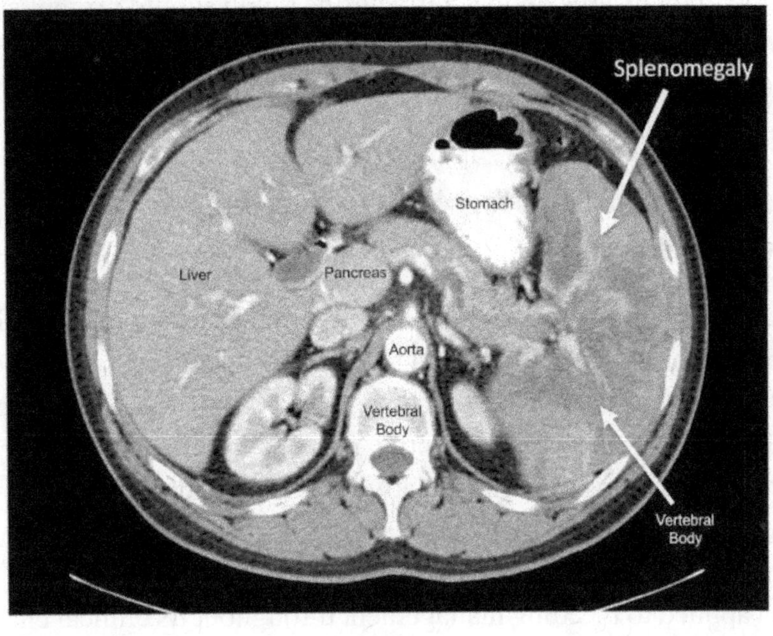

THE PLATELET CRISIS DECISION COMPASS — Refractoriness Recognition Arc

The Presentation: A 34-year-old woman undergoing induction chemotherapy for acute myeloid leukemia shows minimal platelet count increment despite three consecutive apheresis platelet transfusions over one week, each given for a platelet count below the prophylactic threshold.

Mimic Signature: Ongoing consumption from fever and sepsis, splenomegaly, and disseminated intravascular coagulation can each produce a poor transfusion response through nonimmune mechanisms that mimic the appearance of alloimmune refractoriness but require an entirely different management approach.

The Decision: The corrected count increment is calculated and found to be well below the threshold defining refractoriness on both immediate and eighteen-hour post-transfusion counts, and evaluation for nonimmune causes is unremarkable, prompting HLA antibody testing, which returns positive with broad antibody specificity.

Trap Logic: Attributing the poor response to 'just chemotherapy effect' without calculating the corrected count increment and systematically excluding both nonimmune causes and HLA alloimmunization would delay the transition to HLA-matched or crossmatch-compatible platelet products this patient's confirmed alloimmunization requires.

Crisis Anchor: A corrected count increment below the refractoriness threshold on two consecutive ABO-compatible, fresh platelet transfusions defines refractoriness and should prompt systematic evaluation for nonimmune causes first, then HLA and platelet-specific antibody testing, since confirmed alloimmunization requires HLA-matched or crossmatch-compatible platelet products rather than continued standard random-donor transfusion.

Therapeutic Platelet Transfusion for Active Bleeding

Thresholds for Active Bleeding

Therapeutic platelet transfusion, given for active bleeding rather than prophylactically, generally targets a higher platelet count threshold than the prophylactic thresholds discussed above, with most guidelines recommending maintaining the platelet count above 50 x10^9/L for active bleeding in most clinical contexts and above 100 x10^9/L for active central nervous system bleeding, reflecting the increased hemostatic demand active bleeding presents relative to the bleeding prevention goal of prophylactic transfusion. The specific bleeding severity, site, and trajectory should inform the precise target and transfusion frequency in active bleeding, following the same individualized, severity-proportionate approach this book has applied to bleeding management throughout its clinical chapters rather than a rigid, universally applied threshold regardless of the specific bleeding scenario.

Massive Transfusion and Trauma Resuscitation

Massive transfusion protocols, activated for patients with severe traumatic or surgical hemorrhage requiring large-volume blood product resuscitation, incorporate platelet transfusion in a fixed ratio alongside red blood cells and plasma, typically approximating a 1:1:1 ratio, reflecting evidence that balanced, ratio-based resuscitation reduces the dilutional coagulopathy and dilutional thrombocytopenia discussed in the critical illness context of Chapter 14 more effectively than a red blood cell-predominant resuscitation strategy that addresses platelet and coagulation factor deficits only reactively rather than proactively. This balanced resuscitation approach represents a substantial evolution in trauma and massive hemorrhage management, reflecting the recognition that early, proactive platelet and coagulation factor support, rather than sequential, laboratory-triggered replacement after a dilutional coagulopathy has already developed, produces superior outcomes in this specific high-acuity clinical scenario.

Viscoelastic-Guided Transfusion in Active Bleeding

Viscoelastic testing, introduced in its periprocedural monitoring context in Chapter 18, has an increasingly established role in guiding targeted blood product resuscitation during active bleeding, allowing rapid, integrated assessment of the specific hemostatic deficit, whether primarily platelet-mediated, coagulation factor-mediated, or fibrinolytic, and directing correspondingly targeted platelet, plasma, cryoprecipitate, or antifibrinolytic therapy rather than a fixed-ratio approach applied without regard to the specific hemostatic deficit an individual bleeding patient presents. This viscoelastic-guided approach has demonstrated particular value in cardiac surgery and liver transplantation, two clinical contexts involving substantial and often multifactorial hemostatic derangement, where targeted, test-guided resuscitation has been associated with reduced overall blood product utilization relative to empiric, formula-based transfusion strategies.

Complications and Risks of Platelet Transfusion

Transfusion Reactions

Febrile nonhemolytic transfusion reactions, presenting with fever and chills during or shortly after transfusion without hemolysis, represent the most common platelet transfusion reaction and have become substantially less frequent with universal leukoreduction discussed earlier in this chapter, reflecting the reaction's primary mechanism involving cytokines accumulated during platelet storage and residual leukocyte-mediated immune activation, both of which leukoreduction and, to a lesser degree, fresher product use mitigate. Allergic transfusion reactions, ranging from mild urticaria to, rarely, severe anaphylaxis, reflect recipient sensitization to donor plasma proteins and are managed with antihistamines for mild reactions and, for recurrent or severe reactions, the washed platelet products discussed earlier in this chapter, while transfusion-related acute lung injury, a rare but serious complication presenting with acute hypoxemic respiratory failure within hours of transfusion, requires prompt recognition and supportive respiratory management given its potential severity.

Transfusion-associated circulatory overload, presenting with signs of volume overload and pulmonary edema, particularly in patients with underlying cardiac or renal dysfunction, represents a distinct complication from transfusion-related acute lung injury requiring careful clinical distinction given their overlapping respiratory presentation but differing underlying mechanism and management approach, with transfusion-associated circulatory overload responding to diuresis and volume management in contrast to the primarily supportive respiratory management transfusion-related acute lung injury requires.

Infectious Risk

Bacterial contamination represents the most significant infectious risk specific to platelet transfusion given the room-temperature storage requirement discussed earlier in this chapter, and current blood banking practice incorporates bacterial detection testing of platelet products before release, substantially reducing though not entirely eliminating this risk, with clinical suspicion for a transfusion-associated bacterial infection, presenting with fever, chills, and hemodynamic instability during or shortly after platelet transfusion, warranting prompt notification of the blood bank, discontinuation of the implicated product, and blood culture from both the patient and the remaining product for investigation. Viral transmission risk, including hepatitis B, hepatitis C, and HIV, has become extremely low with current donor screening and nucleic acid testing protocols, though this residual risk, however small, should still be included in informed consent discussions regarding platelet transfusion, following the same transparent risk communication principle this book has emphasized throughout its discussion of transfusion and other blood product-based therapies.

Alloimmunization and Platelet Transfusion Refractoriness

Defining and Diagnosing Refractoriness

Platelet transfusion refractoriness is defined by a corrected count increment below an established threshold, typically less than 7,500 to 10,000 depending on the specific institutional definition, on two consecutive transfusions of ABO-compatible, appropriately stored platelet products, a definition specifically requiring exclusion of ABO incompatibility and product-related factors before refractoriness is diagnosed, since transfusing ABO-incompatible platelets or platelets nearing the end of their storage shelf life can each independently produce a poor increment that does not reflect true alloimmune or consumptive refractoriness. The corrected count increment calculation, incorporating the platelet count increment, patient body surface area, and platelet dose transfused, provides a standardized metric that allows meaningful comparison across transfusions and patients of different sizes, distinguishing genuine refractoriness from a simply inadequate platelet dose or an expected, size-appropriate increment that might otherwise be misinterpreted as a poor response.

Nonimmune Causes of Poor Transfusion Response

Nonimmune causes account for the substantial majority of poor platelet transfusion responses and should be systematically evaluated before pursuing alloimmunization testing, including fever and sepsis, splenomegaly producing increased splenic platelet sequestration as discussed in the context of hypersplenism throughout earlier chapters, disseminated intravascular coagulation and other consumptive coagulopathies, amphotericin B and certain other medications associated with reduced platelet survival, and graft-versus-host disease in the post-transplant setting, each of which produces a poor transfusion response through accelerated platelet consumption or destruction rather than through the antibody-mediated mechanism alloimmunization involves.

Figure 19.3: Anatomical Distribution of Splenic Platelet Sequestration

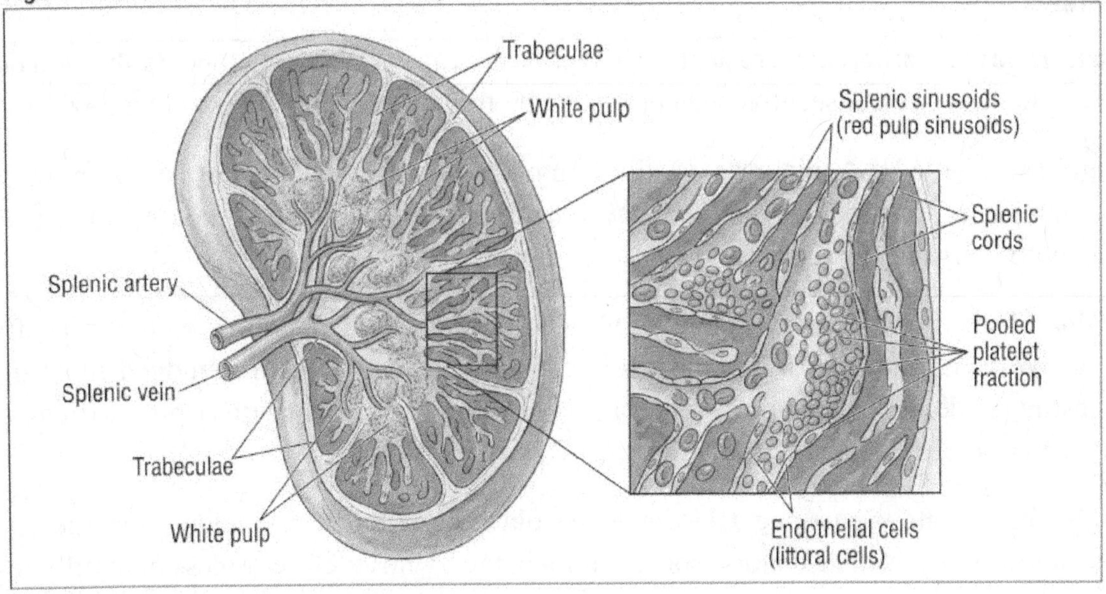

Systematic evaluation for these nonimmune causes, including clinical assessment for fever, splenomegaly on examination or imaging, and laboratory assessment for disseminated intravascular coagulation, should precede or accompany alloimmunization testing given both the greater prevalence of nonimmune causes and their distinct management implications, which center on addressing the underlying consumptive process rather than modifying the platelet product source.

HLA and Platelet-Specific Antibody Testing

Human leukocyte antigen antibody testing, most commonly performed using solid-phase or bead-based immunoassays, identifies the antibody specificities responsible for immune-mediated refractoriness in patients where nonimmune causes have been reasonably excluded, and platelet-specific antibody testing, directed against platelet-specific alloantigens distinct from the HLA system, should be considered when HLA antibody testing is negative or does not fully explain the observed refractoriness, given that platelet-specific alloimmunization, while less common than HLA alloimmunization, can independently produce transfusion refractoriness through a distinct antibody-antigen system. Identifying the specific antibody profile, rather than simply confirming alloimmunization is present, provides the essential information needed to select HLA-matched or, where platelet-specific antibodies are implicated, crossmatch-compatible platelet products for the management strategies discussed in the following section.

THE PLATELET CRISIS DECISION COMPASS — Nonimmune Versus Alloimmune Refractoriness Arc

The Presentation: A febrile, septic patient with hypoproliferative thrombocytopenia shows a poor platelet count increment after two consecutive apheresis platelet transfusions given for active oozing.

Mimic Signature: True HLA alloimmunization can produce an identical pattern of poor corrected count increment on repeated transfusion, making the fever and sepsis alone insufficient to confirm a nonimmune mechanism without further evaluation.

The Decision: The corrected count increment is calculated and confirmed low on both transfusions, and given the active fever and sepsis, a nonimmune consumptive mechanism is judged most likely; HLA antibody testing is deferred pending resolution of the acute infection, with a plan to reassess if poor increment persists once the patient is afebrile.

Trap Logic: Immediately pursuing HLA-matched platelets without first addressing the active sepsis would consume scarce matched-donor resources for a patient whose refractoriness may fully resolve once the nonimmune consumptive process is treated.

Crisis Anchor: A febrile or septic patient with poor transfusion increment should have the nonimmune cause treated first, with HLA and platelet-specific antibody testing reserved for refractoriness that persists once fever, sepsis, and other consumptive processes have resolved.

Management of the Alloimmunized, Refractory Patient

HLA-Matched and Crossmatch-Compatible Platelet Products

HLA-matched platelet products, selected from donors whose HLA type closely matches the recipient's, provide the most definitive management strategy for HLA alloimmunized, refractory patients, though identifying a suitably matched donor requires access to an HLA-typed donor registry and may involve delays or limited donor availability, particularly for patients with less common HLA types or broad antibody specificities, making this strategy more readily implementable at larger transfusion services with established HLA-matched donor programs. Platelet crossmatching, in which the patient's serum is tested against platelets from specific potential donors to identify compatible products without requiring full HLA matching, provides an alternative or complementary strategy that can be implemented more rapidly than identifying a fully HLA-matched donor, particularly useful in urgent clinical scenarios where the delay inherent in arranging HLA-matched product would be clinically unacceptable.

Epitope-based HLA matching algorithms, which identify donors sharing critical antibody-binding epitopes with the recipient's HLA type rather than requiring full antigen-level matching, have expanded the pool of potentially compatible donors for alloimmunized patients, improving practical donor availability relative to strict full-match requirements while maintaining acceptable transfusion response rates, representing an important refinement in the management of this challenging patient population.

Adjunctive and Alternative Strategies

For patients where HLA-matched or crossmatch-compatible platelets are unavailable or insufficiently effective, adjunctive strategies including antifibrinolytic therapy to reduce bleeding risk independent of platelet count correction, and, in select cases, intravenous immunoglobulin, though with more limited and less consistent evidence supporting its use for platelet transfusion refractoriness compared to its established role in immune thrombocytopenia discussed in Chapter 9, may provide additional bleeding risk mitigation while definitive compatible platelet products are sought. Minimizing further alloimmunization risk in patients who remain transfusion-dependent, through continued leukoreduced product use and judicious, evidence-based application of the transfusion thresholds discussed earlier in this chapter rather than unnecessarily frequent transfusion, represents an important preventive strategy for reducing the breadth of antibody specificities an already-alloimmunized patient may develop over time.

CLINICAL CASE: A 19-year-old woman with newly diagnosed acute lymphoblastic leukemia undergoing induction chemotherapy develops poor platelet count increment after her fourth apheresis platelet transfusion over ten days, with a corrected count increment well below the refractoriness threshold on both the most recent transfusion and the one preceding it. Applying the diagnostic framework developed in this chapter, clinical evaluation reveals no fever, no splenomegaly on examination, and coagulation studies excluding disseminated intravascular coagulation, making a nonimmune cause unlikely. HLA antibody testing returns positive with multiple antibody specificities, consistent with alloimmunization likely related to prior pregnancy exposure given her obstetric history. The transfusion service arranges HLA-matched apheresis platelets, and subsequent transfusions with matched product show a substantially improved corrected count increment, confirming the alloimmune mechanism and the effectiveness of the matched product strategy. The patient and her family are counseled regarding the alloimmunization diagnosis, its likely relationship to her prior pregnancy, and the ongoing need for HLA-matched platelet support throughout her chemotherapy course, with continued leukoreduced product use to minimize further antibody development. This case illustrates the complete refractoriness diagnostic and management arc developed in this chapter: corrected count increment calculation confirming true refractoriness, systematic exclusion of nonimmune causes, HLA antibody testing confirming the alloimmune mechanism, and successful transition to HLA-matched platelet support.

Blood Bank and Transfusion Service Logistics

Inventory Management and Platelet Product Availability

The short shelf life of platelet products discussed earlier in this chapter creates ongoing inventory management challenges for blood banks and transfusion services, requiring careful forecasting of anticipated demand, coordination with donor collection centers, and, particularly at smaller hospitals without an on-site apheresis collection program, reliable supply chain relationships with regional blood suppliers to ensure adequate platelet product availability without excessive product expiration and waste, a logistical challenge distinct from the longer-shelf-life red blood cell products this chapter's transfusion medicine framework can be contrasted against. Platelet shortages, which occur periodically at both regional and national levels related to donor availability fluctuations, seasonal donation patterns, and, at times, broader public health disruptions to the blood donation system, may require transfusion services to implement more conservative transfusion thresholds temporarily, underscoring the clinical relevance of the evidence-based, judicious transfusion threshold framework this chapter has developed throughout, which becomes particularly valuable during periods of constrained platelet product supply.

Hospital transfusion committees, incorporating representation from hematology, transfusion medicine, nursing, and relevant procedural specialties, play an important role in developing and periodically reviewing institutional platelet transfusion policies, ensuring these policies reflect current evidence-based thresholds and appropriately balance patient safety with judicious resource utilization, extending the systems-level, multidisciplinary governance principle this book has emphasized in other high-stakes clinical contexts to the specific institutional oversight of platelet transfusion practice.

ABO and Rh Considerations in Platelet Transfusion

ABO compatibility, while less absolutely required for platelet transfusion than for red blood cell transfusion given platelets' comparatively low expression of ABO antigens, still meaningfully affects transfusion response, with ABO-identical platelet transfusion generally producing a superior corrected count increment relative to ABO-incompatible transfusion, and this consideration should specifically inform interpretation of a poor transfusion response, as discussed earlier in this chapter's refractoriness evaluation framework, ensuring ABO incompatibility is excluded before more extensive alloimmunization evaluation is pursued. Rh sensitization risk from Rh-positive platelet products transfused to Rh-negative recipients, though platelet products themselves are essentially Rh antigen-negative, relates to trace red blood cell contamination that may be present in platelet products, and Rh-negative female patients of reproductive potential receiving Rh-positive platelet products may be considered for Rh immune globulin administration to prevent Rh sensitization, extending the Rh alloimmunization prevention framework discussed in the pregnancy context of Chapter 13 to this related transfusion medicine consideration.

Emergency Release and Urgent Platelet Availability

Emergency release protocols, allowing platelet transfusion to proceed before completion of the standard pretransfusion testing process in genuinely life-threatening bleeding scenarios, represent an important safety valve within the broader transfusion service framework, balancing the urgency of life-threatening hemorrhage against the generally lower but nonzero risk this expedited process entails relative to standard, fully verified transfusion, and appropriate use of emergency release protocols requires clear institutional criteria and documentation to ensure this expedited pathway is reserved for genuinely urgent scenarios rather than used as a routine convenience measure. Massive transfusion protocol activation, discussed earlier in this chapter, typically incorporates pre-established emergency release provisions specifically because the balanced, proactive resuscitation approach this protocol requires would be undermined by delays awaiting standard pretransfusion testing completion in the acute trauma or massive hemorrhage scenario this protocol addresses.

Product	Preparation	Typical Volume	Shelf Life	Key Indication
Whole blood-derived (pooled)	Pooled from 4-6 donors	~250-300 mL	5-7 days	Standard adult therapeutic dose, general use
Apheresis (single-donor)	Single-donor apheresis collection	~200-300 mL	5-7 days	Reduced donor exposure; preferred for chronic transfusion
Irradiated	Gamma/x-ray irradiated	Same as source product	Same as source product	Prevention of transfusion-associated graft-versus-host disease
Washed	Plasma removed, replaced with additive solution	Reduced from source	Shortened post-wash	Recurrent severe allergic reaction, IgA deficiency

Platelet Transfusion in Specific Procedural Contexts

Cardiac Surgery and Cardiopulmonary Bypass

Cardiac surgery requiring cardiopulmonary bypass produces a distinctive, multifactorial platelet dysfunction through mechanical shear stress within the bypass circuit, activation and subsequent exhaustion of the circulating platelet population, and hemodilution from the bypass circuit's priming volume, together producing a clinically significant bleeding tendency that platelet transfusion, guided increasingly by viscoelastic testing discussed earlier in this chapter, addresses as part of a broader, algorithm-based bleeding management approach specific to this surgical context. This viscoelastic-guided, algorithm-based approach to cardiac surgical bleeding management has been associated with reduced blood product utilization relative to empiric, formula-based transfusion strategies, reflecting the same targeted resuscitation principle discussed earlier in this chapter's active bleeding management section applied specifically to this common and resource-intensive surgical context.

Liver Transplantation

Liver transplantation presents a complex, evolving hemostatic picture across the surgical course, with the anhepatic phase, during which the diseased liver has been removed but the donor liver has not yet been implanted and become functional, representing a period of particularly pronounced coagulopathy and thrombocytopenia requiring close, phase-specific hemostatic monitoring and targeted blood product support, again increasingly guided by viscoelastic testing given the rapid, dynamic changes in hemostatic status this surgery involves. Platelet transfusion thresholds during liver transplantation are generally individualized based on active bleeding and viscoelastic findings rather than a fixed prophylactic threshold, reflecting the surgery's dynamic hemostatic course and the recognition that rigid threshold-based transfusion, appropriate for the more stable hypoproliferative thrombocytopenia scenarios discussed earlier in this chapter, does not adequately capture the rapidly evolving hemostatic needs this specific surgical context presents.

Traumatic Brain Injury

Traumatic brain injury with intracranial hemorrhage warrants a specifically elevated platelet transfusion threshold, generally 100 x10^9/L, reflecting the severe consequences of even modest ongoing intracranial bleeding within the closed cranial vault, extending the closed-space bleeding risk principle discussed in the neuraxial anesthesia context of Chapter 18 to this related high-stakes anatomic scenario, with platelet transfusion considered even in patients not on antiplatelet therapy given the direct traumatic platelet dysfunction that can accompany significant traumatic brain injury independent of any preexisting antiplatelet medication effect. Coordination with neurosurgery regarding the specific platelet count target and any additional hemostatic support needs, individualized to the severity and trajectory of the intracranial hemorrhage on serial imaging, represents essential practice in this high-acuity clinical scenario given the narrow margin for hemostatic error traumatic brain injury with ongoing intracranial hemorrhage presents.

Cost, Sustainability, and Judicious Platelet Utilization

The Resource Burden of Platelet Transfusion

Platelet products carry a substantially higher per-unit cost than red blood cell products, reflecting the more resource-intensive collection, processing, and short-shelf-life-related wastage this chapter has discussed throughout, and this cost consideration, while never the primary driver of an individual transfusion decision, provides additional support for the evidence-based, judicious transfusion threshold framework this chapter has developed, since unnecessary platelet transfusion carries both direct clinical risk to the individual patient and a genuine, quantifiable resource cost to the broader healthcare system and blood supply. Judicious platelet utilization, guided by the evidence-based thresholds this chapter has developed throughout rather than either historical, less-restrictive practice patterns or reflexive transfusion avoidance that might compromise patient safety, represents the appropriate balance this chapter's overall framework has aimed to establish.

Patient Blood Management Programs

Patient blood management programs, incorporating evidence-based transfusion guidelines, clinical decision support, and structured audit and feedback regarding institutional transfusion practice patterns, have been associated with meaningful reductions in unnecessary platelet and other blood product transfusion without compromising patient outcomes, extending the systems-level quality improvement principle this book has emphasized throughout to the specific institutional context of transfusion practice governance. These programs typically incorporate the same evidence-based thresholds and individualized risk assessment framework this chapter has developed, translated into institutional policy, electronic decision support prompts, and ongoing clinician education, ensuring the evidence-based principles this chapter addresses are consistently applied across an institution's clinical practice rather than varying unpredictably based on individual clinician practice patterns.

Sustaining Adequate Clinical Support Within a Judicious Framework

Judicious platelet utilization and adequate clinical hemostatic support are not competing goals but rather complementary components of the same evidence-based transfusion medicine framework this chapter has developed throughout, in which appropriately applied thresholds simultaneously protect patients from the risks of unnecessary transfusion discussed earlier in this chapter and ensure adequate platelet support is provided when genuinely clinically indicated, reflecting the same balanced, evidence-based philosophy this book has applied consistently across its treatment of platelet disorders from the most severe inherited conditions through the routine, common clinical scenarios this transfusion medicine chapter addresses.

Neonatal, Pediatric, and Massive Transfusion Considerations

Neonatal Platelet Transfusion

Neonatal platelet transfusion thresholds, discussed in the specific context of neonatal alloimmune thrombocytopenia in Chapter 13, follow evidence from randomized trials suggesting that a more restrictive prophylactic threshold, generally 25 x10^9/L for stable preterm neonates without additional bleeding risk factors, produces outcomes at least as favorable as, and possibly superior to, a more liberal threshold, reflecting a specific evidence base distinct from the adult prophylactic thresholds discussed earlier in this chapter and underscoring that pediatric and neonatal transfusion practice should not simply extrapolate adult thresholds without population-specific evidence consideration. Volume-reduced platelet products, discussed earlier in this chapter, are frequently used in neonatal transfusion given neonates' small total blood volume and correspondingly increased vulnerability to volume overload from standard-volume adult platelet products, requiring close coordination with the transfusion service to ensure appropriately volume-adjusted products are available for this population.

Pediatric Platelet Transfusion Beyond the Neonatal Period

Platelet transfusion thresholds for children beyond the neonatal period generally follow the same evidence-based framework developed for adults, with weight-based dosing adjustments discussed earlier in this chapter, though pediatric-specific considerations including smaller vascular access, the psychological impact of frequent transfusion in a pediatric patient undergoing prolonged treatment such as chemotherapy, and family-centered communication regarding the ongoing transfusion needs a child's treatment course may require warrant specific attention beyond the technical transfusion medicine framework this chapter has developed. Extending the family-centered, developmentally appropriate communication principles emphasized for the inherited thrombocytopenia syndromes in Chapter 15 to the transfusion medicine context addressed in this chapter ensures that pediatric patients and their families receive support appropriate to the ongoing, sometimes prolonged, transfusion needs a pediatric hematologic or oncologic diagnosis may involve.

Documentation, Monitoring, and Quality Metrics

Post-Transfusion Documentation and Response Assessment

Systematic documentation of each platelet transfusion episode, including the specific indication, product type and volume transfused, pre- and post-transfusion platelet counts with the timing of each assessment specified, and any observed transfusion reaction, provides the essential data foundation for the corrected count increment calculation and refractoriness evaluation discussed earlier in this chapter, and incomplete or inconsistent documentation, particularly regarding the precise timing of post-transfusion count assessment, can meaningfully undermine the accuracy of subsequent refractoriness evaluation, extending the documentation rigor principle this book has emphasized throughout its discussion of longitudinal disease monitoring to this specific transfusion medicine context. Standardized institutional documentation templates specifically prompting for this complete data set at the time of each transfusion, rather than relying on ad hoc, inconsistent documentation practices, support both individual patient care and the broader quality metric tracking discussed in the following subsection.

Institutional Quality Metrics for Platelet Transfusion Practice

Institutional tracking of platelet transfusion quality metrics, including the proportion of transfusions given at platelet counts above the evidence-based prophylactic thresholds discussed earlier in this chapter, the incidence of transfusion reactions, and the prevalence of confirmed refractoriness within the transfused patient population, provides an important mechanism for identifying practice patterns warranting targeted quality improvement intervention, extending the systems-level quality improvement principle this book has applied throughout to this specific transfusion medicine context. These institutional metrics, when tracked longitudinally and benchmarked against published evidence-based standards, allow a transfusion service and its associated clinical departments to identify whether local practice has drifted from the evidence-based framework this chapter has developed, prompting targeted education or policy revision where meaningful deviation is identified.

Research and the Evolving Evidence Base

The evidence base underlying the platelet transfusion thresholds and management strategies this chapter has developed continues to evolve through ongoing clinical trials addressing remaining areas of uncertainty, including the optimal threshold for specific less-studied clinical scenarios and further refinement of viscoelastic-guided transfusion algorithms, and clinicians should maintain awareness that specific numerical thresholds discussed throughout this chapter, while reflecting the best currently available evidence, may be refined as this research base continues to mature, consistent with the currency requirement this book has emphasized throughout its treatment of evidence-based clinical guidelines. Participation in multi-institutional transfusion medicine research networks and registries, particularly for the less common but clinically important scenarios such as refractory alloimmunization management discussed earlier in this chapter, supports the continued evidence generation this rapidly evolving field requires.

Ethical Considerations in Scarce Compatible Product Allocation

Equity in HLA-Matched Donor Availability

HLA-matched and crossmatch-compatible platelet donor pools, discussed earlier in this chapter as the definitive management strategy for alloimmunized refractory patients, are not equally available across all patient populations, with donor registries historically reflecting the demographic composition of the donor pool from which they were built, so that patients from racial and ethnic minority populations underrepresented in donor registries may face disproportionately limited HLA-matched donor availability, an equity consideration that extends the health disparities awareness this book has emphasized throughout its clinical chapters to this specific transfusion medicine context. Targeted donor recruitment efforts aimed at expanding the racial and ethnic diversity of HLA-typed platelet donor registries represent an important, ongoing effort to address this disparity, though meaningful progress requires sustained, dedicated recruitment investment rather than passive reliance on general donor recruitment efforts to organically diversify the available donor pool over time.

Resource Allocation During Platelet Shortage

During periods of platelet product shortage, discussed earlier in this chapter, transfusion services and treating clinicians may face difficult resource allocation decisions regarding prioritization among patients with competing platelet transfusion needs, and institutional policies addressing this scenario should be developed proactively, before an acute shortage occurs, incorporating transparent, ethically grounded prioritization criteria rather than ad hoc decision-making under acute resource constraint, extending the advance-planning principle this book has emphasized throughout to this specific, ethically weighty institutional planning context. These policies should be developed with input from ethics committees alongside the hematology and transfusion medicine expertise this chapter has otherwise centered, reflecting the genuinely ethical, rather than purely clinical or logistical, dimension resource allocation during genuine scarcity presents.

Patient Communication and Informed Consent

Informed Consent for Platelet Transfusion

Informed consent for platelet transfusion should address the specific indication for transfusion, the expected benefit, the recognized risks discussed throughout this chapter including transfusion reactions and infectious risk, and, for patients anticipated to require repeated transfusion, the possibility of alloimmunization and transfusion refractoriness, delivered in a manner appropriate to the clinical urgency of the transfusion and the patient's capacity to engage in this discussion, extending the transparent, balanced risk communication principle this book has emphasized throughout its discussion of blood product and other significant medical interventions. For patients requiring urgent or emergency transfusion where obtaining detailed informed consent before transfusion is not clinically feasible, appropriate documentation of the clinical urgency and, where possible, retrospective discussion of the transfusion and its rationale once the patient is stabilized, represents appropriate practice consistent with the ethical and legal standards governing emergency medical treatment.

Supporting Patients Through Chronic Transfusion Dependence

Patients requiring chronic or recurrent platelet transfusion, whether from a chronic marrow failure condition, ongoing chemotherapy, or refractory alloimmunization requiring specialized product sourcing, benefit from structured education regarding their specific transfusion plan, what to expect from each transfusion episode, and recognition of symptoms warranting prompt medical attention between scheduled transfusions, extending the chronic disease patient education framework developed throughout this book to this population managing an ongoing, often burdensome, transfusion dependence. This chapter has developed platelet transfusion medicine as both a technically precise clinical discipline, governed by evidence-based thresholds and product selection principles, and a patient-centered practice requiring careful attention to the risks, alternatives, and communication needs this common but consequential intervention involves. The chapter that follows closes this book's disease-focused content by addressing the emerging and investigational platelet-directed therapies poised to further reshape the clinical landscape this book has developed throughout.

THE PLATELET CRISIS DECISION COMPASS — Transfusion Refractoriness Diagnostic Arc

Compass Synthesis: This chapter's Decision Compass instance established the corrected count increment as the definitive metric distinguishing true refractoriness from an inadequate dose or expected size-appropriate response, and the systematic sequence of excluding nonimmune causes before pursuing HLA and platelet-specific antibody testing.

Crisis Anchor: A confirmed refractoriness diagnosis based on corrected count increment across two consecutive ABO-compatible transfusions, with nonimmune causes excluded, should prompt HLA and platelet-specific antibody testing to direct the transition to HLA-matched or crossmatch-compatible platelet products.

Summary and Key Concepts

Apheresis platelet products reduce donor exposure relative to pooled whole blood-derived products and are generally preferred for patients anticipated to require repeated transfusion, given their lower cumulative alloimmunization risk.

Leukoreduction reduces febrile transfusion reactions, cytomegalovirus transmission, and HLA alloimmunization risk; irradiation prevents transfusion-associated graft-versus-host disease in at-risk populations.

Prophylactic platelet transfusion thresholds are evidence-based and context-specific: 10 x10^9/L for stable hypoproliferative thrombocytopenia, with higher thresholds for additional bleeding risk factors and specific invasive procedures.

Platelet transfusion refractoriness is defined by a corrected count increment below threshold on two consecutive ABO-compatible transfusions and should prompt systematic evaluation for nonimmune causes before HLA and platelet-specific antibody testing.

HLA-matched and crossmatch-compatible platelet products provide the definitive management strategy for alloimmunized refractory patients, with epitope-based matching algorithms expanding practical donor availability.

Neonatal and pediatric platelet transfusion follow population-specific evidence-based thresholds distinct from adult practice, and massive transfusion protocols incorporate platelets in a balanced ratio alongside red blood cells and plasma.

CHAPTER 20: EMERGING AND INVESTIGATIONAL PLATELET-DIRECTED THERAPIES

Learning Objectives

1. Describe the current landscape of thrombopoietin receptor agonists and their expanding indications beyond immune thrombocytopenia.
2. Explain the rationale and current evidence for novel agents targeting the FcRn pathway and complement system in immune-mediated platelet disorders.
3. Describe gene therapy and gene editing approaches under investigation for inherited platelet disorders.
4. Explain the mechanism and rationale for factor XI inhibitors and other novel antithrombotic strategies in development.
5. Describe advances in ex vivo platelet generation and artificial platelet substitutes under investigation.
6. Apply a framework for critically evaluating emerging platelet-directed therapies before their incorporation into clinical practice.

Chapter Outline

Expanding Applications of Thrombopoietin Receptor Agonists

Established and Emerging Indications

Thrombopoietin receptor agonists, discussed in their established role in immune thrombocytopenia in Chapter 9, have progressively expanded into additional clinical indications as accumulating evidence has clarified their efficacy and safety profile in populations beyond their original approval, including severe aplastic anemia, where thrombopoietin receptor agonist therapy has demonstrated the capacity to stimulate trilineage hematopoietic recovery beyond the platelet-specific effect its mechanism would initially suggest, chemotherapy-induced thrombocytopenia, where these agents offer a potential alternative to the platelet transfusion-dependent management strategies discussed in Chapter 19, and, in earlier-stage investigation, thrombocytopenia associated with chronic liver disease before invasive procedures, extending the mechanistic principle of augmenting endogenous thrombopoietin signaling well beyond the immune thrombocytopenia context where this drug class was first established. This expanding indication landscape reflects a broader pattern in which a therapeutic mechanism initially validated in one specific disease context progressively finds additional application as the underlying biology proves relevant to related clinical scenarios, a pattern this chapter will revisit across several of the emerging therapy classes discussed throughout.

Newer thrombopoietin receptor agonist formulations, including once-weekly dosing options and oral agents with improved pharmacokinetic properties relative to earlier agents in this class, aim to improve treatment convenience and adherence for patients requiring long-term therapy, addressing a practical treatment burden consideration that, while not altering the fundamental mechanism of action, meaningfully affects the real-world treatment experience for patients managing a chronic condition requiring ongoing therapy, extending the treatment burden and adherence considerations this book has emphasized throughout its chronic disease management discussions to this specific pharmacologic evolution.

Thrombopoietin Receptor Agonists in Inherited Thrombocytopenia

Investigation of thrombopoietin receptor agonist therapy in selected inherited thrombocytopenia syndromes discussed in Chapter 15, particularly those in which the underlying molecular defect does not directly impair the thrombopoietin receptor signaling pathway itself, represents an emerging application extending this drug class into a population traditionally managed with the platelet transfusion and general supportive care approach discussed throughout this book's earlier chapters, and early evidence in specific inherited thrombocytopenia syndromes has suggested a meaningful platelet count response in some patients, though this application remains investigational and should not be considered established practice outside of clinical trial or specialized center settings. This investigational application illustrates the broader theme this chapter develops, in which mechanistic understanding of a specific molecular pathway increasingly informs targeted therapeutic application across disease categories that share a relevant point of convergence in the underlying biology, even when the diseases themselves, an autoimmune platelet destruction disorder and an inherited structural platelet disorder, appear clinically distinct.

Appropriate patient selection for this investigational application requires close collaboration between the treating hematologist and the specialized center or clinical trial coordinating this research, given the need to confirm the specific molecular diagnosis and exclude patients whose specific pathway involvement would make a favorable response biologically implausible, extending the molecular diagnosis-directed treatment selection principle developed throughout Chapter 15 into this emerging therapeutic application.

Novel Agents in Immune Thrombocytopenia and Autoimmune Platelet Destruction

FcRn Antagonism

Neonatal Fc receptor antagonists, which block the recycling mechanism that normally extends circulating IgG antibody half-life, accelerate the degradation of pathogenic autoantibodies including the antiplatelet antibodies responsible for immune thrombocytopenia discussed in Chapter 9, offering a mechanistically distinct approach from the immunosuppressive and thrombopoietin receptor agonist strategies that have historically dominated immune thrombocytopenia management, and this mechanism provides the specific advantage of relatively rapid antibody level reduction without the broader immunosuppressive effect that corticosteroids and other traditional immune thrombocytopenia therapies discussed in Chapter 9 entail. Clinical trials of FcRn antagonist therapy in immune thrombocytopenia have demonstrated meaningful platelet count responses in a substantial proportion of treated patients, including some with disease refractory to multiple prior treatment lines, positioning this drug class as a potentially valuable addition to the immune thrombocytopenia treatment algorithm for patients who have not achieved adequate response with the established therapies discussed in Chapter 9.

The relatively rapid antibody-lowering kinetics FcRn antagonism provides make it a mechanistically distinct alternative to the slower-acting immunosuppressive strategies discussed in Chapter 9, and ongoing investigation into optimal treatment duration, whether continuous long-term therapy or intermittent dosing timed to disease flares, will help clarify the most appropriate long-term treatment paradigm for this drug class as clinical experience accumulates beyond the initial registration trials.

Figure 20.1: FcRn-Mediated IgG Recycling and Antagonist Mechanism

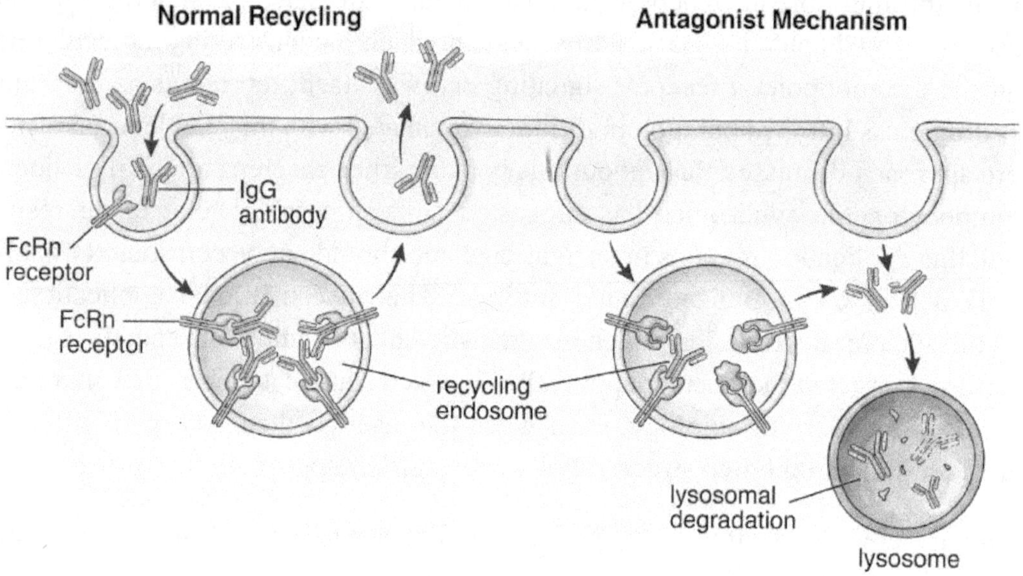

Complement Inhibition

Complement-mediated platelet destruction, increasingly recognized as a contributing mechanism in a subset of immune thrombocytopenia and related autoimmune cytopenias beyond the primarily antibody-mediated Fc receptor-dependent destruction mechanism discussed in Chapter 9, has prompted investigation of complement inhibitor therapy, targeting specific complement pathway components to interrupt this destructive mechanism in patients whose disease appears to involve meaningful complement pathway activation, extending the complement-targeted therapeutic principle already well established in the thrombotic microangiopathy context discussed in Chapter 12 to this related but mechanistically distinct autoimmune platelet destruction context. This complement-targeted approach illustrates the value of mechanistic subtyping within a clinically defined disease category, since immune thrombocytopenia, despite its unifying clinical presentation, likely encompasses a heterogeneous group of underlying immune mechanisms, and future treatment selection may increasingly incorporate mechanistic biomarker assessment to direct patients toward the specific targeted therapy, whether FcRn antagonism, complement inhibition, or the established therapies discussed in Chapter 9, most likely to address their specific underlying disease mechanism.

Identifying which patients have meaningful complement pathway involvement currently requires specialized laboratory assessment not yet widely available outside research or specialized referral center settings, and broader clinical translation of complement-targeted therapy in immune thrombocytopenia will likely depend on the parallel development of practical, accessible biomarker assays capable of identifying appropriate candidates for this specific mechanistic subtype of therapy.

Bruton Tyrosine Kinase Inhibition

Bruton tyrosine kinase inhibitors, which interrupt B-cell receptor signaling and Fc receptor-mediated macrophage activation, both implicated in the antibody-mediated platelet destruction mechanism underlying immune thrombocytopenia, are under investigation as an additional targeted therapeutic approach for this condition, building on this drug class's established role in B-cell malignancies to explore its application in this distinct, though mechanistically related, autoimmune platelet destruction context. Early clinical investigation of Bruton tyrosine kinase inhibitor therapy in immune thrombocytopenia has focused particularly on patients with disease refractory to multiple prior treatment lines, a population for whom the mechanistically diverse emerging therapy landscape this chapter describes offers meaningful additional treatment options beyond what was available when the established treatment algorithm discussed in Chapter 9 represented the full extent of available therapy.

The favorable oral bioavailability of Bruton tyrosine kinase inhibitors, consistent with their established formulation in oncologic use, offers a practical treatment convenience advantage over the parenteral administration many of the other emerging biologic therapies discussed in this chapter require, a consideration that, while secondary to efficacy and safety in treatment selection, meaningfully affects the real-world treatment burden for patients managing a chronic, relapsing autoimmune condition.

THE PLATELET CRISIS DECISION COMPASS — Emerging Therapy Evaluation Arc

The Presentation: A patient with immune thrombocytopenia refractory to corticosteroids, intravenous immunoglobulin, and two thrombopoietin receptor agonists asks about a novel FcRn antagonist she read about online.

Mimic Signature: Enthusiasm for a novel mechanism can lead to premature adoption outside appropriate clinical trial or specialized-center contexts before adequate long-term safety and efficacy data are available, mimicking the appearance of an established, guideline-endorsed treatment option.

The Decision: The treating hematologist reviews the current evidence base, confirms the specific agent's regulatory approval status and the patient's eligibility for either approved use or an active clinical trial, and discusses realistic expectations regarding response likelihood and monitoring requirements.

Trap Logic: Dismissing a legitimate emerging therapy option simply because it is newer than established agents would deny a genuinely refractory patient a potentially effective treatment; conversely, presenting an investigational or recently approved agent without appropriately calibrated evidence-based expectations risks a mismatch between the patient's hopes and the actual, still-maturing evidence base.

Crisis Anchor: Evaluating an emerging platelet-directed therapy requires confirming its specific regulatory and evidence status, matching it to the patient's specific refractory disease characteristics, and delivering balanced, realistic expectations rather than either reflexive dismissal or uncritical enthusiasm.

THE PLATELET CRISIS DECISION COMPASS — Investigational Access Arc

The Presentation: A family of a child with a confirmed severe inherited thrombocytopenia syndrome asks whether gene therapy is available now to cure their child's condition, having read enthusiastic media coverage of early trial results.

Mimic Signature: Early-phase trial press coverage can read as though a therapy is imminently available, mimicking the appearance of an approved, accessible treatment when the underlying evidence is still preliminary and access is restricted to specific trial sites and eligibility criteria.

The Decision: The treating hematologist reviews the specific trial's current phase, eligibility criteria, and enrollment status, and discusses realistic timelines for potential broader availability alongside the family's understandable hope for a curative option.

Trap Logic: Either dismissing the family's question as premature without providing concrete, accurate information about the actual investigational status, or allowing unclarified enthusiasm to stand without correction, both fail this family; honest, specific information serves them best.

Crisis Anchor: When a family asks about an emerging gene therapy or gene editing option, provide the specific current trial phase, eligibility criteria, and realistic timeline rather than either open-ended discouragement or unclarified optimism, and facilitate a specific referral to an enrolling site if the family wishes to pursue it.

Gene Therapy and Gene Editing in Inherited Platelet Disorders

Gene Therapy Approaches for Severe Inherited Disorders

Gene therapy approaches for the most severe inherited platelet disorders discussed in Chapters 15 and 16, including Glanzmann thrombasthenia and selected inherited thrombocytopenia syndromes, are under early-phase clinical investigation, typically employing viral vector-mediated delivery of a functional copy of the affected gene to hematopoietic stem cells, building on the broader gene therapy platform that has achieved regulatory approval for other inherited hematologic conditions and offering the theoretical prospect of durable or potentially curative correction of the underlying molecular defect rather than the lifelong symptomatic and supportive management approach that has historically defined care for these severe inherited disorders. This gene therapy approach, while conceptually promising, remains in early clinical investigation for the platelet disorders specifically, and current evidence does not yet support its use outside specialized clinical trial settings, with substantial questions regarding long-term durability, safety, and the specific patient populations most likely to benefit still requiring further investigation before broader clinical application becomes appropriate.

The conditioning regimens required to prepare a patient's bone marrow for gene-corrected hematopoietic stem cell engraftment carry their own meaningful toxicity, paralleling the risk-benefit considerations already discussed for hematopoietic stem cell transplantation in the severe Glanzmann thrombasthenia context in Chapter 16, and this conditioning-related toxicity represents an important additional consideration, beyond the gene correction technology itself, in determining which patients with severe inherited platelet disorders are appropriate candidates for this investigational approach.

Gene Editing and CRISPR-Based Correction

Gene editing technologies, including CRISPR-based approaches capable of precisely correcting a specific pathogenic variant rather than delivering an additional functional gene copy alongside the existing defective gene as conventional gene therapy does, are under earlier-stage investigation for inherited platelet disorders, offering the theoretical advantage of more physiologic gene regulation since the corrected gene remains under its native regulatory control rather than the potentially less precisely regulated expression conventional gene therapy vector-delivered genes may exhibit. This gene editing approach faces its own distinct technical and safety considerations, including the risk of off-target editing effects and the technical complexity of achieving efficient, precise correction specifically within the hematopoietic stem cell population responsible for sustained megakaryocyte and platelet production, considerations that will require careful evaluation as this technology, still earlier in its clinical development trajectory than the gene therapy approaches discussed above, progresses toward potential clinical application.

Figure 20.2: CRISPR-Based Gene Correction in Hematopoietic Stem Cells

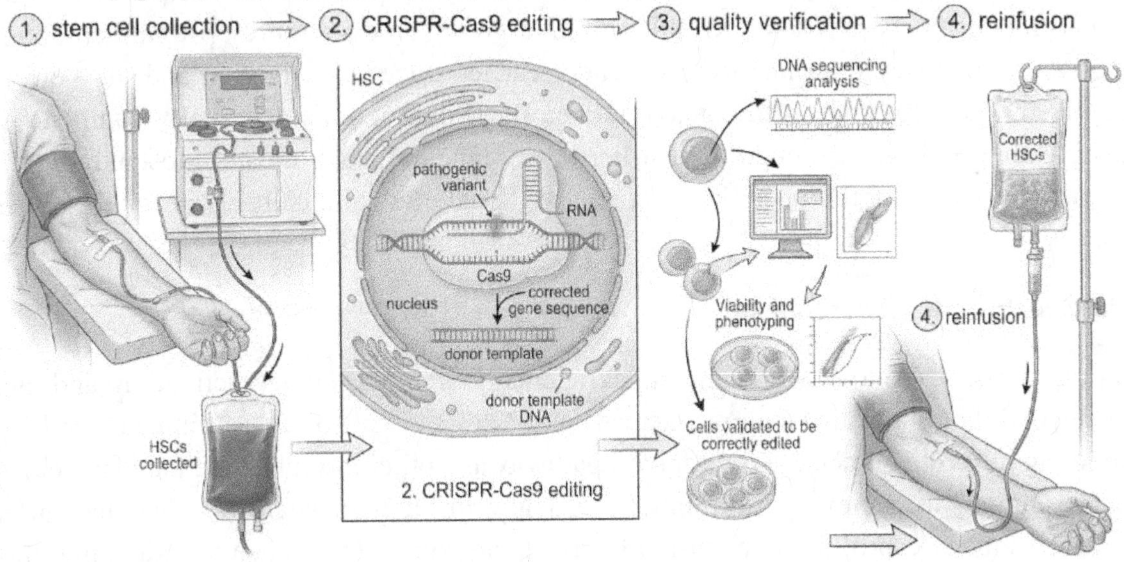

Realistic Timelines and Patient Counseling

Patients and families affected by severe inherited platelet disorders, having often experienced the prolonged diagnostic odyssey discussed in Chapter 16, may reasonably ask about gene therapy and gene editing prospects for their specific condition, and clinicians should provide balanced, accurate information regarding the current early-phase investigational status of these approaches, realistic timelines for potential regulatory approval, which typically span many years even for promising early-phase therapies, and appropriate avenues, such as clinical trial enrollment where eligible and available, for patients interested in pursuing these emerging options, extending the honest, hope-preserving communication framework this book has emphasized throughout its discussion of serious and chronic hematologic diagnoses to this specific emerging therapy counseling context.

Novel Antithrombotic Strategies in Development

Factor XI and Factor XII Inhibition

Factor XI inhibitors, introduced in their emerging pharmacology context in Chapter 18, represent one of the most clinically advanced novel antithrombotic strategies currently in development, with multiple agents, including small molecule inhibitors, antisense oligonucleotides, and monoclonal antibodies, each targeting factor XI through a distinct pharmacologic mechanism, currently progressing through late-phase clinical trials across indications including atrial fibrillation-associated stroke prevention, venous thromboembolism prevention following orthopedic surgery, and secondary stroke prevention, reflecting substantial pharmaceutical industry investment in this therapeutic target given the favorable efficacy-to-bleeding-risk ratio suggested by the contact pathway's disproportionate role in pathologic thrombosis relative to normal hemostasis. Factor XII inhibition, targeting an even more upstream component of the contact activation pathway than factor XI, is under earlier-stage investigation and may offer a further improved bleeding risk profile given congenital factor XII deficiency's essentially complete absence of associated bleeding tendency, though this earlier developmental stage means substantially less clinical evidence currently exists for this specific target relative to the more clinically advanced factor XI inhibitor programs.

Novel Platelet Receptor Antagonists

Investigation continues into novel antiplatelet agents targeting platelet activation and aggregation pathways beyond the established cyclooxygenase and P2Y12 targets discussed in Chapter 18, including agents targeting the protease-activated receptor 4 pathway and other thrombin-mediated platelet activation mechanisms, aiming to achieve antithrombotic efficacy through mechanisms that may offer a more favorable bleeding risk profile than currently available antiplatelet agents, extending the broader therapeutic goal this chapter has developed throughout of achieving improved efficacy-to-bleeding-risk ratios across the antithrombotic therapeutic landscape. These novel platelet receptor antagonists remain earlier in clinical development than the factor XI inhibitor programs discussed above, and their eventual clinical role, if successfully developed, will require careful positioning relative to the established antiplatelet agents and the factor XI inhibitors also under development, given the crowded and rapidly evolving antithrombotic therapeutic landscape this chapter describes.

Combination strategies pairing a novel platelet receptor antagonist with a factor XI inhibitor, targeting complementary points along the platelet activation and coagulation cascade respectively, represent an additional area of early investigation, raising the theoretical prospect of achieving robust antithrombotic efficacy through two mechanistically distinct, lower-intensity interventions rather than a single more intensively dosed agent, though this combination strategy will require its own dedicated safety and efficacy evaluation before any conclusions regarding its comparative merit relative to single-agent approaches can be drawn.

Ex Vivo Platelet Generation and Artificial Platelet Substitutes

Ex Vivo Megakaryocyte Culture and Platelet Production

Ex vivo platelet generation, in which megakaryocytes are cultured and matured outside the body from hematopoietic stem cell or induced pluripotent stem cell sources to ultimately generate transfusable platelets, represents an ambitious long-term research direction aimed at addressing the donor-dependent supply constraints and the alloimmunization and infectious risks discussed in Chapter 19 that characterize conventional donor-derived platelet transfusion, building on the megakaryopoiesis biology introduced in Chapter 1 to attempt to recreate this process at industrial scale outside the human body.

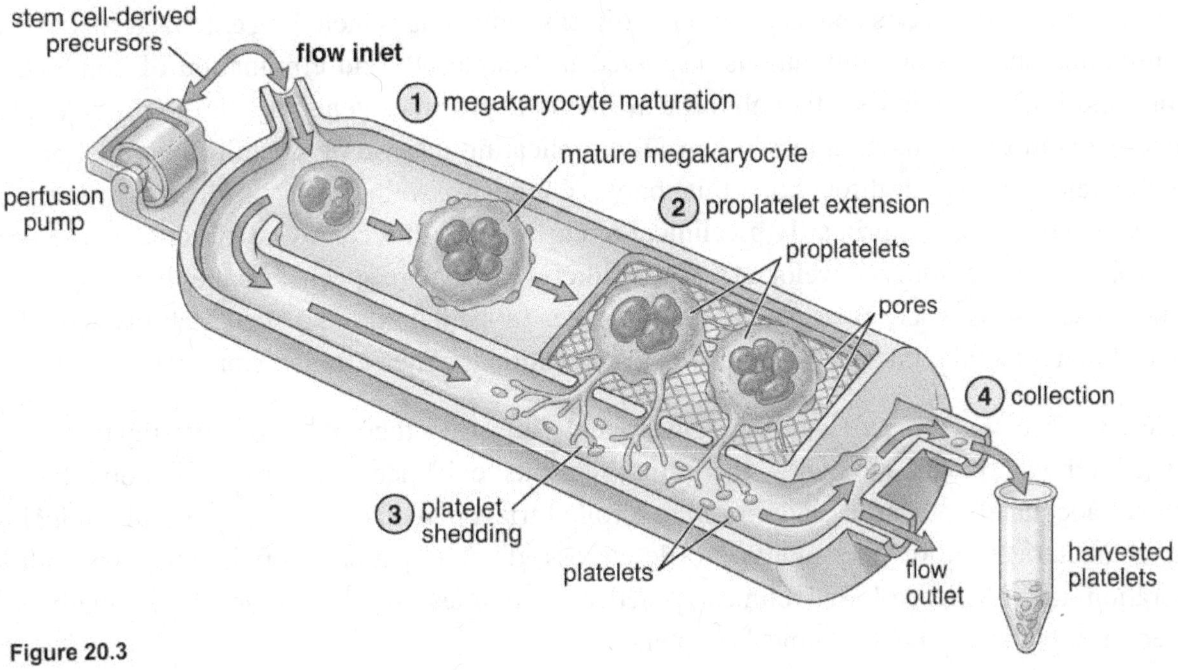

Figure 20.3

Substantial technical challenges remain before ex vivo platelet generation could achieve the scale, cost-effectiveness, and functional quality required for routine clinical use, including achieving adequate platelet yield per cultured megakaryocyte, which remains well below the yield a single megakaryocyte produces in vivo, and confirming that ex vivo-generated platelets achieve fully comparable hemostatic function and survival to conventionally donated platelets, making this technology a longer-term research prospect rather than a near-term clinical reality despite its conceptually attractive potential to address several of the transfusion medicine challenges discussed in Chapter 19.

Induced pluripotent stem cell-derived megakaryocyte lines offer the additional theoretical advantage of establishing a renewable, standardized starting cell population rather than requiring repeated primary hematopoietic stem cell sourcing for each production cycle, potentially addressing the scalability limitations that have constrained earlier ex vivo platelet generation approaches, though establishing that these induced pluripotent stem cell-derived megakaryocyte lines maintain stable, safe genetic and functional characteristics across the extended culture periods industrial-scale production would require remains an active area of investigation.

Artificial and Synthetic Platelet Substitutes

Synthetic and artificial platelet substitutes, including lipid or polymer-based particles engineered to mimic specific platelet hemostatic functions such as fibrinogen-mediated aggregation or subendothelial adhesion, represent an alternative research direction distinct from the biologically-derived ex vivo platelet generation approach discussed above, potentially offering advantages including extended shelf life beyond the room-temperature storage limitations discussed in Chapter 19 and elimination of donor-dependent infectious and immunologic risk, though these synthetic approaches generally aim to provide a bridging or adjunctive hemostatic function rather than fully replicating the complex, multifunctional biology of a genuine platelet discussed throughout this book. Clinical development of these synthetic platelet substitutes remains in early, primarily preclinical or early-phase clinical investigation, and their eventual clinical role, if successfully developed, would likely center on specific acute bleeding or trauma resuscitation scenarios where their potential advantages in availability and shelf stability would provide the greatest incremental clinical value relative to conventional platelet transfusion.

EVIDENCE: The transition of any emerging platelet-directed therapy from investigational status to established clinical practice requires the same rigorous evidence standards this book has applied throughout: adequately powered randomized controlled trials demonstrating meaningful clinical benefit, careful characterization of the safety profile across diverse patient populations, and, ultimately, incorporation into evidence-based clinical practice guidelines from the relevant specialty societies discussed throughout this book's clinical chapters.

Cellular and Antibody-Based Immunotherapy in Autoimmune Platelet Disorders

Beyond the FcRn antagonism, complement inhibition, and Bruton tyrosine kinase inhibition discussed earlier in this chapter, additional cellular and antibody-based immunotherapeutic strategies are under investigation for immune thrombocytopenia and related autoimmune platelet destruction disorders, extending the mechanistically targeted therapeutic approach this chapter has developed throughout to further points along the autoimmune pathogenesis pathway.

Chimeric Antigen Receptor T-Cell and B-Cell Depletion Strategies

Chimeric antigen receptor T-cell approaches targeting B-cell populations, building on this technology's established role in B-cell malignancies and, increasingly, in other antibody-mediated autoimmune conditions, are under early investigation for severe, multiply refractory immune thrombocytopenia, offering the theoretical prospect of more complete and durable B-cell depletion than conventional anti-CD20 monoclonal antibody therapy, discussed in its established role in Chapter 9, achieves, though this approach carries its own distinct toxicity profile, including cytokine release syndrome and neurotoxicity risks well characterized in its oncologic applications, that must be carefully weighed against the potential benefit in a condition, unlike the malignancies where this technology was first established, that is not typically immediately life-threatening. This risk-benefit calculation for chimeric antigen receptor T-cell therapy in immune thrombocytopenia differs meaningfully from its oncologic applications, and appropriate patient selection, likely restricted to the most severely refractory cases with substantial bleeding morbidity despite exhausting other available treatment options discussed throughout this chapter and in Chapter 9, will be essential as this approach progresses through early clinical investigation.

Next-generation anti-CD20 and other B-cell targeted monoclonal antibodies, engineered for more complete or durable B-cell depletion than earlier-generation agents, represent an incremental but potentially clinically meaningful advance building on the established rituximab-based approach discussed in Chapter 9, offering a potentially more accessible alternative to the greater technical complexity and toxicity burden the chimeric antigen receptor T-cell approach discussed above entails.

Antigen-Specific Immune Tolerance Induction

Antigen-specific immune tolerance induction approaches, aiming to selectively suppress the specific pathogenic autoimmune response responsible for platelet destruction while preserving broader immune competence, represent a conceptually attractive but technically challenging research direction distinct from the broader immunosuppressive or B-cell depleting strategies discussed throughout this chapter and in Chapter 9, offering the theoretical advantage of avoiding the infection risk and other toxicities associated with less selective immunosuppression. This antigen-specific approach remains in early preclinical and early clinical investigation for immune thrombocytopenia specifically, building on tolerance induction research more broadly advanced in other autoimmune and transplant immunology contexts, and represents a longer-term research direction relative to the more clinically advanced FcRn antagonist and Bruton tyrosine kinase inhibitor approaches discussed earlier in this chapter.

If successfully developed, antigen-specific tolerance induction would represent a conceptual departure from every other immune thrombocytopenia therapy discussed in this book, offering the theoretical prospect of durable disease remission achieved through immune system recalibration rather than ongoing suppression or antibody clearance, a distinction that, while still speculative given this approach's early developmental stage, illustrates the genuinely transformative potential some of the longer-term research directions this chapter surveys may eventually offer.

Sequencing Emerging Immunotherapies Within the Treatment Algorithm

As the immunotherapeutic landscape for immune thrombocytopenia continues to expand across the mechanistically diverse approaches discussed throughout this chapter, from FcRn antagonism through complement inhibition, Bruton tyrosine kinase inhibition, and the cellular and antibody-based strategies addressed in this section, treatment sequencing decisions for individual refractory patients will increasingly require specialized hematology expertise integrating the specific evidence base, safety profile, and practical accessibility of each option, extending the individualized, specialist-guided treatment sequencing principle already established for the existing immune thrombocytopenia treatment algorithm discussed in Chapter 9 to this expanding array of additional options.

Regulatory Pathways and Health Technology Assessment

The path from an emerging platelet-directed therapy's early clinical investigation to established, widely accessible clinical practice involves regulatory and health technology assessment considerations distinct from, though closely connected to, the clinical evidence evaluation framework discussed elsewhere in this chapter.

Regulatory Approval Pathways

Regulatory approval pathways for platelet-directed therapies, whether through standard approval processes or expedited pathways such as breakthrough therapy or accelerated approval designations available for therapies addressing serious conditions with unmet medical need, directly determine when and under what conditions a given emerging therapy becomes available for clinical use outside a formal clinical trial context, and clinicians should understand the specific regulatory status, including any post-marketing study requirements attached to an accelerated approval, of any emerging therapy they consider incorporating into practice, extending the evidence status verification principle discussed earlier in this chapter to this specific regulatory dimension. Regulatory requirements and approval timelines vary meaningfully across different jurisdictions, and a therapy's approval status in one regulatory jurisdiction does not necessarily indicate similar availability or approval timeline in another, a consideration relevant for clinicians and patients navigating treatment options in an increasingly globalized clinical evidence and pharmaceutical development landscape.

Post-marketing surveillance requirements attached to many accelerated or conditional approvals require the approved therapy's manufacturer to continue generating confirmatory efficacy and safety data after initial approval, and clinicians prescribing a therapy under this pathway should remain aware that continued market availability may, in some circumstances, depend on these confirmatory studies meeting their prespecified endpoints, a regulatory nuance distinct from the more familiar, unconditional approval pathway that governs most established therapies discussed throughout the earlier chapters of this book.

Cost, Access, and Health Technology Assessment

Health technology assessment processes, evaluating a new therapy's cost-effectiveness relative to existing treatment options, increasingly influence practical clinical access to emerging platelet-directed therapies even after regulatory approval has been achieved, particularly for the more expensive biologic and cellular therapy approaches discussed throughout this chapter, and clinicians should recognize that regulatory approval alone does not guarantee immediate, unrestricted clinical access, with insurance coverage determinations, formulary restrictions, and, in some healthcare systems, formal health technology assessment-based coverage decisions each representing additional practical access considerations beyond the clinical evidence and regulatory approval framework this chapter has otherwise emphasized. This access dimension carries genuine equity implications paralleling those discussed in the platelet transfusion resource allocation context in Chapter 19, since the most severely affected or treatment-refractory patients, who stand to benefit most from access to emerging targeted therapies, may face the greatest practical barriers to accessing these therapies given their frequently substantial cost, particularly for the cellular and gene therapy approaches discussed throughout this chapter.

Patient assistance programs, offered by many manufacturers of high-cost emerging therapies, and structured financial counseling incorporated into the treatment planning process can help mitigate, though rarely fully eliminate, the access barriers cost and insurance coverage limitations present, and treating clinicians and their care teams should proactively engage these resources when recommending an emerging therapy with substantial associated cost, extending the practical, resource-aware clinical advocacy this book has emphasized throughout to this specific emerging therapy access context.

Therapeutic Class	Primary Mechanism	Lead Indication(s)	Approximate Development Stage
FcRn antagonists	Accelerated pathogenic IgG degradation	Refractory immune thrombocytopenia	Approved for select indications; expanding investigation
Complement inhibitors	Interruption of complement-mediated destruction	Immune thrombocytopenia with complement activation	Early-to-mid clinical investigation
Bruton tyrosine kinase inhibitors	B-cell receptor and Fc receptor signaling blockade	Refractory immune thrombocytopenia	Early clinical investigation
Gene therapy/editing	Correction of the underlying pathogenic variant	Severe inherited platelet disorders (Glanzmann, others)	Early-phase clinical trials

Factor XI/XII inhibitors	Contact pathway anticoagulation	Atrial fibrillation, VTE prevention	Late-phase clinical trials
Ex vivo platelet generation	Cultured megakaryocyte-derived platelets	Transfusion supply independence	Preclinical/early translational research

CLINICAL CASE: A 29-year-old woman with immune thrombocytopenia refractory to corticosteroids, intravenous immunoglobulin, a thrombopoietin receptor agonist, and rituximab presents for reassessment, with a persistent platelet count of 8 x10^9/L and recurrent mucosal bleeding despite this sequence of established therapies discussed in Chapter 9. Applying the emerging therapy evaluation framework developed in this chapter, the treating hematologist reviews her disease characteristics and confirms eligibility for an FcRn antagonist, now approved for this specific refractory indication. Treatment is initiated with close monitoring, and the platelet count rises to 45 x10^9/L within several weeks, accompanied by resolution of her mucosal bleeding. Splenectomy, discussed in Chapter 9 as an established option for refractory disease, is deferred given this favorable response, and the patient is counseled that continued FcRn antagonist therapy will likely be required long-term, with ongoing monitoring for response durability and any emerging toxicity. This case illustrates the practical application of the emerging therapy framework developed throughout this chapter: a patient who has exhausted the established treatment algorithm discussed in Chapter 9, a mechanistically distinct emerging therapy matched to her specific refractory disease, and a favorable response achieved within an appropriately monitored, evidence-based clinical context rather than through uncritical adoption of an unproven approach.

Biomarkers and Precision Medicine in Platelet Disorders

Molecular Subtyping and Personalized Treatment Selection

The increasing molecular characterization of platelet disorders discussed throughout this book, from the specific driver mutations underlying essential thrombocythemia discussed in Chapter 17 to the expanding genetic landscape of inherited platelet disorders discussed in Chapters 15 and 16, is progressively enabling a precision medicine approach in which treatment selection incorporates specific molecular or mechanistic disease subtyping rather than a uniform approach applied across a clinically defined but molecularly heterogeneous disease category, paralleling the precision medicine evolution that has transformed treatment selection in oncology and several other fields of medicine over recent decades. This precision medicine trajectory, while most clinically mature in specific contexts such as essential thrombocythemia risk stratification discussed in Chapter 17, is likely to progressively extend into additional platelet disorder categories as the mechanistic and biomarker research discussed throughout this chapter continues to mature, potentially allowing future clinicians to select among the expanding array of targeted therapies this chapter describes based on an individual patient's specific molecular disease profile rather than the largely empiric, sequential treatment trial approach that characterizes much of current practice.

Realizing this precision medicine trajectory fully will require continued investment in accessible, clinically practical molecular and biomarker testing infrastructure extending well beyond the specialized academic and research center settings where much of the underlying research discussed throughout this chapter is currently conducted, an infrastructure and accessibility consideration that parallels the health technology assessment and access equity discussion addressed elsewhere in this chapter and that will meaningfully determine how broadly the precision medicine benefits this section describes are ultimately realized across the full population of patients with platelet disorders rather than concentrated only at the specialized centers where these approaches are first developed and validated.

Pharmacogenomics in Platelet-Directed Therapy

Pharmacogenomic factors, discussed specifically for clopidogrel's CYP2C19-dependent metabolism in Chapter 18, represent an additional dimension of precision medicine application relevant to platelet-directed therapy, and continued research into pharmacogenomic predictors of response and toxicity across the broader antiplatelet, anticoagulant, and emerging targeted therapy landscape this chapter has described may progressively refine treatment selection and dosing beyond the population-based approaches that currently predominate, extending the individualized treatment principle this book has emphasized throughout into this specific pharmacogenomic dimension.

Preparing Clinical Practice for an Evolving Therapeutic Landscape

The pace of emerging therapy development this chapter has surveyed across immune thrombocytopenia, inherited platelet disorders, antithrombotic pharmacology, and platelet supply innovation requires clinical practices and individual clinicians to develop sustainable strategies for remaining current, extending beyond the specific agents this chapter has discussed to the broader practice of continuous learning this rapidly evolving field demands.

Continuing Medical Education and Guideline Currency

Clinical practice guidelines from the relevant specialty societies referenced throughout this book, including hematology, cardiology, and transfusion medicine societies depending on the specific therapeutic area, provide the most reliable mechanism for translating the emerging evidence this chapter has surveyed into practice-ready recommendations, and clinicians should establish a sustainable practice of periodic guideline review, recognizing that guidelines in rapidly evolving areas such as immune thrombocytopenia targeted therapy and antithrombotic pharmacology may be updated more frequently than in more mature, stable areas of clinical practice. Structured continuing medical education specifically addressing emerging platelet-directed therapies, whether through specialty society conferences, peer-reviewed journal continuing education activities, or institutional grand rounds and tumor board-style case conferences incorporating emerging therapy discussion, provides an important complementary mechanism for maintaining current knowledge beyond guideline review alone.

Professional society membership and engagement with the specialty-specific literature also provides earlier awareness of emerging evidence than waiting for formal guideline incorporation alone, since the guideline development and revision process, appropriately rigorous and deliberative given the practice-defining role guidelines serve, typically lags meaningfully behind the earliest publication of pivotal clinical trial results, meaning clinicians who engage directly with the primary literature discussed throughout this chapter's evidence evaluation framework will often be aware of significant emerging evidence before it is formally reflected in updated practice guidelines.

Institutional Frameworks for Emerging Therapy Adoption

Individual clinical practices and health systems benefit from establishing structured institutional frameworks for evaluating and, where appropriate, adopting emerging platelet-directed therapies, incorporating pharmacy and therapeutics committee review, multidisciplinary case conference discussion for complex or novel treatment decisions, and structured outcome tracking for patients receiving emerging therapies outside the more rigorously monitored clinical trial context, extending the systems-level quality and safety framework this book has emphasized throughout to this specific emerging therapy adoption context. These institutional frameworks help ensure that emerging therapy adoption proceeds in a structured, evidence-informed manner consistent with the critical evaluation framework this chapter has developed, rather than through unstructured, individual clinician-driven adoption decisions that may vary considerably in their rigor and evidence basis across a given institution's clinical practice.

Smaller community-based practices without the infrastructure to support a dedicated institutional framework of this kind can achieve many of the same benefits through affiliation with a larger academic medical center or regional hematology network, extending access to specialized emerging therapy expertise and multidisciplinary case discussion without requiring each individual smaller practice to independently develop the full institutional infrastructure larger academic centers maintain, an affiliation model that helps extend the benefits of structured emerging therapy evaluation beyond the largest academic centers alone.

Critical Evaluation of Emerging Therapies

A Framework for Assessing New Evidence

Clinicians encountering claims regarding emerging platelet-directed therapies, whether through the peer-reviewed literature, conference presentations, industry communication, or patient inquiries prompted by media coverage or online information, should apply a systematic evaluation framework incorporating the evidence hierarchy discussed throughout this book, specifically distinguishing preliminary, uncontrolled, or single-arm study findings from adequately powered randomized controlled trial evidence, assessing whether the study population and outcomes are relevant to the specific clinical question at hand, and considering the therapy's current regulatory approval status, which directly determines whether use outside a clinical trial context is currently appropriate. This systematic evaluation framework protects against both premature adoption of insufficiently validated therapies and unwarranted dismissal of genuinely promising emerging treatments, striking the same evidence-based, appropriately skeptical but genuinely open-minded balance this book has aimed to model throughout its treatment of both established and emerging platelet-directed therapeutics.

Applying this framework consistently also requires honest acknowledgment of publication bias and the tendency for positive, industry-favorable results to reach publication and media attention more readily than negative or neutral findings, a general evidence interpretation principle this book has referenced throughout its treatment of clinical evidence but that carries particular relevance for emerging therapies still in active, commercially significant clinical development, where the incentive structure surrounding evidence generation and dissemination differs meaningfully from that surrounding the long-established therapies this book has otherwise addressed.

Clinical Trial Access and Referral

Patients with platelet disorders refractory to established therapy, or with rare conditions for which established therapy options remain limited, may benefit from referral to specialized academic centers with active clinical trial programs relevant to their specific condition, providing potential access to the emerging therapies discussed throughout this chapter within the structured, safety-monitored context clinical trial participation provides, extending the specialized referral principle this book has emphasized throughout its discussion of rare and complex platelet disorders to this specific emerging therapy access context. Clinicians should maintain awareness of relevant ongoing clinical trials for the platelet disorders they commonly encounter and should proactively discuss clinical trial participation as a treatment option, where genuinely appropriate and available, rather than reserving this discussion only for patients who specifically inquire about it themselves.

Publicly accessible clinical trial registries provide the standard mechanism for identifying relevant, currently enrolling trials for a specific platelet disorder, and clinicians should familiarize themselves with searching these registries efficiently by disease category and geographic region, extending practical clinical trial navigation skills that complement the underlying scientific and evidence evaluation literacy this chapter has otherwise emphasized, ensuring that patients who might benefit from clinical trial participation are not overlooked simply because the referring clinician lacked familiarity with how to identify appropriate, actively enrolling trial options.

CLINICAL PEARL: The rapid evolution of the platelet-directed therapeutic landscape means the specific agents and evidence discussed throughout this chapter will continue to develop after this book's publication. The mechanistic and evaluative framework this chapter provides, rather than the specific agent names and current evidence status alone, represents its most durable teaching: understanding why a given mechanism is biologically plausible and how to critically evaluate emerging evidence will remain relevant even as specific agents progress through, or fail to complete, clinical development.

Synthesis: The Future of Platelet-Directed Clinical Practice

Integrating Emerging Therapies Into Established Clinical Frameworks

The emerging therapies this chapter has surveyed, spanning immune thrombocytopenia, inherited platelet disorders, antithrombotic pharmacology, and platelet supply innovation, will not replace but rather progressively integrate into the established diagnostic and management frameworks this book has developed throughout its preceding chapters, requiring clinicians to maintain both mastery of current evidence-based standard practice and ongoing awareness of the evolving evidence base this chapter has described, a dual competency this book's overall structure, building from foundational platelet biology through clinical diagnosis and management to this closing survey of the emerging therapeutic landscape, has aimed to support. This integration process will likely proceed unevenly across the different therapeutic areas this chapter has addressed, with some emerging therapies, such as the FcRn antagonists and expanding thrombopoietin receptor agonist applications in immune thrombocytopenia, likely achieving broader clinical practice integration on a nearer-term timeline than the more nascent gene therapy and ex vivo platelet generation research directions, reflecting their differing current stages of clinical development and evidence maturity.

Clinicians should therefore expect the practical clinical relevance of this chapter's content to evolve unevenly over time, with the sections addressing FcRn antagonism and expanding thrombopoietin receptor agonist indications likely requiring the earliest revisiting and practical application, while the sections addressing gene therapy, gene editing, and ex vivo platelet generation are more appropriately understood as an orientation to a longer-term research trajectory whose eventual clinical translation timeline remains genuinely uncertain, a distinction that should inform how each reader prioritizes their own ongoing engagement with the specific emerging therapy areas this chapter has surveyed.

Closing Perspective

This book has developed platelet biology, disorders, and their management as an integrated clinical discipline spanning foundational megakaryopoiesis and platelet ultrastructure through the full range of quantitative and qualitative platelet disorders, transfusion medicine, and antithrombotic pharmacology, consolidated throughout by the Platelet Crisis Decision Compass framework this book's chapters have applied to the recurring diagnostic and management decision points this field presents. The emerging therapies surveyed in this closing chapter represent not an endpoint but a continuation of the same evidence-based, mechanistically grounded clinical reasoning this book has modeled throughout, and the clinician who has internalized this book's cumulative framework, from the platelet activation sequence introduced in Chapter 1 through the precision medicine and emerging therapy landscape addressed in this final chapter, is well equipped to continue integrating new evidence into clinical practice as this dynamic field continues to evolve.

THE PLATELET CRISIS DECISION COMPASS — Emerging Therapy Evaluation and Closing Synthesis

Compass Synthesis: Across this book's twenty chapters, the Decision Compass has consistently directed the clinician from a presenting clinical pattern through mimic exclusion and trap logic to a definitive decision anchor; this closing chapter's instance extends that same structured reasoning to the evaluation of emerging evidence itself.

Crisis Anchor: Evaluating any emerging platelet-directed therapy requires the same rigor this book has applied throughout: confirm the evidence tier, confirm regulatory and clinical trial status, and match the specific mechanism to the specific patient's disease biology before incorporating a new therapy into clinical decision-making.

Summary and Key Concepts

Thrombopoietin receptor agonists are expanding beyond immune thrombocytopenia into severe aplastic anemia, chemotherapy-induced thrombocytopenia, and investigational inherited thrombocytopenia applications.

FcRn antagonism, complement inhibition, and Bruton tyrosine kinase inhibition offer mechanistically distinct approaches to immune thrombocytopenia, particularly for disease refractory to established first- and second-line therapy.

Gene therapy and gene editing approaches for severe inherited platelet disorders remain in early clinical investigation, offering the theoretical prospect of durable correction but requiring further evidence before broader clinical application.

Factor XI and factor XII inhibitors represent the most clinically advanced novel antithrombotic strategies, targeting a pathway with a favorable efficacy-to-bleeding-risk ratio suggested by congenital deficiency phenotypes.

Ex vivo platelet generation and synthetic platelet substitutes remain longer-term research directions aimed at addressing donor-dependent transfusion supply constraints, alloimmunization risk, and shelf-life limitations.

Critical evaluation of emerging therapies requires applying the evidence hierarchy consistently, distinguishing preliminary from randomized controlled trial evidence, and confirming regulatory approval status before clinical adoption outside trial settings.

THE PLATELET CRISIS MASTER COMPASS

The Platelet Crisis Master Compass consolidates the named proprietary feature developed throughout this book's twenty chapters into a single dedicated reference. Each Rhythm Layer instance embedded within a chapter followed the same five-part structure — The Presentation, Mimic Signature, The Decision, Trap Logic, and Crisis Anchor — designed to move the reader from a recognizable clinical pattern through the reasoning most likely to go wrong to the single decision rule that resolves it. This Anchor Section does not introduce new clinical content; it reorganizes and indexes the forty Compass instances already developed within their respective chapters so they can be located and reviewed quickly, independent of the chapter in which they first appeared.

The Platelet Crisis Master Compass: Indexed Pattern Atlas

This Atlas consolidates every Crisis Compass instance introduced across the twenty chapters of this book into a single, cross-referenced navigator organized by the same five-part structure this book has followed. Each entry restates the presenting clinical pattern, the Trap Logic that most commonly leads a clinician astray, and the Crisis Anchor, the single decision rule that resolves the pattern. The Atlas is designed as a scanning reference for clinic, the wards, or the moments before a call-night decision, not as a substitute for the fuller clinical reasoning developed within each chapter, to which every entry is cross-referenced.

Entries are grouped by Part and, within each Part, by the chapter in which the pattern was first introduced, so that a reader working through a specific clinical question can move directly to the relevant section rather than scanning the full forty-entry index. A consolidated quick-lookup table by presenting problem follows the Part-by-Part Atlas for readers who prefer to navigate by clinical scenario rather than by book structure.

Part I: Foundational Platelet Biology

Isolated Thrombocytosis on a Routine Panel — Chapter 1 Presentation: A platelet count above the upper reference limit, discovered incidentally on a routine or preoperative complete blood count, in a patient who is otherwise asymptomatic and has no prior hematologic history. Trap Logic: The absence of symptoms is not evidence against a myeloproliferative neoplasm; early essential thrombocythemia is frequently asymptomatic, and the danger of dismissing an incidental thrombocytosis as benign is that clonal thrombocytosis carries a meaningful long-term risk of arterial and venous thrombosis that is not mitigated by reassurance. Crisis Anchor: Persistent thrombocytosis without an identified reactive cause after a basic screening evaluation should proceed to molecular testing, not to a default diagnosis of reactive thrombocytosis by exclusion of history alone.

A Disappointing Platelet Count Rise After Transfusion — Chapter 1 Presentation: A platelet transfusion is administered for thrombocytopenia, and the post-transfusion platelet count, measured at ten minutes to one hour or at eighteen to twenty-four hours, rises far less than the calculated corrected count increment predicts for the dose given and the patient's body surface area. Trap Logic: Ordering an HLA antibody panel after a single refractory transfusion, before excluding sepsis, active bleeding, or splenomegaly, delays identification of the far more common and often more urgent non-immune cause and can commit a patient to an unnecessary search for HLA-matched platelet products. Crisis Anchor: One low corrected count increment is a consumptive-cause screen; a pattern of low corrected count increments across multiple ABO-compatible transfusions is what should trigger an alloimmunization workup.

Prolonged Bleeding Time with a Normal Platelet Count — Chapter 2 Presentation: A patient with mucocutaneous bleeding symptoms and a normal platelet count on complete blood count, in whom a screening bleeding time or platelet function analyzer closure time returns prolonged. Trap Logic: Ordering aggregometry before excluding von Willebrand disease inverts the correct diagnostic sequence, since von Willebrand disease is far more prevalent than any inherited platelet receptor disorder and aggregometry itself can be secondarily abnormal in von Willebrand disease, producing a confusing result that delays the correct diagnosis. Crisis Anchor: Von Willebrand factor testing precedes platelet function testing in the evaluation of mucocutaneous bleeding with a normal platelet count, not the reverse.

A Platelet Function Panel Suggesting a Storage Pool Disorder — Chapter 2 Presentation: Light transmission aggregometry shows a normal primary wave of aggregation to multiple agonists but an absent or blunted secondary wave, particularly to adenosine diphosphate and epinephrine, with normal aggregation to ristocetin. Trap Logic: Diagnosing an inherited storage pool disorder from a single aggregometry tracing obtained without confirming an adequate medication washout risks a false inherited-disorder label that follows the patient for life and can affect future perioperative and obstetric management unnecessarily. Crisis Anchor: A blunted secondary aggregation wave is confirmed as a genuine storage pool disorder only after medication-related and uremic causes have been excluded and, ideally, after direct granule content quantification supports the diagnosis.

Bleeding on Dual Antiplatelet Therapy — Chapter 3 Presentation: A patient established on dual antiplatelet therapy, typically aspirin plus a P2Y12 inhibitor after coronary stenting, develops a bleeding complication ranging from minor mucocutaneous bleeding to a major gastrointestinal or intracranial hemorrhage. Trap Logic: Reflexively and unilaterally discontinuing dual antiplatelet therapy for a bleeding complication, without cardiology input on stent thrombosis timing, can convert a manageable bleeding problem into a fatal stent thrombosis, particularly within the first month after placement of a coronary stent. Crisis Anchor: Antiplatelet therapy is modified only after weighing bleeding severity against stent thrombosis risk together with the prescribing cardiologist; it is never stopped unilaterally on hematology's initiative alone outside of immediately life-threatening hemorrhage.

Early Recognition of Platelet-Driven Microvascular Thrombosis — Chapter 3 Presentation: A patient develops new thrombocytopenia together with early signs suggesting diffuse microvascular platelet consumption: unexplained neurologic symptoms, evolving renal dysfunction, or a rapidly falling platelet count without an obvious bleeding source or overt disseminated intravascular coagulation picture. Trap Logic: Waiting for a comprehensive coagulation and hemolysis laboratory panel before requesting an urgent peripheral smear delays recognition of a thrombotic microangiopathy, in which the correct intervention, addressed fully in Chapter 12, is time-critical and should not be deferred pending laboratory confirmation once clinical suspicion is high. Crisis Anchor: An urgent peripheral smear for schistocytes is obtained the moment a thrombotic microangiopathy is suspected, in parallel with, not after, the remainder of the diagnostic workup.

Unexplained Easy Bruising with Normal Platelet Studies — Chapter 4 Presentation: A patient reports easy bruising or recurrent petechiae, but platelet count, peripheral smear, von Willebrand factor testing, and platelet function testing are all normal. Trap Logic: Repeating platelet count, aggregometry, and von Willebrand factor testing multiple times in a patient whose initial evaluation was normal and adequately performed delays recognition of a vascular, nutritional, or non-hematologic explanation and can create the false impression that a hematologic cause simply has not yet been found. Crisis Anchor: A normal, adequately performed platelet and von Willebrand factor evaluation should redirect, not repeat, the workup toward vascular, nutritional, and non-hematologic causes of a bruising or purpuric phenotype.

Periprocedural Assessment of a Mild, Borderline Platelet Count — Chapter 4 Presentation: A patient with a platelet count in the borderline range, generally 50 to 100 x10^9/L, is scheduled for an elective procedure, and the proceduralist requests hematology input on whether the procedure can proceed safely. Trap Logic: Applying a single, universal platelet count threshold to every procedure regardless of bleeding risk category either exposes a patient to unnecessary bleeding risk for a high-risk procedure or subjects a patient to unnecessary delay and platelet transfusion for a low-risk procedure that did not require it. Crisis Anchor: Periprocedural platelet threshold recommendations are procedure-specific and account for concurrent hemostatic risk factors, never a single universal number applied uniformly across all procedure types.

Part II: Clinical Evaluation and Diagnostic Approach

Recognizing a Bleeding History That Requires Same-Day Evaluation — Chapter 5 Presentation: A patient reports a bleeding history during a routine or urgent care visit, and the clinician must decide whether this can be evaluated through routine outpatient referral or requires same-day hematologic assessment. Trap Logic: Deferring a same-day complete blood count in a patient with new, spontaneous, unexplained bruising or bleeding because the history sounds similar to a chronic, benign pattern risks missing an acute, rapidly evolving process such as immune thrombocytopenia, acute leukemia, or a thrombotic microangiopathy, each of which can progress rapidly if evaluation is delayed. Crisis Anchor: New-onset spontaneous bruising or mucosal bleeding, as distinct from a chronic, stable bleeding pattern, warrants a same-day complete blood count and smear review, not routine outpatient scheduling.

A Markedly Low Platelet Count in an Asymptomatic Patient — Chapter 5 Presentation: A platelet count in the range of 10 to 30 x10^9/L is reported on a routine or incidental complete blood count in a patient who denies any bleeding symptoms and appears clinically well. Trap Logic: Treating an asymptomatic presentation as evidence that a markedly low reported count can safely wait for routine follow-up conflates the patient's current symptom status with the count's underlying accuracy and risk, when in fact a genuinely severe, confirmed thrombocytopenia carries substantial near-term bleeding risk regardless of whether symptoms have yet appeared. Crisis Anchor: A platelet count below 30 x10^9/L is confirmed via smear review for clumping and evaluated urgently the same day, regardless of the patient's current symptom status.

An Analyzer Flag Accompanying a Low Platelet Count — Chapter 6 Presentation: An automated complete blood count reports a platelet count of 45 x10^9/L accompanied by an instrument flag for possible platelet clumping. Trap Logic: Accepting a flagged platelet count at face value because the flag seems like a routine laboratory technicality, rather than treating it as a specific instruction to confirm the result before clinical action, risks initiating an unnecessary and potentially invasive workup for an artifactual finding. Crisis Anchor: Any platelet count accompanied by a clumping flag is confirmed by smear review before it is treated as clinically actionable.

Resolving a Suspected Pseudothrombocytopenia Result — Chapter 6 Presentation: Smear review of a patient with an automated platelet count of 32 x10^9/L reveals prominent platelet clumping at the feathered edge with associated platelet satellitism around several neutrophils. Trap Logic: Assuming that clumping fully explains the low count without obtaining a corrected value risks missing a mixed picture in which a genuinely low, clinically significant platelet count is present beneath the artifact, particularly in a patient with an independent reason for thrombocytopenia. Crisis Anchor: A confirmed clumping artifact is resolved with a corrected count from an alternative anticoagulant, not simply disregarded as falsely low without verification of the true value.

An Aggregometry Pattern Suggesting Glanzmann Thrombasthenia — Chapter 7 Presentation: A young patient with a lifelong severe mucocutaneous bleeding history undergoes aggregometry, which shows absent aggregation to adenosine diphosphate, collagen, epinephrine, and arachidonic acid, with a normal ristocetin-induced response. Trap Logic: Accepting a flat, pan-agonist aggregometry tracing as diagnostic of Glanzmann thrombasthenia without confirming technical validity of the preparation risks a false-positive diagnosis when the true explanation is a technically inadequate specimen rather than a genuine inherited defect. Crisis Anchor: A near-absent response to all agonists except ristocetin, in a technically valid preparation, is the aggregometry signature of Glanzmann thrombasthenia and warrants confirmatory glycoprotein IIb/IIIa flow cytometry.

A Discordant Point-of-Care Closure Time in a Patient on Antiplatelet Therapy — Chapter 7 Presentation: A patient on chronic low-dose aspirin therapy undergoes point-of-care platelet function testing before a planned procedure, and the closure time returns within the normal reference range despite the known antiplatelet exposure. Trap Logic: Treating a normal point-of-care closure time as proof that a patient's aspirin therapy carries no periprocedural bleeding risk overstates the sensitivity of this specific assay for the cyclooxygenase-mediated mechanism and risks underestimating true bleeding risk before an invasive procedure. Crisis Anchor: A normal point-of-care closure time on aspirin does not reliably exclude clinically relevant antiplatelet effect; arachidonic acid-specific aggregometry is the more direct confirmatory test when the clinical stakes require certainty.

New Thrombocytopenia with Accompanying Cytopenias — Chapter 8 Presentation: A previously well adult presents with new thrombocytopenia (platelet count 62 x10^9/L) accompanied by a new mild anemia and mild leukopenia on the same complete blood count. Trap Logic: Attributing multilineage cytopenia to a single presumed cause, such as a mild concurrent viral illness, without pursuing the smear morphology and marrow-directed evaluation this presentation warrants risks delaying diagnosis of a marrow infiltrative process for which early diagnosis meaningfully affects outcome. Crisis Anchor: New thrombocytopenia accompanied by unexplained anemia or leukopenia is evaluated with smear review and, when morphology is abnormal, urgent hematology referral for marrow examination — not attributed to a single presumed benign cause without this evaluation.

Sequencing the Evaluation of New Thrombocytopenia in a Hospitalized Patient — Chapter 8 Presentation: A patient hospitalized for pneumonia and started on prophylactic heparin six days ago develops a new platelet count decline from 240 to 95 x10^9/L. Trap Logic: Attributing hospital-acquired thrombocytopenia reflexively to 'sepsis' without constructing the specific exposure timeline this chapter emphasizes risks missing a time-sensitive, specifically treatable diagnosis such as heparin-induced thrombocytopenia, for which continued heparin exposure carries substantial thrombotic risk. Crisis Anchor: New thrombocytopenia in a hospitalized patient is evaluated against a specific exposure and procedure timeline, with heparin-induced thrombocytopenia pretest probability formally assessed whenever heparin exposure and compatible timing are present.

Part III: Thrombocytopenia — Immune, Drug-Induced, Consumptive, and Special-Population Disorders

Determining Urgency of First-Line Treatment in Newly Diagnosed Immune Thrombocytopenia — Chapter 9 Presentation: A 34-year-old woman is newly diagnosed with immune thrombocytopenia, platelet count 8 x10^9/L, with scattered petechiae and mild gingival bleeding but no wet purpura, retinal hemorrhage, or major bleeding. Trap Logic: Delaying first-line treatment for a platelet count this severe because the patient currently lacks major bleeding conflates current symptom absence with future risk, when a count this low carries substantial risk of a bleeding complication developing before treatment can take effect if initiation is delayed. Crisis Anchor: A confirmed platelet count below approximately 20-30 x10^9/L in newly diagnosed immune thrombocytopenia warrants prompt first-line treatment initiation, regardless of whether major bleeding is yet present.

Sequencing Second-Line Therapy After First-Line Treatment Failure — Chapter 9 Presentation: A 41-year-old man with immune thrombocytopenia relapses to a platelet count of 15 x10^9/L with recurrent bruising during corticosteroid taper, three months after initial diagnosis. Trap Logic: Repeating additional corticosteroid courses indefinitely in a corticosteroid-dependent relapsing pattern, rather than transitioning to a second-line strategy at the appropriate point, exposes the patient to cumulative corticosteroid toxicity without addressing the underlying pattern of dependency this presentation demonstrates. Crisis Anchor: A corticosteroid-dependent relapse pattern meeting criteria for persistent immune thrombocytopenia prompts transition to second-line therapy selection rather than indefinite repeated corticosteroid courses.

Recognizing the Characteristic Timing Pattern of Drug-Induced Thrombocytopenia — Chapter 10 Presentation: A patient develops an abrupt platelet count drop from 220 to 12 x10^9/L with new petechiae and gum bleeding eight days after starting a new medication for a urinary tract infection, with no other clear explanation. Trap Logic: Continuing a newly started medication because the temporal association 'could be coincidental' while pursuing an extensive alternative workup delays the single intervention, discontinuation, most likely to resolve a severe, high-risk thrombocytopenia. Crisis Anchor: Abrupt severe thrombocytopenia occurring one to two weeks after a new medication exposure is treated as drug-induced until proven otherwise, with prompt discontinuation of the suspected agent regardless of whether alternative causes have been fully excluded.

Managing an Inadvertent Rechallenge with a Previously Implicated Medication — Chapter 10 Presentation: A patient with a documented history of vancomycin-induced thrombocytopenia two years ago is inadvertently started on vancomycin again during a new hospitalization, and the platelet count begins falling within six hours of the first dose. Trap Logic: Continuing to monitor rather than immediately discontinuing a medication with a documented prior causative history in this specific patient, on the assumption that this episode might follow a milder course, disregards the anamnestic response principle that generally predicts a more rapid and severe reaction upon reexposure to a previously sensitizing drug. Crisis Anchor: A documented prior drug-induced thrombocytopenia episode with a specific medication is an absolute contraindication to future rechallenge; any inadvertent rechallenge warrants immediate discontinuation upon recognition, not observation pending confirmation of severity.

Applying the 4Ts Score to Guide Immediate Management — Chapter 11 Presentation: A patient receiving therapeutic unfractionated heparin for seven days develops a platelet count decline from 260 to 95 x10^9/L, with no new thrombosis identified and several other plausible alternative explanations including recent surgery and a concurrent infection. Trap Logic: Continuing heparin while awaiting laboratory confirmation in a patient with an intermediate or high 4Ts score, on the reasoning that alternative explanations seem equally or more plausible, disregards the asymmetric risk this chapter has emphasized: the consequence of continued heparin exposure in true heparin-induced thrombocytopenia is thrombosis, a risk too severe to accept while awaiting confirmatory testing in an intermediate-or-higher probability patient. Crisis Anchor: An intermediate or high 4Ts score prompts immediate heparin discontinuation and transition to alternative anticoagulation, with laboratory testing sent concurrently rather than management decisions deferred until results return.

Managing Confirmed Heparin-Induced Thrombocytopenia with Thrombosis — Chapter 11 Presentation: A patient with a high 4Ts score and strongly positive immunoassay develops acute lower extremity deep vein thrombosis, with platelet count 45 x10^9/L. Trap Logic: Withholding or reducing anticoagulation intensity because the platelet count appears to indicate bleeding risk applies the wrong mental model to this condition — heparin-induced thrombocytopenia thrombocytopenia does not reflect the bleeding-prone state typical of the destructive thrombocytopenias discussed elsewhere in this book, and under-anticoagulating in this setting substantially increases, rather than decreases, patient risk. Crisis Anchor: Confirmed heparin-induced thrombocytopenia with thrombosis is treated with full therapeutic-dose non-heparin anticoagulation regardless of platelet count severity — thrombocytopenia in this specific condition is not a reason to withhold or reduce anticoagulation intensity.

Recognizing Thrombotic Microangiopathy as Requiring Same-Day Treatment — Chapter 12 Presentation: A 38-year-old woman presents with fatigue and mild confusion, and initial laboratory testing reveals a platelet count of 18 x10^9/L, hemoglobin 7.8 g/dL, and schistocytes on peripheral smear. Trap Logic: Deferring plasma exchange initiation until ADAMTS13 results return, when the clinical and laboratory picture and PLASMIC score already support a high probability of thrombotic thrombocytopenic purpura, exposes the patient to a delay that meaningfully increases mortality risk in a condition where each day of delayed treatment carries measurable additional risk. Crisis Anchor: Thrombocytopenia with microangiopathic hemolytic anemia (schistocytes, elevated lactate dehydrogenase, low haptoglobin) and a high PLASMIC score triggers same-day plasma exchange initiation, not deferral until ADAMTS13 confirmation returns.

Distinguishing TTP from Atypical HUS While ADAMTS13 Results Are Pending — Chapter 12 Presentation: A 45-year-old man presents with thrombocytopenia, microangiopathic hemolytic anemia, and acute kidney injury requiring dialysis, with no preceding diarrheal illness; ADAMTS13 activity results are pending and expected to take three days. Trap Logic: Withholding plasma exchange while awaiting ADAMTS13 results because the renal predominance and absent prodrome seem to favor atypical hemolytic uremic syndrome over thrombotic thrombocytopenic purpura risks withholding effective therapy from a patient who, in fact, has thrombotic thrombocytopenic purpura with an atypical presentation — clinical pattern alone cannot reliably exclude thrombotic thrombocytopenic purpura before ADAMTS13 confirmation. Crisis Anchor: Empiric plasma exchange is initiated for any patient meeting thrombotic microangiopathy criteria regardless of which specific variant clinical pattern initially suggests, continuing until ADAMTS13 results definitively exclude severe deficiency and allow transition to variant-specific therapy.

Distinguishing Benign Gestational Thrombocytopenia from a Pregnancy Emergency — Chapter 13 Presentation: A woman at 34 weeks gestation is found to have a platelet count of 88 x10^9/L on routine prenatal laboratory testing, with no prior thrombocytopenia history. Trap Logic: Reassuring a pregnant patient that a mildly low platelet count 'is probably just pregnancy' without obtaining the blood pressure, urine protein, and hemolysis assessment this chapter requires risks missing early preeclampsia or HELLP syndrome, both of which can progress rapidly once initially subtle laboratory abnormalities become clinically apparent. Crisis Anchor: Any new thrombocytopenia identified during pregnancy triggers same-visit assessment of blood pressure, urine protein, and hemolysis markers before a benign gestational thrombocytopenia diagnosis is accepted, regardless of how mild or reassuring the presentation initially appears.

Recognizing Neonatal Alloimmune Thrombocytopenia Risk in a Subsequent Pregnancy — Chapter 13 Presentation: A woman whose first child was born with severe thrombocytopenia and a grade 2 intracranial hemorrhage, later confirmed as neonatal alloimmune thrombocytopenia, presents now pregnant with her second child by the same partner. Trap Logic: Treating this pregnancy as routine because the mother herself is asymptomatic and her own platelet count is normal overlooks that neonatal alloimmune thrombocytopenia is a fetal, not maternal, hematologic condition — normal maternal platelet count provides no reassurance regarding fetal risk given the alloimmune, rather than autoimmune, mechanism this condition reflects. Crisis Anchor: A prior pregnancy affected by neonatal alloimmune thrombocytopenia mandates specialized antenatal referral for any subsequent pregnancy with the same partner, regardless of normal maternal platelet count, given the substantially elevated recurrence risk this history establishes.

Recognizing Evolving Disseminated Intravascular Coagulation Before Overt Criteria Are Met — Chapter 14 Presentation: A patient with severe sepsis shows a platelet count declining from 180 to 95 x10^9/L over 24 hours, prothrombin time mildly prolonged, and fibrinogen declining from 480 to 220 mg/dL, though not yet meeting formal overt disseminated intravascular coagulation scoring criteria. Trap Logic: Waiting for a formal overt disseminated intravascular coagulation score before recognizing the clinical significance of a consistently worsening trend across multiple coagulation parameters ignores the dynamic, evolving nature of this condition and delays the heightened monitoring and source-control urgency this trajectory warrants. Crisis Anchor: A consistent worsening trend across platelet count, coagulation studies, and fibrinogen in a patient with a disseminated intravascular coagulation-predisposing condition warrants intensified monitoring and aggressive treatment of the underlying trigger, regardless of whether a formal overt scoring threshold has yet been met.

Distinguishing Chronic Liver Disease Thrombocytopenia from a Superimposed Acute Process — Chapter 14 Presentation: A patient with known, stable cirrhosis and a chronically low platelet count around 70 x10^9/L presents with a new decline to 35 x10^9/L over the preceding week, without an obvious precipitant identified on initial review. Trap Logic: Attributing a new, more rapid decline in a chronically thrombocytopenic cirrhotic patient to simple progression of known liver disease, without systematically screening for a new superimposed precipitant, risks missing a specifically treatable acute process such as infection or evolving disseminated intravascular coagulation that a stable chronic baseline would not itself explain. Crisis Anchor: A new, more rapid platelet count decline in a patient with known chronic liver disease thrombocytopenia is evaluated for a superimposed acute precipitant (infection, new medication, evolving coagulopathy) rather than attributed reflexively to progression of the known chronic baseline.

Part IV: Inherited Platelet Disorders

Recognizing a Macrothrombocytopenia Pattern Warranting Genetic Evaluation — Chapter 15 Presentation: A 26-year-old man is found to have a platelet count of 95 x10^9/L on routine testing, with smear review showing giant platelets and mean platelet volume markedly elevated; he reports a lifelong history of a similarly low platelet count with only mild bruising. Trap Logic: Diagnosing and treating this presentation as immune thrombocytopenia based on the platelet count and giant platelet morphology alone, without recognizing the lifelong stable history as a specific clue pointing toward an inherited macrothrombocytopenia syndrome, risks both ineffective immune-directed therapy and a missed opportunity for the renal surveillance this specific category of syndrome requires. Crisis Anchor: Macrothrombocytopenia with a lifelong, stable history prompts genetic evaluation for an inherited syndrome and baseline renal function assessment, rather than default classification as acquired immune thrombocytopenia.

Establishing Malignancy Surveillance After Confirming a Predisposition Syndrome — Chapter 15 Presentation: Genetic testing confirms a pathogenic RUNX1 variant in a 22-year-old woman evaluated for mild, lifelong thrombocytopenia with a family history of two relatives who developed acute myeloid leukemia in their thirties and forties. Trap Logic: Treating this as 'just mild thrombocytopenia' and discharging the patient to routine primary care without establishing structured hematology surveillance disregards the substantial malignancy risk this specific confirmed genetic diagnosis carries, a risk the family history in this case further reinforces rather than merely coincides with. Crisis Anchor: A confirmed pathogenic variant in a malignancy-predisposing inherited thrombocytopenia gene establishes lifelong structured surveillance and family cascade testing, regardless of how mild the patient's own current hematologic presentation appears.

Aggregometry Pattern Recognition Arc — Chapter 16 Presentation: A neonate develops severe bleeding from the umbilical stump and circumcision site, prompting hematology referral. Platelet count is normal, but bleeding time and closure times are markedly prolonged. Trap Logic: The preserved ristocetin response is the critical discriminator: because ristocetin agglutination depends on GPIb-von Willebrand factor interaction rather than GPIIb/IIIa-mediated aggregation, its preservation distinguishes Glanzmann thrombasthenia from Bernard-Soulier syndrome, in which ristocetin-induced agglutination is characteristically absent or markedly reduced alongside giant platelets and a low-normal platelet count. Crisis Anchor: Absent aggregation to all agonists except ristocetin, in a patient with a normal platelet count and normal platelet size, is the aggregometry signature of Glanzmann thrombasthenia and should prompt GPIIb/IIIa flow cytometric confirmation and genetic counseling for this autosomal recessive disorder.

Acquired Dysfunction Recognition Arc — Chapter 16 Presentation: A 68-year-old man with essential thrombocythemia and a platelet count of 1,450 x10^9/L presents with epistaxis and easy bruising despite having no prior bleeding history. Trap Logic: The temptation to attribute new bleeding in essential thrombocythemia solely to antiplatelet therapy, if the patient is taking aspirin, would miss the count-dependent acquired von Willebrand syndrome mechanism, which requires cytoreductive therapy targeting the platelet count itself rather than antiplatelet therapy adjustment alone. Crisis Anchor: New bleeding at a markedly elevated platelet count in a myeloproliferative neoplasm should prompt von Willebrand factor multimer analysis for acquired von Willebrand syndrome, and cytoreductive therapy lowering the platelet count, rather than platelet transfusion, is the mechanistically appropriate corrective measure.

Part V: Thrombocytosis, Pharmacology, Transfusion Medicine, and Emerging Therapies

Reactive Versus Clonal Recognition Arc — Chapter 17 Presentation: A 45-year-old woman has a platelet count of 620 x10^9/L identified incidentally on routine bloodwork, with no symptoms and an unremarkable examination. Trap Logic: Attributing persistent, unexplained thrombocytosis to a presumed but unidentified reactive cause without pursuing molecular testing risks delaying the essential thrombocythemia diagnosis and the thrombotic risk assessment this chapter's management framework depends upon. Crisis Anchor: Persistent thrombocytosis without an identifiable reactive trigger, confirmed on repeat testing, warrants JAK2, CALR, and MPL mutation testing before further reactive causes are pursued, since a positive result establishes essential thrombocythemia and directs the risk-stratified management pathway.

Extreme Count Dual-Risk Arc — Chapter 17 Presentation: A 52-year-old man with known essential thrombocythemia on hydroxyurea presents with new epistaxis and bruising, and his platelet count is found to be 1,420 x10^9/L, up from 780 x10^9/L at his last visit three months ago. Trap Logic: Increasing aspirin or adding an additional antiplatelet agent in response to the marked platelet count elevation, without first recognizing the bleeding phenotype as a signal for acquired von Willebrand syndrome, would worsen rather than improve this patient's hemostatic status. Crisis Anchor: New bleeding accompanying a rising platelet count at extreme levels should prompt von Willebrand factor multimer testing before any antiplatelet therapy escalation, since cytoreductive therapy intensification to lower the platelet count, not additional antiplatelet therapy, is the mechanistically appropriate correction.

Antiplatelet Recovery Timeline Arc — Chapter 18 Presentation: A 66-year-old man on clopidogrel following a coronary stent placed four months ago requires an elective inguinal hernia repair, and the surgical team asks hematology for periprocedural antiplatelet guidance. Trap Logic: Focusing exclusively on the pharmacologic recovery timeline for clopidogrel discontinuation, without first establishing whether discontinuation is appropriate at all given the specific stent thrombosis risk this patient's recent drug-eluting stent placement confers, risks a catastrophic stent thrombosis and myocardial infarction that would far outweigh the bleeding risk the hernia repair itself presents. Crisis Anchor: Before addressing how long to hold a P2Y12 inhibitor before a procedure, first establish whether holding it at all is safe given the specific indication, stent type, and time since placement — cardiology co-management is mandatory whenever a recent coronary stent is present, and elective surgery should be deferred rather than the antiplatelet therapy discontinued when the minimum dual antiplatelet therapy duration has not yet elapsed.

Reversal Agent Selection Arc — Chapter 18 Presentation: A patient on rivaroxaban for atrial fibrillation presents with major gastrointestinal bleeding and hemodynamic instability, and the emergency team asks whether to give fresh frozen plasma, prothrombin complex concentrate, or a specific reversal agent. Trap Logic: Reflexively reaching for fresh frozen plasma because it is the traditional 'reversal' product risks both delaying effective factor Xa inhibitor reversal and unnecessarily exposing the patient to a large-volume infusion that provides little specific benefit for this particular anticoagulant class. Crisis Anchor: Reversal strategy must match the specific anticoagulant mechanism: andexanet alfa for factor Xa inhibitors, idarucizumab for dabigatran, and four-factor prothrombin complex concentrate with vitamin K for vitamin K antagonist therapy — fresh frozen plasma is not the default reversal agent for direct oral anticoagulants.

Refractoriness Recognition Arc — Chapter 19 Presentation: A 34-year-old woman undergoing induction chemotherapy for acute myeloid leukemia shows minimal platelet count increment despite three consecutive apheresis platelet transfusions over one week, each given for a platelet count below the prophylactic threshold. Trap Logic: Attributing the poor response to 'just chemotherapy effect' without calculating the corrected count increment and systematically excluding both nonimmune causes and HLA alloimmunization would delay the transition to HLA-matched or crossmatch-compatible platelet products this patient's confirmed alloimmunization requires. Crisis Anchor: A corrected count increment below the refractoriness threshold on two consecutive ABO-compatible, fresh platelet transfusions defines refractoriness and should prompt systematic evaluation for nonimmune causes first, then HLA and platelet-specific antibody testing, since confirmed alloimmunization requires HLA-matched or crossmatch-compatible platelet products rather than continued standard random-donor transfusion.

Nonimmune Versus Alloimmune Refractoriness Arc — Chapter 19 Presentation: A febrile, septic patient with hypoproliferative thrombocytopenia shows a poor platelet count increment after two consecutive apheresis platelet transfusions given for active oozing. Trap Logic: Immediately pursuing HLA-matched platelets without first addressing the active sepsis would consume scarce matched-donor resources for a patient whose refractoriness may fully resolve once the nonimmune consumptive process is treated. Crisis Anchor: A febrile or septic patient with poor transfusion increment should have the nonimmune cause treated first, with HLA and platelet-specific antibody testing reserved for refractoriness that persists once fever, sepsis, and other consumptive processes have resolved.

Emerging Therapy Evaluation Arc — Chapter 20 Presentation: A patient with immune thrombocytopenia refractory to corticosteroids, intravenous immunoglobulin, and two thrombopoietin receptor agonists asks about a novel FcRn antagonist she read about online. Trap Logic: Dismissing a legitimate emerging therapy option simply because it is newer than established agents would deny a genuinely refractory patient a potentially effective treatment; conversely, presenting an investigational or recently approved agent without appropriately calibrated evidence-based expectations risks a mismatch between the patient's hopes and the actual, still-maturing evidence base. Crisis Anchor: Evaluating an emerging platelet-directed therapy requires confirming its specific regulatory and evidence status, matching it to the patient's specific refractory disease characteristics, and delivering balanced, realistic expectations rather than either reflexive dismissal or uncritical enthusiasm.

Investigational Access Arc — Chapter 20 Presentation: A family of a child with a confirmed severe inherited thrombocytopenia syndrome asks whether gene therapy is available now to cure their child's condition, having read enthusiastic media coverage of early trial results. Trap Logic: Either dismissing the family's question as premature without providing concrete, accurate information about the actual investigational status, or allowing unclarified enthusiasm to stand without correction, both fail this family; honest, specific information serves them best. Crisis Anchor: When a family asks about an emerging gene therapy or gene editing option, provide the specific current trial phase, eligibility criteria, and realistic timeline rather than either open-ended discouragement or unclarified optimism, and facilitate a specific referral to an enrolling site if the family wishes to pursue it.

Presenting Scenario	Relevant Compass Instance(s)	Chapter
Incidental thrombocytosis, asymptomatic	Isolated Thrombocytosis on a Routine Panel; Reactive	1, 17

	Versus Clonal Recognition Arc	
Poor platelet increment after transfusion	A Disappointing Platelet Count Rise After Transfusion; Refractoriness Recognition Arc; Nonimmune Versus Alloimmune Refractoriness Arc	1, 19, 19
Mucocutaneous bleeding, normal platelet count	Prolonged Bleeding Time with a Normal Platelet Count; Unexplained Easy Bruising with Normal Platelet Studies	2, 4
Aggregometry with blunted secondary wave	A Platelet Function Panel Suggesting a Storage Pool Disorder	2
Bleeding on antiplatelet or anticoagulant therapy	Bleeding on Dual Antiplatelet Therapy; Reversal Agent Selection Arc	3, 18
New thrombocytopenia with neurologic or renal findings	Early Recognition of Platelet-Driven Microvascular Thrombosis; Recognizing Thrombotic Microangiopathy as Requiring Same-Day Treatment	3, 12
Preprocedural platelet count assessment	Periprocedural Assessment of a Mild, Borderline Platelet Count; Antiplatelet Recovery Timeline Arc	4, 18
New spontaneous bruising or bleeding	Recognizing a Bleeding History That Requires Same-Day Evaluation	5
Markedly low platelet count, asymptomatic	A Markedly Low Platelet Count in an Asymptomatic Patient	5
Low platelet count with analyzer clumping flag	An Analyzer Flag Accompanying a Low Platelet Count; Resolving a Suspected Pseudothrombocytopenia Result	6, 6

Aggregometry suggesting Glanzmann or Bernard-Soulier pattern	An Aggregometry Pattern Suggesting Glanzmann Thrombasthenia; Aggregometry Pattern Recognition Arc	7, 16
Discordant point-of-care platelet function result	A Discordant Point-of-Care Closure Time in a Patient on Antiplatelet Therapy	7
New thrombocytopenia, multilineage or hospital-acquired	New Thrombocytopenia with Accompanying Cytopenias; Sequencing the Evaluation of New Thrombocytopenia in a Hospitalized Patient	8, 8
Newly diagnosed or relapsing immune thrombocytopenia	Determining Urgency of First-Line Treatment in Newly Diagnosed Immune Thrombocytopenia; Sequencing Second-Line Therapy After First-Line Treatment Failure	9, 9
Abrupt severe thrombocytopenia after new medication	Recognizing the Characteristic Timing Pattern of Drug-Induced Thrombocytopenia; Managing an Inadvertent Rechallenge with a Previously Implicated Medication	10, 10
Thrombocytopenia on heparin	Applying the 4Ts Score to Guide Immediate Management; Managing Confirmed Heparin-Induced Thrombocytopenia with Thrombosis	11, 11
Thrombocytopenia with microangiopathic hemolysis	Recognizing Thrombotic Microangiopathy as Requiring Same-Day Treatment; Distinguishing TTP from Atypical HUS While ADAMTS13 Results Are Pending	12, 12
Thrombocytopenia in pregnancy or neonate	Distinguishing Benign Gestational Thrombocytopenia from a	13, 13

	Pregnancy Emergency; Recognizing Neonatal Alloimmune Thrombocytopenia Risk in a Subsequent Pregnancy	
Thrombocytopenia in sepsis, DIC, or liver disease	Recognizing Evolving Disseminated Intravascular Coagulation Before Overt Criteria Are Met; Distinguishing Chronic Liver Disease Thrombocytopenia from a Superimposed Acute Process	14, 14
Lifelong macrothrombocytopenia or malignancy predisposition	Recognizing a Macrothrombocytopenia Pattern Warranting Genetic Evaluation; Establishing Malignancy Surveillance After Confirming a Predisposition Syndrome	15, 15
Marked thrombocytosis with new bleeding	Acquired Dysfunction Recognition Arc; Extreme Count Dual-Risk Arc	16, 17
Life-threatening bleeding on a direct oral anticoagulant	Reversal Agent Selection Arc	18
Emerging or investigational therapy inquiry	Emerging Therapy Evaluation Arc; Investigational Access Arc	20, 20

Using the Master Compass in Practice

The Master Compass is organized for two complementary modes of use. A reader working systematically through a clinical topic can locate the relevant Part and chapter grouping directly, reviewing the full set of Compass instances associated with that topic area as a consolidated recap. A reader facing an active clinical decision, whether on the wards, in clinic, or during a call-night consultation, can instead start from the quick-lookup table above, matching the presenting scenario to the relevant instance and chapter, then referring back to the fuller chapter discussion when the clinical situation requires reasoning beyond the Crisis Anchor rule itself.

The Master Compass is not a substitute for the clinical reasoning, evidence synthesis, and management detail developed within each chapter, and it is not designed to be used in isolation from the surrounding clinical judgment a specific patient's full presentation requires. Trap Logic entries in particular describe the most common reasoning error associated with each pattern, not an exhaustive account of every way a given clinical scenario can be misjudged, and the Crisis Anchor for each instance states a general decision rule that, like every general rule in medicine, requires application with attention to the individual patient's full clinical context rather than as a mechanical, context-free algorithm.

KEY POINT: Forty Crisis Compass instances span this book's five Parts: eight in Part I (foundational platelet biology), eight in Part II (clinical evaluation and diagnostic approach), twelve in Part III (thrombocytopenia across its immune, drug-induced, consumptive, and special-population causes), four in Part IV (inherited platelet disorders), and eight in Part V (thrombocytosis, antithrombotic pharmacology, transfusion medicine, and emerging therapies). Every instance is question-free by design, ending in a stated clinical decision anchor rather than a question with answer choices, consistent with this book's framework-wide commitment to teaching clinical reasoning through narrative pattern recognition rather than through examination-style testing.

This Atlas closes the book's core content. The appendices, formulary, and index that follow provide additional supplementary reference material organized in the conventional back-matter format familiar from other clinical references, while the Master Compass above remains this book's distinguishing structural asset: a single, consolidated, cross-referenced navigator through the recurring decision points a clinician managing platelet disorders will repeatedly encounter across a career in clinical practice.

CONCLUSION

A platelet count is a number. What this book has argued, chapter by chapter, is that the number means nothing until it is placed inside a clinical context — the patient's age, the acuity of presentation, the drugs on the medication list, the peripheral smear, the trend over hours rather than the value at one moment. From the molecular choreography of megakaryopoiesis through the final chapters on emerging platelet-directed therapies, the throughline of this text has been the same: platelet disorders are rarely solved by a single test result. They are solved by a clinician who knows which question the count is actually answering.

The early chapters built that foundation deliberately. Understanding how a megakaryocyte fragments into thousands of platelets, how dense and alpha granules store the machinery of activation, and how the glycoprotein receptors translate vessel injury into aggregation is not academic throat-clearing — it is what allows a clinician to reason forward from mechanism to phenotype rather than backward from a memorized list of diagnoses. A clinician who understands why ADAMTS13 deficiency causes ultra-large multimers to shear platelets from circulation will never mistake thrombotic thrombocytopenic purpura for a bleeding disorder, because the physiology itself rules out the wrong differential before a laboratory test confirms it.

The middle chapters of this book carried that physiology into the territory where most clinical error actually occurs: the undifferentiated patient with a low or high platelet count and no diagnosis yet attached to it. Pseudothrombocytopenia from EDTA-dependent clumping, drug-induced thrombocytopenia from a medication started two weeks earlier, heparin-induced thrombocytopenia in a postoperative patient whose count is falling while a clinician is reassured by a normal absolute number, immune thrombocytopenia in a patient who looks otherwise well — each of these conditions can present with a nearly identical number and an entirely different next step. The clinical cases threaded through this text were chosen because they preserve that ambiguity rather than resolving it prematurely, the same ambiguity a clinician faces at the bedside before the full picture assembles itself.

The later chapters extended this reasoning into populations and settings where the stakes compound: the pregnant patient whose gestational thrombocytopenia must be distinguished from preeclampsia and HELLP syndrome before delivery, the septic patient whose falling platelet count may be the earliest laboratory signal of disseminated intravascular coagulation, the inherited platelet disorder that has masqueraded as a bleeding diathesis of unclear etiology for a decade before genetic testing names it. Antithrombotic pharmacology and platelet transfusion medicine closed the therapeutic arc, and the final chapter on investigational platelet-directed therapies was included deliberately — this is a field still in active motion, and a clinician trained only on today's algorithms will be undertrained within a decade.

The Platelet Crisis Decision Compass that has run through every chapter of this book was built for exactly this kind of decision pressure. Its five-part structure — the presentation, the mimic signature, the decision, the trap logic, and the crisis anchor — exists because the moment a clinician most needs clarity is rarely the moment a full literature review is possible. The Platelet Crisis Master Compass at the end of this book consolidates all forty of those instances into a single navigable reference, organized so that a specific clinical scenario can be matched to its governing pattern in the time it takes to flip to an index rather than to reconstruct reasoning from first principles under pressure.

KEY POINT: The competent management of platelet disorders is not the accumulation of diagnostic labels but the disciplined narrowing of possibility — from an abnormal number, to a clinical pattern, to a decision that changes what happens to the patient next.

Hematology as a discipline rewards this kind of pattern discipline more than almost any other area of internal medicine, because the platelet count is one of the few laboratory values that a clinician encounters daily, in nearly every patient population, and because the differential behind an abnormal count spans mechanisms as different as marrow failure, immune destruction, consumption, dilution, and clonal proliferation. This book was written on the premise that the clinician who understands why each of these mechanisms produces the number it does will manage the patient in front of them better than the clinician who has simply memorized which drug to start. That understanding, applied consistently at the bedside, is the actual practice of platelet medicine — and it is the standard this book was written to serve.

www.ingramcontent.com/pod-product-compliance
Lightning Source LLC
LaVergne TN
LVHW060439061126
851857LV00016B/1672
9780557978403